Transfusion-Free Medicine and Surgery

To my wife Nadine

Transfusion-Free Medicine and Surgery

EDITED BY

Nicolas Jabbour, MD

Associate Director, Liver Transplantation Service
Director, Transfusion-Free Medicine and Surgery
University of Southern California University Hospital
Los Angeles, USA

Blackwell
Publishing

© 2005 by Blackwell Publishing Ltd
Blackwell Publishing, Inc., 350 Main Street, Malden, Massachusetts 02148-5020, USA
Blackwell Publishing Ltd, 9600 Garsington Road, Oxford OX4 2DQ, UK
Blackwell Publishing Asia Pty Ltd, 550 Swanston Street, Carlton, Victoria 3053, Australia

First published 2005

Library of Congress Cataloging-in-Publication Data

Transfusion-free medicine and Surgery/edited by Nicolas Jabbour.
    p. ; cm.
  Includes bibliographical references.
  ISBN 1-4051-2159-9 (alk. paper)
  1. Transfusion-free surgery. 2. Blood–Transfusion–Complications. 3. Blood–Transfusion–Law and legislation. 4. Blood substitutes–Therapeutic use. 5. Blood–Collection and preservation.
  [DNLM: 1. Blood Substitutes–therapeutic use. 2. Blood Loss, Surgical–prevention & control. 3. Blood Transfusion–adverse effects. WH 450 T772 2005] I. Jabbour, Nicolas.
  RD33.35.T736 2005
  615'.39–dc22   2005004900

ISBN-13: 978-1-405-1599
ISBN-10: 1-4051-599

A catalogue record for this title is available from the British Library

Set in 9.5/12pt Meridien by SPI Publisher Services, Pondicherry, India
Printed and bound in the United Kingdom by TJ International Ltd, Padstow, Cornwall

Commissioning Editor: Maria Khan
Development Editor: Claire Bonnett
Production Controller: Kate Charman

For further information on Blackwell Publishing, visit our website:
http://www.blackwellpublishing.com

The publisher's policy is to use permanent paper from mills that operate a sustainable forestry policy, and which has been manufactured from pulp processed using acid-free and elementary chlorine-free practices. Furthermore, the publisher ensures that the text paper and cover board used have met acceptable environmental accreditation standards.

Contents

Contributors, vii

Preface, ix

Acknowledgments, xi

1 Legal and Administrative Issues Related to Transfusion-Free Medicine and Surgery, 1
Randy Henderson, Nicolas Jabbour, Gary Zeger

2 Transfusion Therapy – Balancing the Risks and Benefits, 24
Roslyn A Yomtovian, Katharine A Downes, Ira A Shulman

3 Preoperative Management and Preparation for Transfusion-Free Surgery, 60
Lawrence T Goodnough

4 Intraoperative Strategies for Transfusion-Free Surgery, 75
Joseph D Tobias

5 Current View of the Coagulation System, 114
Yoogoo Kang, Paul Audu

6 The Physiology of Anemia and the Threshold for Blood Transfusion, 144
Joseph D Tobias

7 Postoperative Management in Transfusion-Free Medicine and Surgery in the ICU, 158
Jean-Louis Vincent

8 Anemia and Blood Conservation in the Critically Ill Patient, 170
Aryeh Shander, Tanuja Rijhwani, Nimish Nemani, Carmine Gianatiempo

9 Feasibility of Transfusion-Free Medicine and Surgery in Clinical Practice, 185
Nicolas Jabbour, Ryan Young, S Ram Kumar, Rick Selby, Yuri Genyk

10 The Changing Transfusion Practice of Neonatal and Pediatric Surgery, 218
Pamela J Kling, Nicolas Jabbour, S Ram Kumar

11 The Cost of Blood Product Transfusion, 237
Gary Zeger, Nicolas Jabbour

12 Oxygen Therapeutics – The Quest for Artificial Blood, 254
Robert Bartlett

13 Basic Principles of Bloodless Medicine and Surgery, 283
Nicolas Jabbour

Index, 293

Contributors

Paul Audu, MD
Clinical Assistant Professor
Department of Anesthesiology
Thomas Jefferson University, Jefferson
  Medical College
Director, Neuroanesthesiology
Thomas Jefferson University Hospital
Philadelphia, USA

Robert Bartlett MD, FACEP, CIME
Edward Teller Chair for Hyperbolic
  Medicine
Palmetto Richland Hospital/USC School
  of Medicine
Columbia, South Carolina, USA

Katharine A Downes, MD
Assistant Professor of Pathology
Case Western Reserve University
Director of Regulatory and Quality
  Affairs
Associate Director of Blood Banking and
  Transfusion Medicine
Department of Pathology
University Hospitals of Cleveland
Cleveland, Ohio, USA

Yuri Genyk, MD
Assistant Professor of Surgery
Hepatobiliary/Pancreas and Abdominal
  Organ Transplant Surgery
Keck School of Medicine
University of Southern California
Los Angeles, California, USA

Carmine Gianatiempo, MD
Assistant Clinical Professor of Surgery
Mount Sinai School of Medicine, New York
Director, Cardiothoracic Intensive Care
  Unit
Associate Director, Critical Care Medicine
Englewood Hospital and Medical Center
Englewood, New Jersey, USA

Lawrence T Goodnough, MD
Professor of Pathology and Medicine
Stanford University
Director, Transfusion service, Stanford
  Medical Center
Stanford, California, USA

Randy Henderson
Program Manager, Department of
  Transfusion-Free Medicine and Surgery,
  USC University Hospital and USC Norris
  Cancer Hospital
Los Angeles, California, USA

Nicolas Jabbour, MD
Associate Professor of Surgery
Associate Director of Hepatobiliary/
  Pancreas and Abdominal Organ
  Transplant
Director Transfusion Free Medicine and
  Surgery Program
Keck School of Medicine
University of Southern California
Los Angeles, California, USA

Yoogoo Kang, MD
Professor & Vice Chair
Department of Anesthesiology
Thomas Jefferson University, Jefferson
  Medical College
Director, Hepatic Transplantation
  Anesthesiology
Thomas Jefferson University Hospital
Philadelphia, USA

Pamela J Kling, MD
Assistant Professor
Department of Pediatrics
University of Wisconsin and Meriter
  Hospital
Madison, Wisconsin, USA

Nimish Nemani, MD
Clinical Research Assistant
Department of Anesthesiology and Critical
  Care Medicine
Englewood Hospital and Medical Center
Englewood, New Jersey, USA

Tanuja Rijhwani, MBBS, MPH
Director, Clinical Research
Department of Anesthesiology and Critical
  Care Medicine
Englewood Hospital and Medical Center
Englewood, New Jersey, USA

S Ram Kumar, MD
Resident, Department of Surgery
Keck School of Medicine of the University of
  Southern California
Los Angeles, California, USA

R Rick Selby, MD
Professor of Surgery
Surgical Director of Hepatobiliary/Pancreas
  and Abdominal Organ Transplant surgery
Keck School of Medicine
University of Southern California
Los Angeles, California, USA

Aryeh Shander, MD, FCCM, FCCP,
Clinical Professor of Anesthesiology and
  Medicine
Mount Sinai School of Medicine, New York
  Chief, Department of Anesthesiology,
  Critical Care Medicine, Pain Management
  and Hyperbaric Medicine
Englewood Hospital and Medical Center
New Jersey, USA

Ira A Shulman, MD
Director of Transfusion Medicine / Professor
  and Vice Chair of Pathology
Keck School of Medicine of the University of
  Southern California
Director of Laboratories and Pathology, LAC
  +USC Medical Center
Los Angeles, California, USA

Joseph D Tobias, MD
Vice-Chairman, Department of
  Anesthesiology
Chief, Division of Pediatric Anesthesiology
Professor of Anesthesiology & Pediatrics
Russell and Mary Shelden Chair in Pediatric
  Critical Care
University of Missouri
Columbia, Missouri, USA

Jean-Louis Vincent, MD, PhD
Professor of critical care medicine
Free University of Brussels
Head, Dept of Intensive Care
Erasme Hospital, Brussels, Belguim

Roslyn A Yomtovian, MD
Professor, Department of Pathology
Case Western Reserve University School of
  Medicine
Director, Blood Bank Transfusion Medicine
  Service
University Hospitals of Cleveland
Cleveland, Ohio, USA

Ryan Young
Keck School of Medicine
University of Southern California
Los Angeles, California, USA

Gary Zeger, MD
Associate Professor of Pathology
Keck School of Medicine, USC University of
  Southern California
Co-Medical Director, University Hospital
  Clinical Laboratories
Medical Director, Blood Bank,
  USC University Hospital
Medical Director, USC Blood Donor Center
Los Angeles, California, USA

Preface

Bloodless or transfusion-free surgery was introduced to serve the Jehovah's Witness community who, for religious reasons, refused transfusion of blood products even at the risk of their own lives. Historically, the issues associated with blood transfusion focused on ethical, legal and religious topics and not on the real problem, which is the liberal use of blood products. The medical community perceives blood as plentiful, safe and inexpensive, and thus little effort is paid to conservation, improvement or development of alternatives. This view of blood is somewhat analogous to the view of energy: oil is seen by the public as plentiful, safe and inexpensive; however, like blood, oil is a limited resource, is expensive and carries significant health risks.

As far as blood is concerned, our lack of interest is no longer an option, given that the discovery of HCV and HIV as viruses potentially transmitted by blood and the anxiety surrounding potential diseases such as West Nile, mad cow disease and SARS have increased the awareness of the risks of transfusion.

The principles of transfusion-free surgery were originally driven by the Jehovah's Witness community, but it should be a nidus for a wide change in the practice of medicine and surgery. Despite the stringent criteria for ever-safe blood donor screening, collection and administration, blood will never be absolutely safe, and even a small percentage of risk will translate into major health care problems.

Since 50% of blood transfusions is prescribed by surgeons, physicians in general and surgeons specifically have the responsibility of objectively assessing the risks, availability and cost of blood products. They should be at the forefront of adopting strategies to limit blood loss, to decrease the risk of transfusion and to develop alternatives to blood products. Wide adoption of these innovations will yield higher standards of patient care.

I hope this manuscript will serve as a guide for blood conservation in medical and surgical practices. If every physician adopts part or all of these principles, less blood would be needed, and despite the ongoing shortage of potential blood donors, no elective surgery should ever need to be cancelled due to the lack of blood.

Nicolas Jabbour, 2005

CHAPTER 1

Legal and Administrative Issues Related to Transfusion-Free Medicine and Surgery

Randy Henderson, Nicolas Jabbour, Gary Zeger

Introduction

Few would argue that patient rights should be protected and respected. However, when this right involves a patient's refusal of potentially lifesaving treatment, serious issues come to the fore. In this chapter we will discuss the rights of patients to refuse blood transfusion, and the right and duty of the physician assuming care for such patients. We will also review how the implementation and establishment of bloodless medicine and surgery programs evolved from Jehovah's Witnesses' position on blood, and the lessons that science has learned in the process.

History of Jehovah's Witnesses and blood

The issue involving Jehovah's Witnesses and blood transfusions became most prominent in the 1940s at the height of World War II [1]. Blood was liberally transfused into wounded soldiers, and this led to an increased demand for blood donors. Most individuals in the medical profession, as well as members of the lay community, regarded the practice of blood transfusion as an accepted therapeutic method. But those who were members of the religious organization known as Jehovah's Witnesses did not. And the passage of time has not changed their point of view.

The Witnesses' belief is that God, the Creator of life, views blood as sacred and holy, and therefore it should not be used for the purpose of transfusion, regardless of the consequences [2]. They cite several Bible passages found in both the Old and New Testaments. One such passage is found in Genesis 9:3–4: 'Every moving animal that is alive may serve as food for you. As in the case of green vegetation, I do give it all to you. Only flesh with its soul – its blood – you must not eat.' Leviticus 17:10 says: 'As for any man of the house of Israel or some alien resident who is residing as an alien in their midst *who eats any sort of blood*, I shall certainly set my face against the soul that is eating the blood, and *I shall indeed cut him off* from among his people.' Furthermore, Acts 15:28–29 states: 'The holy spirit and we ourselves have favored adding no further burden to you, except these necessary things, to keep *abstaining...from...blood*.' Although no mention is made of transfusing blood, Jehovah's Witnesses view this directive to 'not eat blood' or 'to abstain from blood' as something that applies to both *oral* and *intravenous* feeding.

While it is true that Jehovah's Witnesses refuse blood, they are not averse to medical and surgical treatment. On the contrary, many of them are physicians, even surgeons. However, as already stated, their position on blood is unequivocal and absolute [3].

Acceptable products, treatments and procedures

Although Jehovah's Witnesses do not accept blood transfusions, accepting products *derived* from red cells, white cells, platelets or plasma is viewed as a decision that individual Witness patients must make for themselves. In a recent issue of *The Watchtower*, the principal journal of Jehovah's Witnesses, a distinction is made between whole blood and its *primary components* (i.e. red cells, white cells, platelets and plasma) and *fractions* [4]. These primary components are unacceptable to devout Jehovah's Witnesses. However, acceptable blood fractions may include plasma proteins such as immune globulins, albumin and cryoprecipitate. Platelet-derived wound-healing factors may also fall into this category of acceptable blood fractions. The rationale of Jehovah's Witnesses in regard to products fractionated from blood is partly based on the complexity of blood itself. Medical practitioners recognize that plasma, for example, consists of many substances such as hormones, inorganic salts, enzymes and nutrients. Plasma also carries proteins such as albumin, clotting factors and antibodies. Jehovah's Witnesses believe that the Bible does not give details about these products that, medically speaking, are not typically defined as blood. Therefore, each individual Witness is instructed to use their conscience in making a decision to accept or refuse these products.

The availability of recombinant growth factors such as erythropoietin (EPO) to stimulate hematopoiesis has been very helpful in minimizing or eliminating a patient's exposure to allogeneic blood. However, while the majority of Jehovah's Witnesses will accept recombinant EPO, since all formulations of the product available in the USA are packaged with a stabilizer that includes trace amounts of human serum albumin, consent must be obtained prior to its use. There are some Witness patients who refuse to accept any blood-derived product, regardless of the amount. Therefore, health care providers should utilize a specific form that allows patients to choose the products, treatments and procedures that are acceptable to them (see Figure 1.1).

Autologous procedures and equipment

Citing other Biblical statements that discuss the use of blood, Jehovah's Witnesses do not allow the preoperative collection and storage of their own

TRANSFUSION-FREE MEDICINE & SURGERY PROGRAM
(PERSONAL DIRECTIVES)

Patient: _____   Attending Physician: _____
                    (Please Print)

I direct that **no blood transfusion** (including whole blood, red cells, white cells, platelets, or blood plasma) are to be given me under any circumstances, even if physicians deem such necessary to preserve my life or health. I will accept non-blood volume expanders (such as dextran, saline or Ringer's solution, or hetastarch) and other non-blood management.

I hereby fully and unconditionally release physicians, anesthesiologists, hospitals and their personnel from liability for any damages, claim or liability related to my refusal of blood or blood products, despite their otherwise competent care.

The following are my wishes and directions regarding procedures, treatments and blood fractions (initial ALL boxes):

PRODUCT/TREATMENT/PROCEDURE	Accept	Refuse
Albumin (minor blood fraction)		
Erythropoietin (contains albumin)		
Immune Globulins (e.g., minor blood fractions, RhoGAM, antivenoms)		
Hemophiliac Preparations (clotting factors)		
Tissue Adhesives (e.g., fibrinogen, fibrin glue, thrombin, etc.)		
Cryoprecipitate (intravenous infusion)		
Dialysis & Heart-Lung equipment (non-blood primed)		
Intraoperative Blood Salvage ("Cell Saver") where extracorporeal circulation is a closed circuit without blood storage (non-blood primed)		
Intraoperative Hemodilution (where extracorporeal circulation is a closed circuit)		
Plasmapheresis (similar to dialysis)		

Dated this: _____ day of _____, year _____

Signature: _____
                    (Patient, Parent or Guardian)

Witness: _____

Figure 1.1 USC Transfusion-Free Medicine and Surgery Program: Personal Decision and Release.

blood for later infusion. For example, Leviticus 17:13 says what a man should do if he killed an animal for food: 'He must in that case pour its blood out and cover it with dust.' According to some Biblical scholars, this act of pouring out blood is best understood as an act of reverence demonstrating respect for the life of the animal and, thus, respect for God who created and continues to care for that life [5]. Again, Jehovah's Witnesses' principal journal *The Watchtower* addressed the therapeutic and surgical use of procedures or equipment involving autologous blood. As with fractions of primary components of blood, this too is a matter for personal decision. If the intraoperative cell-saver machine is not primed with blood, and is set up in a closed circuit that is in constant contact with the patient's circulatory system, this is acceptable to many Witness patients. The same principle would apply to the use of dialysis and heart-lung machines, as well as acute normovolemic hemodilution (ANH) (see Figure 1.1).

Organ transplantation

There has been a great deal of confusion over the fact that the doctrine of Jehovah's Witnesses prohibits them from receiving blood transfusions but not organ transplants. Blood itself is often viewed as a 'liquid organ transplant'. Why then do Jehovah's Witnesses view organ transplants differently than they do blood?

About 24 years ago, *The Watchtower* briefly discussed this issue [6]. The principle guiding Jehovah's Witnesses' decision to accept organ transplants or human tissue focuses on their view that while the Bible specifically forbids consuming blood, there is no Biblical command or injunction proscribing the 'taking in' of other human tissue. They mention that meat is not prohibited for human consumption as long as it is properly bled, and therefore this principle can be applied to organ transplantation. However, each member of the Jehovah's Witness faith is instructed to weigh all relevant factors and make a personal, conscientious decision about accepting an organ transplant. In the main, if a human organ transplant does not involve blood or blood products, it is left up to each individual Witness to decide for himself or herself.

Overview of legal principles related to refusal of blood

Refusal of blood as life-sustaining treatment

Does a patient have the right to refuse blood transfusion at the risk of his or her life? Before we address that question, it is important to understand the legal rights of patients to refuse *any* type of medical or surgical treatment.

The basic common law right of bodily self-determination establishes that every person of sound mind is master over his own body. Therefore, such an individual is free to prohibit surgery or medical treatment deemed by others as potentially lifesaving. Over 100 years ago, the US Supreme Court upheld the notion of individual autonomy. It stated that 'no right is held more sacred, or is more carefully guarded, by the common law, than the right of every individual to the possession and control of his own person, free from all restraint or interference of others, unless by unquestionable authority of law' [7].

This fundamental legal principle of bodily self-determination serves as the basis for the doctrine of informed consent. The right to privacy dovetails with informed consent. No doctor or hospital should subject patients to medical and/or surgical treatment without informed consent. The patient must be informed of the name, means and likely consequences of the proposed treatment in order to 'knowingly' determine what should or should not be done to his or her body.

Informed consent

The US President's Commission for the Study of Ethical Problems in Medicine was charged with preparing a report about making health care decisions. The report revealed that informed consent rests on two very important values: (1) the patient's own conception of his personal well being; and (2) the patient's right to self-determination. This commission also concluded that the principle of self-determination 'is best understood as respecting people's right to define and pursue their own view of what is good' [7].

In *Cobbs v. Grant*, a landmark California Supreme Court decision, it was determined that physicians have had a duty to obtain the informed consent of patients before performing certain medical procedures [8]. Over 90 years ago, Justice Benjamin Cardozo stated: 'Every human being of adult years and sound mind has a right to determine what shall be done with his own body; and a surgeon who performs an operation without his patient's consent, commits an assault, for which he is liable in damages.' Justice Cardozo's statement was in response to the case of a woman who was admitted to the hospital with abdominal pain and a palpable lump. She gave her doctors consent to physical examination, but she refused surgical examination. However, while under general anesthetic (ether) for further physical examination, surgeons surgically removed a fibroid tumor. Subsequently, gangrene developed in her left arm, and two fingers were amputated. The physicians were held liable for negligence and battery [9,10].

Therefore, doctors who administer treatment or perform surgery without a patient's consent are liable for battery (i.e. for nonconsensual interference with the patient's person). A surgical operation on the body of a person is a technical battery or trespass unless that person or some other authorized person consented to it, regardless of the skill and care employed in the performance of the operation. In addition, a case of battery is established where a physician obtains consent to perform one type of treatment and thereafter performs a substantially different treatment for which consent was not obtained [9,11].

In the precedent setting case of *Cruzan v. Missouri Department of Health*, 497 US 261 (1990), the Supreme Court determined that 'the logical corollary of the doctrine of informed consent is that the patient generally possesses the right not to consent, that is the right to refuse treatment' [7]. Even if a patient refuses treatment that a physician views as life-sustaining, 'the primacy of a patient's interest in self-determination and in honoring the patient's own view of well-being warrant leaving with the patient the final authority to decide'.

Specific issues related to refusal of blood in Jehovah's Witnesses
Competent adults

In view of clearly established laws regarding informed consent, any competent adult has the right to refuse blood. However, Jehovah's Witnesses' refusal of blood should be based on a clear understanding of the *consequences* involved in not receiving blood.

At least three high courts have found that the 1st Amendment Free Exercise Clause protects religion-based refusals of medical treatment from state interference [7,12–14]. The fact that Jehovah's Witnesses' refusal of blood may be viewed as a nonact or refusal to act rather than a positive, affirmative act is a significant point to consider. Whereas some states have exercised their 'law enforcement' authority to limit or prohibit religiously motivated action in order to protect public health, safety or welfare, there is no precedent for prohibiting action motivated by religion when there is no grave or pressingly imminent danger to the public [7,15–18].

Example 1
In re Brown [9,19]

Mrs Brown was a Jehovah's Witness who was shot by her daughter and consequently required surgery. The doctors recommended a blood transfusion, which she refused to consent to. Thereafter, the state sought and obtained a court order to force a transfusion due to the fact that Mrs Brown was the only eyewitness to the shooting, and if she died from lack of a blood transfusion, she would not be able to testify for the state in the prosecution. The surgery did take place and Mrs Brown did receive blood transfusions.

Mrs Brown required further surgery and again her surgeon recommended blood transfusions. She refused and made an appeal to the court to stop the order. The decision of the court was that the order be vacated and Mrs Brown not be required to submit to, or receive, a blood transfusion against her will. The Supreme Court made the following statement regarding her common law right to privacy:

Each individual has a right to the inviability and integrity of the person, freedom to choose or bodily self-determination. . . . The right to be left alone . . . which is the most comprehensive of rights and the right most valued by civilized man. Violation of this rule constitutes a battery.

The court also stated that 'the factual information available to us makes clear that Brown's position has been consistent throughout: that she wants to live, that she wants the benefits of all that medical science can do for her with the sole and only exception that she rejects any treatment proscribed by the tenets of her religious faith'.

Emergency/incompetent adults (patients known to be Jehovah's Witnesses refusing blood)

Generally speaking, the fundamental right of bodily self-determination does not vanish when a patient loses consciousness or becomes incompetent. That right remains intact even when the patient is no longer able to assert the right [9,20,21]. In addition, when a patient has religious views against certain forms of medical treatment that predate, and are unaltered by, their incapacity, physicians and health care providers are not justified in substituting their own judgment for the patients at the time of treatment.

When refusals of treatment are religiously motivated they are 'usually considered more thoroughly and less likely to change than nonreligious ones because they are not dependent upon predictions of future circumstances, available medical treatment, or preferences' [9,22].

In reality, the main question is whether there is evidence of the patient's previously expressed wishes or refusal, not whether incompetent or unconscious adults in general have the right to refuse treatment.

Example 1
In re Dorone [7,9,23]

Mr Dorone was a 22-year-old Jehovah's Witness man who was seriously injured in an automobile accident and thus rendered unconscious. After being taken to a New Jersey hospital, his medical alert card indicating that he wanted nonblood treatment was found. Thereafter, Mr Dorone was transferred to a Pennsylvania hospital but his personal effects, including his medical alert card, were left behind. He required two more emergent surgeries, one for a subdural hematoma and another to remove a blood clot in his brain.

In each case, the hospital sought and received oral, telephonic court orders to allow blood transfusions against Mr Dorone's previously expressed refusal and over the objections of his family. His family had been excluded from the judicial hearings. The Pennsylvania Supreme Court upheld the prior orders to allow blood transfusions for Mr Dorone. The Supreme Court stated:

When evidence of this nature is measured against third party speculation as to what an unconscious patient would want, there can be no doubt that medical intervention is required. Indeed, in a situation like the present, where there is an emergency calling for an immediate decision, nothing less than a fully conscious contemporaneous decision by the patient will be sufficient to override evidence of medical necessity.

Example 2
Werth v. Taylor [7]

Mrs Werth, a Jehovah's Witness and mother of two children, became pregnant with twins in 1985. In preparation for delivery, she filled out a 'Refusal to Permit Blood Transfusion' form with the hospital. A few months later, she went into labor and upon admission to the hospital her husband filled out another 'Refusal to Permit Blood Transfusion' form in her behalf.

Subsequent to the birth of her twins, Mrs Werth required an emergency D&C due to bleeding. Prior to performing the procedure, the attending physician again confirmed her refusal of blood with Mr Werth. The D&C was completed but after she continued to bleed and became hemodynamically unstable, Dr Taylor, the anesthesiologist, believed that a transfusion should be given to save her life. Mrs Werth remained unconscious. Despite being informed that Mrs Werth was one of Jehovah's Witnesses, and therefore refused blood, Dr Taylor proceeded with the order for transfusion. In his opinion, this was a life-threatening emergency.

Mrs Werth and her husband did file a medical malpractice and battery suit against Dr Taylor but the trial court accepted his defense that her refusal was not binding. His argument was similar to the Dorone case; he argued that Mrs Werth's refusal was not a conscious, competent, contemporaneous, fully informed refusal made in contemplation of the life-threatening situation that arose. In July 1991, Mrs Werth appealed the trial court's decision to the Michigan Court of Appeals but they upheld the decision in favor of Dr Taylor. The court of appeals did acknowledge that competent adults can refuse medical treatment, but they determined that a life-threatening emergency was different from a routine elective surgery. Applying the Dorone case to Mrs Werth's condition, they believed that the lack of a fully informed, contemporaneous decision was sufficient to override evidence of medical necessity.

These cases raise several legal/ethical questions. Is the requirement of a contemporaneous, fully informed or fully conscious refusal truly practical and realistic? How can an unconscious or noncommunicative patient be able to satisfy this standard?

Example 3
In re Hughes [7]
Mrs Hughes was scheduled for an elective hysterectomy. Before consenting to the surgery, she spoke to her doctor, Dr Ances, about her refusal of blood transfusions due to her religious beliefs. He agreed to perform the surgery without blood. On the morning that Mrs Hughes was admitted to the hospital, she filled out the hospital's standard refusal-of-blood form. The form released the doctor and the hospital from liability for respecting her wishes that no blood products be used. It also stated that she 'fully understood the possible consequences' of her refusal of blood – a key phrase.

Unfortunately the surgery was not uneventful and Mrs Hughes experienced massive bleeding. Despite the conversation she had with Dr Ances before the surgery, and the refusal form she filled out at the hospital, he felt that a blood transfusion was necessary. Mrs Hughes' husband was contacted and after being told that his wife would likely die if she did not receive a blood transfusion, he gave permission. Mr Hughes was not a Jehovah's Witness. Mrs Hughes' sister (who was a Jehovah's Witness) was at the hospital and she eventually discovered that a transfusion had been recommended for her sister. She objected to the use of blood and decided to contact the Philadelphia Hospital Liaison Committee for Jehovah's Witnesses. This conflict came to the attention of hospital administration and therefore a court hearing was arranged.

Dr Ances testified that Mrs Hughes discussion with him regarding her refusal of blood, though clear and competent, was not in anticipation of such complications that led to massive blood loss. Although Mrs Hughes husband agreed to the use of blood for his wife after being called by the doctor, he stated in court that he knew his wife would not want blood. Mrs Hughes' sister and teenage daughter, testifying on behalf of Mrs Hughes, said that she would not want blood under any circumstances.

The trial court's decision was to grant the hospital authority to transfuse until Mrs Hughes regained consciousness and could again speak for herself. Mrs Hughes was transfused and after regaining consciousness she reiterated her refusal of blood. As stipulated by the terms of the court, the order for transfusion was then terminated.

Mrs Hughes did appeal to the New Jersey Superior Court but the earlier decision of the trial court was upheld. The appellate court did not base their decision on the requirement of a contemporaneous, fully informed or fully conscious refusal. Rather, they ruled that in an emergency involving a refusal of allegedly lifesaving treatment, the refusal will be honored only if there is 'clear, convincing, unequivocal evidence' that the patient's refusal was 'fully informed'. Furthermore, they stated that such a refusal could be established by the patient's 'oral directives, actions or writings'. They also indicated that if there exists even a 'glimmer of uncertainty' about the patient's wishes, the refusal would not be honored.

Indirectly, the court criticized Dr Ances and the hospital. Dr Ances failed to thoroughly discuss with Mrs Hughes all the possible consequences of the surgery. And the hospital's refusal form was lacking in that it did not accomplish its intended purpose.

Example 4
In re Duran [7]
In 1996 Ms Duran was diagnosed with liver failure. As one of Jehovah's Witnesses, Ms Duran sought treatment at the University of Pittsburgh Medical Center since they were known to have successfully performed 'bloodless' liver transplants on Jehovah's Witnesses. Ms Duran and her husband (who was not one of Jehovah's Witnesses) traveled to Pittsburgh in early 1997 to be evaluated for liver transplantation. The transplant team accepted her as a candidate with the stipulation that blood transfusions would not be given under any circumstances.

To ensure that her wishes would be respected, Ms Duran executed a health care durable power of attorney (DPA) form and appointed an elder from a Pittsburgh area congregation of Jehovah's Witnesses to be her health care agent. Ms Duran and her husband moved to Pittsburgh in 1999 after being informed that a liver would soon become available. She was transplanted in July 1999. Just a few days later, however, she experienced an episode of organ rejection. Since she was still unconscious, the doctors sought and gained consent for another transplant from her health care agent. 1 week later she was retransplanted. However, her body once again rejected the liver organ.

Ms Duran remained unconscious and despite the poor prognosis for recovery, her doctors recommended blood transfusions as a means to improve her chances of survival. A court hearing was quickly arranged in order to appoint her husband as emergency guardian for the purpose of granting consent for blood to be given. Her health care agent was not informed. The court heard testimony from Ms Duran's attending physician, her husband and her adult sister who was in favor of giving her blood transfusions. Mr Duran was granted authority as her emergency guardian and over a period of 3 weeks multiple blood transfusions were given. Ms Duran died having never regained consciousness.

Ms Duran's health care agent was eventually informed about what transpired and he filed an appeal with the Pennsylvania Superior Court. He challenged the trial court's order on several grounds, namely (1) overriding Ms Duran's oral and written refusals of blood; (2) circumventing her personally appointed health care agent and appointing a guardian with authority to consent to blood; and (3) failing to notify the health care agent of the guardianship petition and trial court hearing. The superior court's decision was to uphold the agent's challenges and it unanimously reversed the trial court's order.

In commenting on its decision, the superior court noted that the right of a patient to 'refuse medical treatment is deeply rooted' in common law. They further explained that Ms Duran's DPA was unequivocal in its pointed refusal of blood transfusions under any circumstance. Furthermore, in regard to the appointment of her husband as emergency guardian, the superior court agreed that since Ms Duran had already appointed a health care representative when she executed her DPA, her husband 'should not have been appointed emergency guardian for the express purpose of consenting to a blood transfusion because his beliefs conflicted with [his wife's] regarding blood transfusion therapy'. They also stated that the trial court should have taken into consideration her unequivocal directions when the very situation contemplated by her DPA arose. Regarding the failure of the trial court to notify her self-appointed health care agent, the superior court ruled that in view of the fact that both Ms Duran's husband and the hospital staff knew where to find her health care agent in an emergency situation, it was 'reasonable under these circumstances' to afford the agent notice of the hearing.

The above case illustrates that despite a patient's right to refuse blood transfusions, certain situations put physicians in hesitation mode, especially when confronted by other family members. This enforces the necessity of clear policies and procedures within a transfusion-free program to clearly delineate such possibilities in advance. This is mostly true when electively treating adult patients undergoing high-risk procedures. The refusal of blood in such situations should equate with any other consent between physician and patient prior to initiating therapy. Refusal of blood transfusions should not be different from any other directive given by the patient. The consent form developed in a transfusion-free program should clearly stipulate that the patient's wishes should not be questioned, even if the patient becomes incapacitated and even if their life is endangered due to lack of transfusion (see Figures 1.1 and 1.2).

In the case of an emergency, health care providers should do their best to ascertain whether or not the patient has previously expressed his or her position either verbally or in writing. Exercising such due diligence can greatly reduce, if not eliminate, liability and possible legal action.

Emergency/incompetent adults (no information available)

What is the responsibility or duty of the physician/hospital staff when there is no information available?

No physician or hospital is subject to liability based solely on failure to obtain consent in rendering emergency medical, surgical, hospital or health services to any patient regardless of age if (1) the patient is unable to consent; (2) no other person is reasonably available to legally authorize consent; and (3) the hospital and medical staff have acted in good faith and without any knowledge of facts that would negate the consent [7]. However, if it is discovered that a patient's religious status is Jehovah's Witness, reasonable efforts should be made to abort a transfusion and to proceed in a manner that accords with the patient's religious beliefs.

What if questions arise about the patient's Jehovah's Witness status?

Most Jehovah's Witness patients carry a wallet-sized advance medical directive/release card that documents their refusal of blood. However, due to negligence or perhaps unforeseen circumstances, some Jehovah's Witness patients may not always have this document with them. In cases where the patient was previously a patient at the hospital, chart notes can be checked [7,9]. There may also be a family member or friend previously appointed by the patient as health care agent or surrogate decision-maker. In regard to adults who are viewed as incompetent, if they never had decision-making capacity, the law views them as the same as minor children lacking capacity. However, the law is different for those who have had such capacity but are currently incapacitated.

If prior to losing capacity the adult was rational and capable of expressing his or her views and opinions regarding unacceptable treatment, a doctor or hospital is obligated to honor the patient's decision even if the patient is

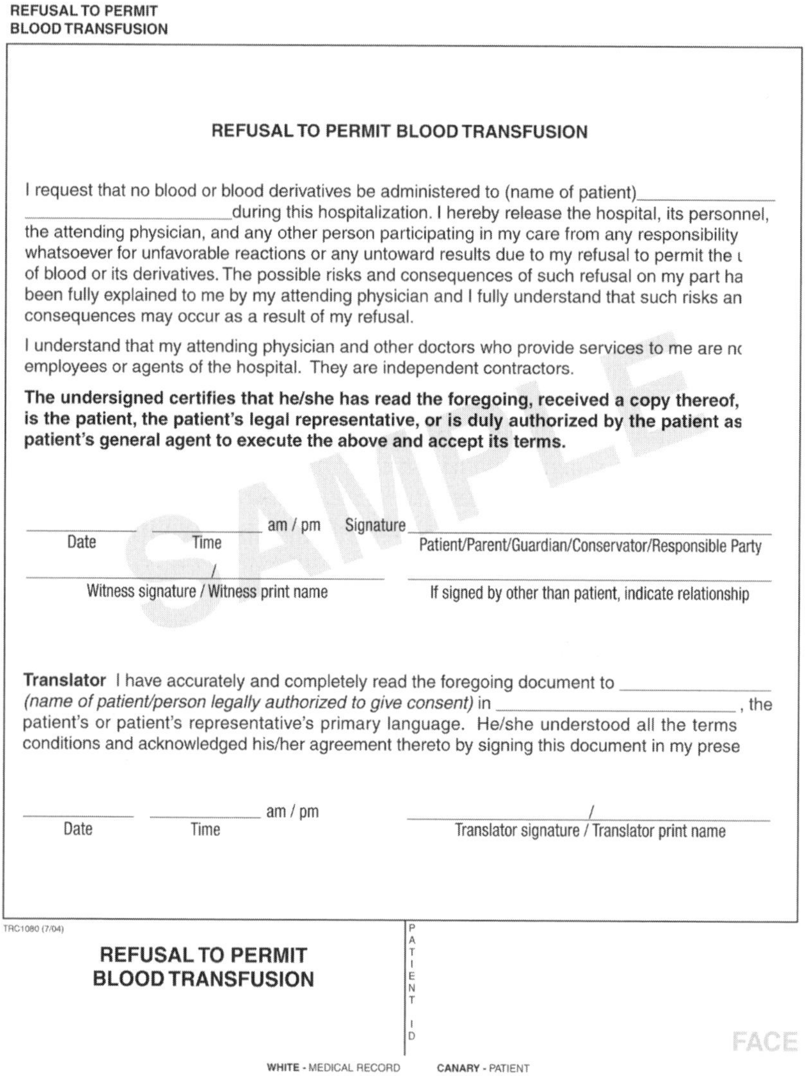

REFUSAL TO PERMIT
BLOOD TRANSFUSION

REFUSAL TO PERMIT BLOOD TRANSFUSION

I request that no blood or blood derivatives be administered to (name of patient)_____
_____during this hospitalization. I hereby release the hospital, its personnel,
the attending physician, and any other person participating in my care from any responsibility
whatsoever for unfavorable reactions or any untoward results due to my refusal to permit the ʋ
of blood or its derivatives. The possible risks and consequences of such refusal on my part ha
been fully explained to me by my attending physician and I fully understand that such risks an
consequences may occur as a result of my refusal.

I understand that my attending physician and other doctors who provide services to me are nc
employees or agents of the hospital. They are independent contractors.

**The undersigned certifies that he/she has read the foregoing, received a copy thereof,
is the patient, the patient's legal representative, or is duly authorized by the patient as
patient's general agent to execute the above and accept its terms.**

_____ _____ am / pm   Signature _____
    Date   Time   Patient/Parent/Guardian/Conservator/Responsible Party

                                    /
_____   _____
    Witness signature / Witness print name   If signed by other than patient, indicate relationship

Translator   I have accurately and completely read the foregoing document to _____
(name of patient/person legally authorized to give consent) in _____ , the
patient's or patient's representative's primary language. He/she understood all the terms
conditions and acknowledged his/her agreement thereto by signing this document in my prese

_____ _____ am / pm   /
    Date   Time   Translator signature / Translator print name

TRC1080 (7/04)

REFUSAL TO PERMIT
BLOOD TRANSFUSION

PATIENT ID

FACE

WHITE - MEDICAL RECORD   CANARY - PATIENT

Figure 1.2 Refusal To Permit Blood Transfusion.

incapable of speaking for himself or herself. This applies especially in cases
where the incapacitated patient's treatment preferences are based on deeply
held religious beliefs. The basic standard for dealing with incompetent or
unconscious adults is: What would the patient choose if able to communicate
his or her choice? Acceptable evidence of the patient's previously expressed

refusal would be: (1) prior written or oral direction; (2) advance medical directive/release card; (3) living will and medical power of attorney; (4) chart notes; and (5) testimonial evidence from others, that is surrogate decision-makers. While the rest may be questioned, a medical DPA is the best legal document to outline the incapacitated patient's treatment preferences [7,9].

Unlike the situation of an incapacitated patient where the consent clearly expresses the patient's wishes and is obtained prior to the patient's being incapacitated during the same hospital stay, in a situation where the physician is faced for the first time with an incapacitated patient or emergency situation, the standard of care is to administer blood transfusions. This may pose a dilemma for the physician regardless of any available information from a third party or family members. If the patient has a medical alert card, this should be considered as strong evidence of the patient's wishes to refuse transfusion. Having verbal information from family members or friends does not completely satisfy the physician's decision to transfuse or not, since people may change their mind regarding issues related to consent or refusal of blood. Therefore, a hospital policy should be in place to prepare for this dilemma if and when it arises.

More often than not, physicians and hospital staff will favor the voice of a surrogate decision-maker to clarify the issue and mitigate confusion or uncertainty. In regard to surrogate decision-makers, the state statute (RCW 7.70.065 a–f) establishes the following order of priority that should be followed in descending order [9,24]:

1 Appointed guardian
2 Attorney in fact: DPA
3 Spouse
4 Children at least 18 years of age
5 Parents
6 Adult brothers and sisters

The surrogate decision-maker's duty is to use good faith in determining the decision the patient would make if competent and able to speak for himself or herself.

Disagreeing family members

One of the most challenging scenarios arises when a patient's spouse, family member, relative or friend disagrees with the patient's refusal of blood. As previously mentioned, every competent adult has the constitutional right and freedom to determine what shall be done to their bodies. Therefore, courts have uniformly upheld that competent persons have the legal right to accept or refuse medical treatment absent of consent from their spouse or other relatives [7]. It is viewed as a natural corollary to an individual's rights of self-determination and personal autonomy to honor a patient's choice of treatment regardless of the views of the family.

For example, regarding a non-Witness husband's 'consent' to blood transfusion for his Witness wife, a Florida Supreme Court stated that 'marriage does not destroy one's constitutional right to personal autonomy' [7,25]. The basic rule on spousal consent is that patients who are conscious, mentally capable of consent and who give their consent do not require consent from their spouse, nor is it otherwise material [7,26]. Another reason for the uniformity of case law that supports a patient's choice of treatment despite the disapproval of family or relatives is that family members may have a bias against the patient's interest due to conflicting interests [7,27]. In addition, some family members may base their actions on their own religious beliefs. This may cause them to request treatment that contradicts the patient's wishes or desires [7,28].

In summary, the patient's decision should control their medical treatment. The fundamental rights of personal privacy, bodily self-determination (informed consent) and, for Witness patients, religious freedom would be rendered void if respect for a patient's health care decisions were contingent upon the unanimous agreement of the patient's spouse or relatives. Health care providers should not be unduly concerned about litigation whenever these rights are upheld [7].

Minors

By California statutory definition, a minor is a person under the age of 18 and is not legally able to consent to medical treatment unless the law designates him or her as an emancipated minor [29]. The same law applies in most other states. In most cases, a minor's parents have the legal authority to consent to treatment for their child and consent must be obtained prior to treatment. There is a caveat, however, to such consent. If the minor objects to the treatment, the case should be referred to the hospital attorney if doubt exists about proceeding with treatment. For instance, if the objection is by a minor who is 14 years or older, it may be appropriate to seek legal advice if the parents consent to a procedure that involves significant risk of severe adverse consequences.

Most Witness families recognize the delicate balance between their rights and the legal obligations of the physicians. The US Constitution protects the fundamental right of parents to make decisions concerning the care, custody and control of their children. Therefore, with the exception of an emergency, if a surgeon operates on a child without the parents' consent, the surgeon will be liable for assault [7,9].

Issues arise when the state seeks to interfere with the parents' right to make decisions regarding their child's medical treatment due to the state's interest in protecting those who are disabled or who are unable to protect themselves. If the state perceives that a minor child's life or health is in danger because of a parent's refusal to consent to blood transfusion, they may grant a court order for the transfusion. However, such an order will only be granted if the state's interest in the protection of an innocent third party is 'compelling'. For the state's interest to be compelling it must be proven that there are no alternative nonblood treatments available. When the state's interest is viewed as compelling and there is risk of imminent harm or death, the court will order that blood be given. The physician or hospital may otherwise be held liable.

Mature and emancipated minors

An exception is sometimes made in the case of a mature minor. A mature minor is one who is able to understand the nature and extent of his or her condition. The patient should also understand the recommended alternatives to blood and should be able to appreciate the consequences of the blood refusal. The decision is not solely dependent on the parents but is based on the patient's clear understanding of the facts.

California Legislature has enacted a series of statutes that authorize particular classes of minors to consent to various medical services [29]. However, a minor who would otherwise have the legal authority to consent to medical treatment may not be permitted to do so if he or she does not fully understand and appreciate the nature and consequences of the proposed health care, including its significant benefits, risks and alternatives. In such a scenario, consultation with legal counsel should be arranged to eliminate any doubt that may exist.

According to the California Health Care Association, when a minor of 15 years or older is living separate and apart from his or her parent(s) or legal guardian, whether with or without the consent or acquiescence of his or her parent(s) or legal guardian, and manages his or her own financial affairs, regardless of the source of income, the minor is capable of giving a valid consent for medical or dental care without parental or guardian consent, knowledge or financial liability. 'Medical care' means 'X-ray examination, anesthetic, medical or surgical diagnosis or treatment, and hospital care' under the supervision and upon the advice of a licensed physician. This is the definition of an emancipated minor.

When dealing with emancipated or mature minors who are Jehovah's Witnesses, physicians do well to have a clear understanding of the laws pertaining to their rights and to proceed in a manner that accords them with the same respect and dignity as they would give to an adult patient. However, decisions made by mature minors should be followed by the hospital only after a court decision is rendered regarding their ability to refuse treatment such as blood transfusion. This will protect health care providers from any potential liability.

Evolution of bloodless programs

Initially Jehovah's Witnesses' adamant refusal of blood and blood products was met with much controversy and frustration by members of both the medical and legal community. Most doctors viewed Jehovah's Witnesses' position as one that 'tied their hands' and prevented them from rendering adequate care under circumstances where profound anemia or significant surgical blood loss might compromise their patient's life. They were proponents of the accepted 'rule' to transfuse a patient if their hemoglobin was below 10 g/dl or their hematocrit was below 30%. Many physicians flatly refused to treat Jehovah's Witnesses due to their refusal of blood. However, due to the continued growth of the Witness community, others recognized that this issue was not going away soon, and a few physicians saw a unique opportunity in caring for these patients.

Early pioneers of bloodless medicine and surgery

Everyone wants effective medical care of the highest quality. To that end, a few members of the medical community began to ask the question: 'Are there legitimate and effective ways to manage serious medical problems without using blood?' Fortunately for Jehovah's Witnesses, the answer was yes.

As early as the 1950s, a handful of physicians began to view the Witnesses' refusal of blood not as 'tying their hands', but as just one more complication challenging their skill. Noteworthy among this group of pioneers was Dr Denton Cooley of the Texas Heart Institute. In 1957, Cooley pioneered open-heart surgery without blood support [30,31–34]. Dr Cooley led a team of cardiovascular surgeons who performed thousands of cardiovascular operations on adults and children. In those days, most open-heart surgeries required 20–30 units of blood. In fact, as many as 12 units of blood were used just to prime the heart-lung bypass machine. However, Dr Cooley and his colleagues used innovative methods to prime the bypass machine with nonblood fluids. In time, other techniques were developed to obviate the need for blood. Dr Cooley's experience revealed that 'the risk of surgery in patients of the Jehovah's Witness group was not substantially higher than for others'. This was indeed the genesis of 'bloodless surgery'.

In 1995, Dr Hiram C. Polk Jr, editor-in-chief of the *American Journal of Surgery*, recognized Dr Cooley's outstanding accomplishments [35]. He commented on the trailblazing efforts of Dr Cooley in performing some 1250 'bloodless' open-heart surgeries on patients who requested it due to their religious beliefs. He stated that 'Dr Cooley's blood conservation techniques are applicable to every operation and, therefore, meaningful to all 17 000 readers of *The American Journal of Surgery*'.

Genesis of bloodless medicine and surgery programs

As more and more physicians began to respect Jehovah's Witnesses' position on blood, the atmosphere became less adversarial and much more cooperative. In fact, doctors and hospital administrators learned that the key to managing patients without blood transfusion required proper planning and good coordination between all members of the hospital staff, including nursing, laboratory, pharmacy and social services. Although there are more doctors and hospitals who are willing to cooperate with patients who choose not to accept blood transfusion, a *promise* not to give blood is often not good enough to satisfy some patients. Thus the concept of a structured, formalized 'bloodless' program was born. A bloodless or transfusion-free program offers a group of experienced and skilled physicians, surgeons, anesthesiologists and nurses who are dedicated and committed to 'quality' medical care, without the use of blood. The hospital administration must fully support this program and make it clear to all staff that once a patient is admitted to the hospital, the patient's refusal of blood should no longer be an issue.

USC University Hospital Program Experience
The administrative team in concert with several key physicians decided to launch the Bloodless Medicine and Surgery Program at USC University Hospital and USC/Norris Cancer Hospital. With a large population of Jehovah's Witnesses residing in California, they came to realize the importance of providing these patients with alternatives to traditional medical and surgical techniques that require transfusions.

In early 1994, the representatives of hospital administration held several meetings with members of the local Hospital Liaison Committee for Jehovah's Witnesses (HLC). Working under the direction of the Hospital Information Services of Jehovah's Witnesses (HIS), headquartered in Brooklyn, New York, the HLC's role is to seek out physicians and hospitals that will offer nonblood management to the Witness community. Presentations about Jehovah's Witnesses' position on health care, specifically blood and blood products, were given to members of the USC faculty.

Subsequently, personal contact was made with individual physicians to determine their willingness to treat Witness patients without blood. The goal of these one-on-one interviews was to ascertain each doctor's comfort level and experience in providing elective and emergent treatment to adults and minors without blood product support.

The program was officially launched in 1997 under the direction of Dr Nicolas Jabbour. The program was promoted using newsletters, seminars, health fairs and medical conferences, and media outlets.

Legal structure of bloodless program

Consent: liability of physician and hospital
The Paul Gann Blood Safety Act, based on California State Law, Health & Safety Code puts the onus on the physician to talk with patients facing the possibility of receiving allogeneic blood, and explain to them the risks, benefits and alternatives. The Paul Gann Act emphasizes alternatives such as preoperative autologous donation, directed donor blood, intraoperative cell-salvage and hemodilution. The physician must note in the patient's medical record that a standardized written summary produced by the State Department of Health Services (DHS) is given to the patient (see Figures 1.3 and 1.4). No other pamphlet, other than the DHS pamphlet, will satisfy the physician's obligation under the law.

Upon admission to the hospital, patients must sign a release-of-liability form that clearly documents their refusal of blood and releases the physician and all hospital personnel from any untoward consequences of such refusal (see Figure 1.2).

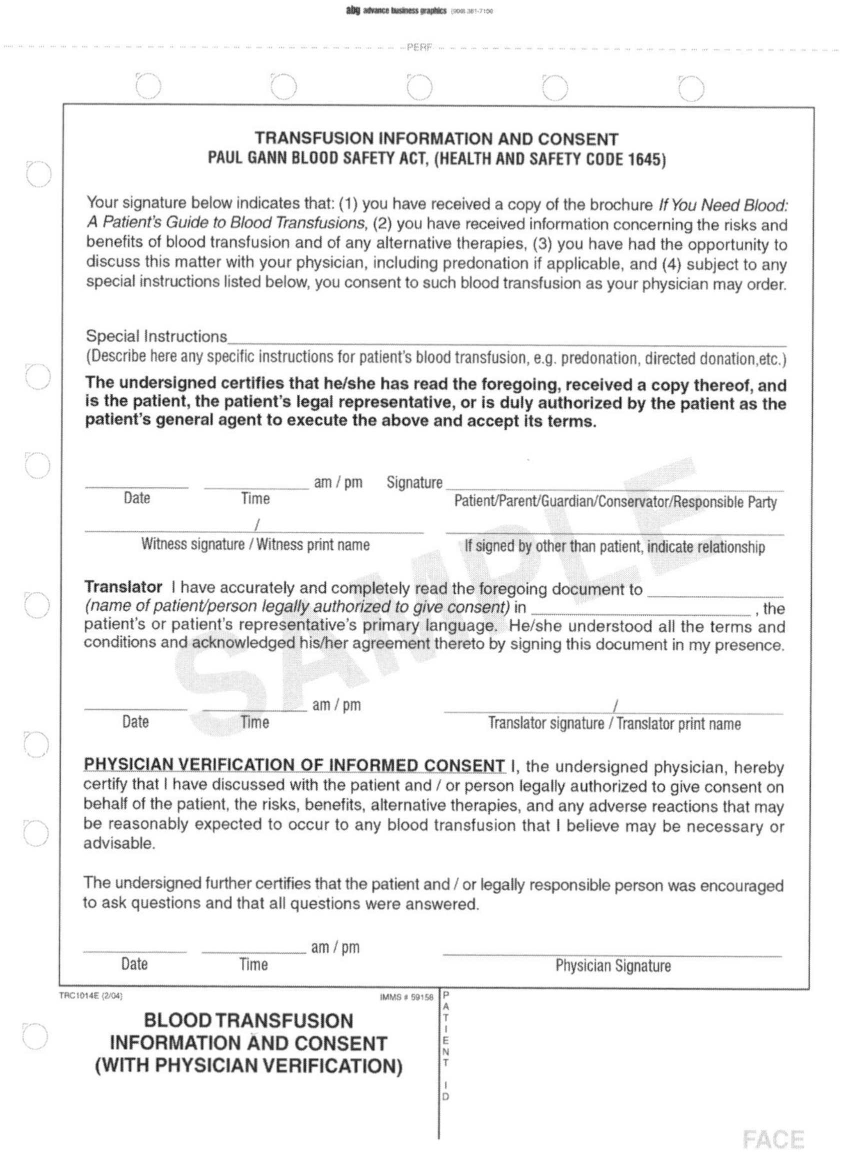

--- PERF ---

TRANSFUSION INFORMATION AND CONSENT
PAUL GANN BLOOD SAFETY ACT, (HEALTH AND SAFETY CODE 1645)

Your signature below indicates that: (1) you have received a copy of the brochure *If You Need Blood: A Patient's Guide to Blood Transfusions*, (2) you have received information concerning the risks and benefits of blood transfusion and of any alternative therapies, (3) you have had the opportunity to discuss this matter with your physician, including predonation if applicable, and (4) subject to any special instructions listed below, you consent to such blood transfusion as your physician may order.

Special Instructions_____
(Describe here any specific instructions for patient's blood transfusion, e.g. predonation, directed donation,etc.)

The undersigned certifies that he/she has read the foregoing, received a copy thereof, and is the patient, the patient's legal representative, or is duly authorized by the patient as the patient's general agent to execute the above and accept its terms.

_____ _____ am / pm   Signature _____
　　Date　　　　Time　　　　　　　　　　　　Patient/Parent/Guardian/Conservator/Responsible Party
_____ / _____　　　_____
　Witness signature / Witness print name　　　　If signed by other than patient, indicate relationship

Translator I have accurately and completely read the foregoing document to _____
(name of patient/person legally authorized to give consent) in _____ , the
patient's or patient's representative's primary language. He/she understood all the terms and conditions and acknowledged his/her agreement thereto by signing this document in my presence.

_____ _____ am / pm   _____
　　Date　　　　Time　　　　　　　　　　　Translator signature / Translator print name

PHYSICIAN VERIFICATION OF INFORMED CONSENT I, the undersigned physician, hereby certify that I have discussed with the patient and / or person legally authorized to give consent on behalf of the patient, the risks, benefits, alternative therapies, and any adverse reactions that may be reasonably expected to occur to any blood transfusion that I believe may be necessary or advisable.

The undersigned further certifies that the patient and / or legally responsible person was encouraged to ask questions and that all questions were answered.

_____ _____ am / pm   _____
　　Date　　　　Time　　　　　　　　　　　　　　Physician Signature

TRC1014E (2/04)　　　　　　　　　　IMMS # 59158

BLOOD TRANSFUSION
INFORMATION AND CONSENT
(WITH PHYSICIAN VERIFICATION)

PATIENT ID

FACE

Figure 1.3 DHS Pamphlet: Transfusion Information and Consent (Paul Gann Blood Safety Act).

When such due diligence is exercised by the physician and hospital, there is little, if any, need to be concerned about litigation arising from a patient whose refusal of blood leads to morbidity or mortality.

The methods of using your own blood can be used independently or together to eliminate or minimize the need for donor blood, as well as virtually eliminate transfusion risks of infection and allergic reaction.

■ AUTOLOGOUS BLOOD - Using Your Own Blood

Option	Explanation	Advantages	Disadvantages
PRE-OPERATIVE DONATION Donating Your Own Blood Before Surgery	The blood bank draws your blood and stores it until you need it, during or after surgery. For elective surgery only.	✓ Eliminates or minimizes the need for someone else's blood during and after surgery.	• Requires advance planning. • May delay surgery. • Medical conditions may prevent pre-operative donation.
INTRA-OPERATIVE AUTOLOGOUS TRANSFUSION Recycling Your Blood During Surgery	Instead of being discarded, blood lost during surgery is filtered, and put back into your body during surgery. For elective and emergency surgery.	✓ Eliminates or minimizes the need for someone else's blood during surgery. Large amounts of blood can be recycled.	• Not for use if cancer or infection is present.
POST-OPERATIVE AUTOLOGOUS TRANSFUSION Recycling Your Blood After Surgery	Blood lost after surgery is collected, filtered and returned. For elective and emergency surgery.	✓ Eliminates or minimizes the need for someone else's blood after surgery.	• Not for use if cancer or infection is present.
HEMODILUTION Donating Your Own Blood During Surgery	Immediately before surgery, some of your blood is taken and replaced with I.V. fluids. After surgery, your blood is filtered and returned to you . For elective surgery.	✓ Eliminates or minimizes the need for someone else's blood during and after surgery. Dilutes your blood so you lose less concentrated blood during surgery.	• Limited number or units can be drawn. • Medical conditions may prevent hemodilution.
APHERESIS Donating Your Own Platelets and Plasma	Before surgery, your platelets and plasma, which help stop bleeding, are withdrawn, filtered, and returned to you when you need it. For elective surgery.	✓ May eliminate the need for donor platelets and plasma, especially in high blood-loss procedures.	• Medical conditions may prevent apheresis. • Procedure has limited application.

In some cases, you may require more blood than anticipated. If this happens and you receive blood other then your own, there is a possibility of complications, such as hepatitis or AIDS.

■ DONOR BLOOD - Using Someone Else's Blood

Donor blood and blood products can never be absolutely 100% safe, even though testing makes the risk very small.

Option	Explanation	Advantages	Disadvantages
VOLUNTEER BLOOD From the Community Blood Supply	Blood and blood products donated by volunteer donors to a community blood bank.	✓ Readily available. Can be life-saving when your own blood is not available.	• Risk of disease transmission (such as hepatitis or AIDS), and allergic reactions.
Note You may wish to check whether donors are paid or volunteer, since blood from commercial (paid) donors may not, in some cases, be as safe as blood from volunteers.			
DESIGNATED DONOR BLOOD From Donors You Select	Blood and blood donors you select who must meet the same requirements as volunteer donors.	✓ You can select people with your own blood type who you feel are safe donors.	• Risk of disease transmission (such as hepatitis or AIDS), and allergic reactions. • May require several days of advanced donation. • Not necessarily as safe, nor safer, than volunteer donor blood.
Note Care should be taken in selecting donors. Donors should never be pressured into donating. Donations from certain family members may require irradiation of blood			

Figure 1.4 DHS Pamphlet: Transfusion Information and Consent (Paul Gann Blood Safety Act).

Confirming a patient's decision to refuse blood

On occasion, a physician may feel compelled to 'confirm' or 'verify' a patient's decision to refuse blood transfusion. The physician's personal conscience may dictate that he or she *privately* discuss the matter with the patient without any input from family members. Such a discussion is appropriate and usually welcome. However, a physician should be careful not to use this session as an opportunity to pressure the patient to revisit his or her refusal of blood. How far should the physician go in 'confirming' the patient's choice of nonblood management without it being viewed as 'badgering' or coercion? Oftentimes this can be a very subtle issue. The goal of this discussion is to give the physician the confidence and peace of mind that withholding blood products is the absolute decision of the patient. On the other hand, if a family member or friend is present to give advice or moral support to the patient (especially in the case of Jehovah's Witnesses), the medical staff should have it clear in mind that the decision being made is the patient's and not the other persons'. If the patient is looking to another person to answer questions being posed to him or her, it can make a physician quite uneasy, and understandably so. This sort of input should be given to the patient during pre-op or some other more appropriate time.

Policies and procedures

An essential step to ensuring the success of a bloodless program is to develop well-defined policies and procedures that are legally, ethically and clinically sound (see Appendix). They should make absolutely clear the role of every member of the medical and hospital staffs who have direct contact with patients refusing blood or blood products. Distinct methods of identifying patients should be implemented, for example colored armbands, computer codes/symbols and chart stickers. A mechanism should be in place to monitor orders to type and crossmatch blood for patients enrolled in the bloodless program. In addition, laboratory draws for blood testing should be ordered judiciously, not routinely.

Highlights of USC Program

The Transfusion-Free Medicine and Surgery Program at USC University Hospital is supported by a comprehensive dedicated team of over 100 medical and administrative professionals. The program has an appointed medical director and program manager. There is also an advisory committee that is designed to steer the development and management of the program. Its core functions are to revise policies and procedures to support the program, and develop mechanisms to measure compliance. In addition, the advisory committee establishes criteria to identify physicians to be included on a transfusion-free medicine panel for the purpose of referring patients, and to ascertain indicators and develop a database for outcome measurement. The committee members may also assist in examining the feasibility of utilizing specific products and services offered by vendors that are designed to minimize blood loss. All in all, the advisory committee serves as a tool to increase quality of care and patient satisfaction within this specialized area of medicine. The collaborative effort of everyone involved has led to steady growth and noteworthy accomplishments (see Figure 1.5). Most notably in

USC transfusion-free program–surgical admissions

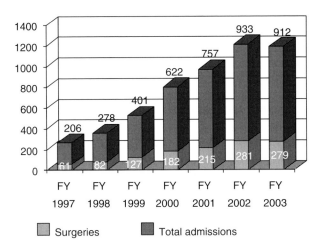

Figure 1.5 USC Transfusion-Free Program growth.

June 1999 the USC liver transplant team led by Dr Nicolas Jabbour, Dr Rick Selby and Dr Yuri Genyk performed the world's first adult-to-adult living-related live-donor liver transplant in a Jehovah's Witness patient without blood product. Not long after that, the team performed their first successful pediatric live-donor liver transplant in a child from a Jehovah's Witness family without blood product transfusion. Other major surgical cases performed at USC University Hospital and the USC Norris Cancer Hospital without blood include prostatectomy, radical nephrectomy, cystectomy, primary and revision hip/knee surgery, neuro-spine and ortho-spine surgery, cardiac bypass and valve replacement surgery, and even heart transplants.

Future extension of transfusion-free programs

When most people hear the words 'bloodless' or 'transfusion-free', they immediately think of Jehovah's Witnesses. Historically Jehovah's Witnesses have been the largest users of bloodless and/or transfusion-free medicine and surgery. However, in recent years the objective of many individuals and organizations, both in the medical community and the lay public, has been to expand this approach to medicine to a much larger population. Religious, ethical and legal issues aside, one must take a hard look at whether or not blood avoidance offers benefits for the community at large.

It is hoped that transfusion-free medicine becomes the standard of care for any medical or surgical patient. One cannot deny that there are many modalities that have been heavily relied upon in the past, even as it relates to the use of blood, that are now considered archaic and unscientific.

With ongoing progress in the area of oxygen-carrying products and synthetic clotting factors such as factor VIIA, the future looks brighter in providing a safe and effective alternative to blood transfusions.

References

1 Bloodless medicine and surgery – the growing demand. *Awake* 2000; **81**: 3–6.
2 *Jehovah's Witnesses and the Question of Blood*. Watchtower Bible and Tract Society of Pennsylvania, 1977.
3 *How Can Blood Save Your Life?* Watchtower Bible and Tract Society of Pennsylvania, 1990.
4 Questions from readers. *The Watchtower* 2000; **121** (Jun 15): 29–31.
5 Questions from readers. *The Watchtower* 2000; **121** (Oct 15): 29–31.
6 Questions from readers. *The Watchtower* 1980; **101**: 31.
7 *Legally Defending Jehovah's Witnesses' View of Blood*. New York: Patterson, 2001.
8 *California Physician's Legal Handbook*. California Medical Association, 1997.
9 Legal Considerations for Balancing Patients' Rights and The Bloodless Medicine and Surgery Program. Ralph A. Leaf, Attorney at Law, 1997.
10 *Schloendorff v. Society of New York Hospital*, 105 N.E. 92, 93 (NY 1914).
11 61 Am Jur 2d. Physicians, Surgeons, and Other Healers 197 (1981).
12 *In re Milton*, 505 N.E.2d 255 (OH 1987).
13 *In re Osborne*, 294 A.2d 372 (DC 1972).
14 *In re Estate of Brooks*, 205 N.E.2d 435 (IL 1965).
15 *Reynolds v. United States*, 98 U.S. 145, 167 (1878).
16 *Harden v. State*, 216 S.W.2d 708 (TN 1948).
17 *The Refused Blood Transfusion*, 10 Nat. L.F. 202, 207–09 (1965).
18 *The Right to Die*, 9 Utah L. Rev. 161, 163–68 (1964).
19 *In re Brown*, 478 So.2d 1033, 1039 (MS 1985).
20 *In re Conroy*, 486 A.2d 1209, 1229 (NJ 1985).
21 *Winters v. Miller*, 446 F.2d 65,69 (2d. Cir 1971)
22 Developments in the Law – Medical Technology and the Law, 103 Harv L Rev 1519, 1670 (1990).
23 535 A.2d 452 (Pa 1987). Informed Refusal: Legal Befuddlement.
24 President's Commission, Deciding to Forego Life-Sustaining Treatment at 132–33.
25 *In re Dubreuil*, 629 So. 2d 819, 827 n.13 (Fla 1993).
26 2 Health Law Center, Hospital Law Manual 180 (P. Young 3d 1989).
27 President's Commission for the Study of Ethical Problems, *Making Health Care Decisions* 183 (1982).
28 Developments in the Law – Medical Technology and the Law, 103 Harv L Rev 1519, 1651 (1990).
29 Consent Manual. California Healthcare Association 2001, 28th edn.
30 Farmer S, Webb D. *Your Body, Your Choice*. Singapore: Media Masters, 2000: 14–15.
31 Cooley DA, Crawford ES, Howell JF, Beall AC Jr. Open heart surgery in jehovah's witnesses. *Am J Cardiol* 1964; **13**: 779–81.
32 Ott DA, Cooley DA. Cardiovascular surgery in Jehovah's Witnesses: report of 542 operations without blood transfusion. *JAMA* 1977; **238**: 1256–8.

33 Henling CE, Carmichael MJ, Keats AS, Cooley DA. Cardiac operation for congenital heart disease in children of Jehovah's Witnesses. *J Thorac Cardiovasc Surg* 1985; **89**: 914–20.

34 Carmichael MJ, Cooley DA, Kuykendall RC, Walker WE. Cardiac surgery in children of Jehovah's Witnesses. *Tex Heart Inst J* 1985; **12**: 57–63.

35 Cooley DA. Conservation of blood during cardiovascular surgery. *Am J Surg* 1995; **170**: 53S–59S.

CHAPTER 2

Transfusion Therapy – Balancing the Risks and Benefits

Roslyn A Yomtovian, Katharine A Downes, Ira A Shulman

> Never go to excess, but let moderation be your guide
>
> –Cicero (106–43 BC)

Introduction/Overview

Throughout recorded history, blood has been a subject of fascination and mystery. Perceptions regarding blood, whether grounded in science or superstition, have engendered intense emotion and ongoing controversy. The Greek concept of the humors, in which blood played so vital a role, is still evident in expressions such as 'hot-blooded', 'cold-blooded' and 'bad-blood' that are used the world over (*www.bloodbook.com*). The word blood is mentioned over 400 times in the Bible (*www.biblegateway.com*) where it is often associated or synonymous with the essence of life.

Following the description of blood circulation by the British physician William Harvey in 1628, animal blood was tried as a human therapeutic modality. In one case, a bad outcome and subsequent notoriety resulted in a French and later British and Italian Parliamentary ban on transfusion therapy, initiated in 1670 and lasting for 150 years [1]. This might be the first, but certainly not the last, instance of the politicalization of blood.

The modern use of blood transfusion as a therapeutic modality is perhaps surprisingly less than 70 years old. The outbreak of World War II catalyzed the need for transfusion therapy and led to the establishment of the first blood bank in Barcelona, Spain, in 1936. In the USA, the 'Blood for Britain' program, an effort to collect and export large quantities of plasma to the war theatre in Great Britain, spearheaded by Dr Charles Drew in 1941, became the model for today's regional blood programs [2]. Following World War II, ongoing developments and innovations in blood collection and storage led to the availability of blood component therapy in which a single blood donation could be separated into several therapeutic products consisting of red blood cells (RBCs), platelets and either frozen plasma or cryoprecipitate (CRYO). Thus, transfusions could be targeted to replace a specific deficient component.

Each year Americans donate an estimated 16 million units of blood, which is processed into more than 26 million units of blood components. About 4.8 million Americans annually receive transfusion therapy of various kinds from these components. Each day approximately 40 000 units of RBC transfusions are used in the USA. While the use of transfusion therapy, over the decades, has grown dramatically to accommodate advances in medical and surgical treatments and practices – and clearly has afforded lifesaving treatment to millions of patients – its use comes at the cost of a variety of adverse complications, some associated with significant morbidity and mortality. This chapter focuses on the scientific basis and medical justification for the administration of blood transfusions. Other chapters will focus on medical, surgical and/or pharmacological strategies that can reduce or eliminate the need for blood transfusions. The decision to refuse blood transfusions altogether, however, may be based on religious, political or personal preference. The fundamental goal of this chapter is to present a model of transfusion practice that focuses on the optimization of blood transfusion therapy. According to this model, blood transfusion therapy is a balancing act – it should neither be used when not indicated nor withheld when indicated. Clearly, the challenge is to decipher the difference. This is made particularly difficult since the contributions on each side of the balance – representing the risks and benefits (Figure 2.1) – are constantly changing based on the ongoing identification of new risks, new benefits, new safety measures to reduce identified risks and new alternatives to transfusion therapy.

Utility of transfusion practice

The utility of a blood transfusion might be judged according to its medical justification and/or the quality of the clinical outcome. One might envision that if the justifications for, and the clinical outcomes of, several hundreds of transfusion events were plotted, one might see a bell-shaped curve like the one displayed in Figure 2.2. Most transfusion events would fall near the center of the bell curve, having been administered for appropriate medical indications and having resulted in a positive outcome (see Cases 1–4 and 6–11). However, some transfusion events fall on either side of the bell curve. Some patients experience harm from receipt of inappropriate transfusion therapy (see Case 20) or suffer adverse consequences, inadvertently, from appropriately administered transfusion therapy (Cases 25–31). Other patients may experience harm when they do not receive transfusion therapy when clinically indicated or fail to receive it in a timely manner (see Cases 12–16) or in an appropriate dose (see Cases 17–19 and Tables 2.3 and 2.4). Thus, such unintended errors of omission and commission may lead to significant morbidity or mortality.

Following an overview of the clinical utility of transfusion therapy – RBCs, platelets, plasma and CRYO – a series of clinical vignettes are provided to illustrate representative examples of appropriate and faulty transfusion prac-

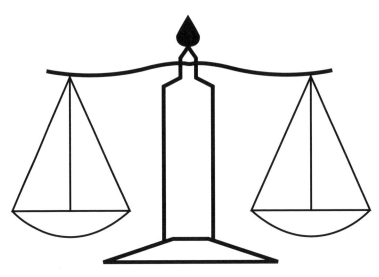

Risks	Benefits
Infectious disease transmission	Provides tissue oxygenation (RBCs)
Incorrect transfusion	Allows blood coagulation (plasma,
Improper Transfusion	cryoprecipitate, platelets)
Metabolic disturbances	Enhances treatment of sepsis (PMNs)
Immune pertubations	Restores hematopoiesis (stem cells)
Infusion of toxic agents	Tumor inhibition (stem cells,
Unknown risks	mononuclear cells)

Figure 2.1 The risks and benefits of transfusion therapy.

tices. This will be followed by a summary of the risks of transfusion practice caused by products as well as processes. Finally, the optimization of transfusion therapy will be established as a balancing act between risks and benefits.

The clinical utility of transfusion therapy

Red blood cell transfusion

The primary purpose of RBC transfusion therapy is to sustain physiologically adequate tissue oxygenation, which is critical for maintenance of life [3,4]. Patients in need of RBC transfusion therapy are those with physiologically important reductions in red cell mass as a result of bleeding (see Cases 1 and 3), hemolysis, lack of production (see Case 2) or profound sequestration. RBC transfusion therapy is also used to replace or exchange abnormal RBCs (see Cases 4 and 5). The use of RBC transfusion therapy should be guided by the combination of patient history, acuteness of developing anemia, symptoms, physical findings and laboratory results. Signs and symptoms of anemia, indicating a possible need for RBC transfusion, include palpitations, anxiety, tinnitus, dizziness, tingling, anorexia, nausea, headaches and scotomata. As the anemia worsens, dyspnea, tachycardia, fatigue and malaise become

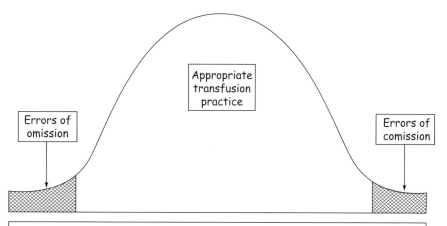

It is envisioned that transfusion practice simulates a bell-shaped curve. In this example, the area in the center represents an estimated 90% of transfusions, which are likely administered for appropriate indications in an appropriate manner and achieve a positive clinical benefit. The area to the right of the center represents the estimated (hypothetical) 5% of transfusions that are associated with errors in commission – transfusions that are administered either inappropriately and are associated with significant adverse consequences; or appropriately but have inadvertent adverse consequence following transfusion. The area to the left of the center, represents the estimated (hypothetical) 5% of transfusions that are associated with errors of omission – transfusions that are not administered when clinically needed or not administered in a timely manner. Both the errors of commission and errors of omission may result in significant morbidity and mortality.

Figure 2.2 Transfusion practices – conceptual overview of errors of commisson and omission.

manifest, though many previously and otherwise healthy patients may remain apparently asymptomatic even with profound anemia as illustrated in Case 14. Dyspnea at rest, if present, is an ominous finding in any patient with diminished RBC mass and requires immediate transfusion therapy [5]. Patients with significant underlying cerebral (see Case 13), coronary or peripheral atherosclerosis, especially the elderly (see Case 15), may instead complain of claudication, angina, syncope or transient ischemic attacks [6].

The etiology and chronicity of anemia determine the compensatory mechanisms in place to assure that the balance of supply and demand of oxygen delivery is maintained. Tissue oxygen extraction increases linearly with decreases in hematocrit (Hct) to 10%, at which point extractions greater than 50% herald anaerobic metabolism. High baseline oxygen extraction percentages (55–70%) in the myocardium and brain limit compensation via this mechanism, relying instead on increased blood flow for increased oxygen delivery [7]. Overall, age, cardiovascular status and clinical circumstances determine the extent to which compensation is possible. Below a certain hemoglobin (Hb) or Hct and/or ability of adequate compensation, demand outpaces supply heralding ischemia and infarction (see Cases 13 and 15). Increased cardiac output, the fundamental compensatory response, begins at an Hb of < 10 g/dl, though significant increases begin only when the Hb is < 7 g/dl [6,8]. Interestingly, nonsurgical, critically ill patients maintained at Hb levels of 7–9 g/dl versus 10–12 g/dl seem to have no increase in mortality or morbidity [9] unless there is underlying coronary atherosclerotic disease [10–14].

With worsening anemia, cardiac output increases steeply, peaking at 180% of normal at an Hb of 6–7 g/dl. Below an Hb of 3–5 g/dl, shifts in coronary blood flow from endocardium to epicardium signal imminent danger in the otherwise healthy patient [8,15,16]. Coexistence of coronary vascular stenoses lowers this tolerance to 7–10 g/dl [17]. The importance of coexisting cardiac disease when determining the tolerance to anemia is further highlighted in a study of the correlation of the baseline Hb level and hospital-based and long-term mortality in male patients undergoing percutaneous coronary interventions (PCIs). Over a median follow-up period of 697 days, patients with Hb levels in the lowest quintile (< 12.9 g/dl) had a mortality rate two to seven times higher than those in other quintiles, even after accounting for the impact of other covariables [18]. A further study demonstrated that mild anemia (Hb < 12 g/dl) was a significant and independent predictor of poor outcome in patients with congestive heart failure (hazard ratio 2.9, 95% confidence interval, 1.2–7.2; $p = 0.02$) over an 18-month period [19]. The authors advocate use of erythropoietin as a potential therapeutic modality in this patient group.

Although numerous efforts have been made to define a broadly applicable 'transfusion trigger' [20–27], the literature emphasizes evaluation of each patient's individual needs as paramount [6,28–37]. Studies of patients refusing transfusion for religious reasons have helped define the absolute lower limit of human tolerance; mortality is 87% at an Hct of 9%. While other studies of Jehovah's Witnesses have found that a decreased Hb or Hct was either a direct or indirect cause of death in only 0.5–1.5% of patients, 91% of the patients who expired had an Hb of < 5 g/dl [34,38]. In identifying and predicting surgical patients at risk for anemia, estimated blood loss (EBL) must be evaluated in concert with the initial and subsequent Hb and/or Hct values. Perioperative mortality in Jehovah's Witness patients was 7% with the Hb > 10 g/dl and 62% with the Hb < 6 g/dl. Of note, when the EBL was < 500 cc, mortality was 8%; this rose to 43% when the EBL was > 2000 cc. No patient with Hb > 8 g/dl and EBL < 500 cc expired [39]. In a similar study, mortality was 75% in patients with a 24% Hct and EBL > 500 cc, while mortality was zero in patients with Hb ≥ 6 g/dl and EBL < 500 cc [40]. A more recent study of 1958 patients confirmed these findings, further noting a 1.3% 30-day mortality in patients with a preoperative Hb ≥ 12 g/dl versus a 33.3% mortality in patients with Hb < 6 g/dl. Mortality was significantly more pronounced in patients with cardiovascular disease; and, the effect of blood loss on mortality was greater in those patients with low preoperative Hb [17].

Table 2.1 Clinical situations where blood transfusion may be harmful.

Blood component	Consequence of transfusion
Red blood cells	
Sickle cell hemolytic transfusion reaction syndrome	May lead to erythroid aplasia in marrow
Platelets	
Thrombotic thrombocytopenic purpura	May exacerbate thrombosis
Posttransfusion purpura	May precipitate severe reaction
Heparin-induced thrombocytopenia	May exacerbate thrombosis
Idiopathic (immune) thrombocytopenic purpura	May further accelerate platelet destruction
Plasma	
Heparin reversal	May exacerbate heparin effect
Factors VIII and IX replacement	Use only if a virally inactivated concentrate is not available
Cryoprecipitate	
Factor VIII replacement	Use only if a virally inactivated concentrate is not available

Although RBC transfusion is clearly lifesaving in most instances where the level of Hb or Hct is at a very low level, in some instances it may do more harm than good (see Table 2.1). For example, Case 31 illustrates a severely anemic patient with sickle cell anemia in whom there was simultaneous hemolysis of the transfused RBCs with the subsequent development of pure red cell aplasia in the bone marrow. By withholding RBC transfusion therapy, despite profound anemia, in this and similar cases, hemolysis ceases and there is reconstitution of bone marrow erythropoiesis. Naturally such patients must be carefully monitored, and receive oxygen and the most compatible RBCs available in case of life-threatening decompensation. In instances of severe anemia due to B_{12}, folate or iron deficiency, where total blood volume is normal or possibly even increased, the patient should be carefully assessed and treated for the specific deficiency. If the clinical signs and symptoms and extreme level of anemia dictate the need for RBC transfusion therapy, it must be given slowly and with extreme care to prevent precipitation of congestive heart failure due to rapid increase in intravascular volume.

A potential important variable in the efficacy of transfusion therapy is the storage age of the blood, especially when administered to critically ill patients [41]. Experimental work in a rat model has suggested that transfusion of older, stored blood may fail to provide improved systemic oxygenation compared to transfusion of fresh blood [42]. Patients' transfused units after prolonged storage have developed evidence of splanchnic ischemia. Increased

viscosity, decreased erythrocyte deformability at the capillary level (sphero-
cyte formation due to reduced ATP), and diminished 2,3-DPG levels in stored
blood (> 15 days) may account for these observations: erythrocytes require
about 6 h to recover enough ATP and 2,3-DPG stores to function adequately.
There are suggestions of possible increased postoperative infectious complications and morbidity with transfusion of blood stored for greater than 21 to
28 days [43–46]. How RBC storage age might interrelate with the role of nitric
oxide and its relationship to RBC hemoglobin as it synergizes with the
exchange of oxygen and carbon dioxide during transfusion therapy remains
to be further defined [47,48].

While there has been a great deal of emphasis in the literature on attempt-
ing to define and limit 'overtransfusion' of RBCs, instances of potential
'undertransfusion' are not usually sought or readily appreciated [49–53].
Yet, as illustrated in Cases 12–16, RBC undertransfusion has been reported
to be associated with clinical harm or high risk [54–56]. Most recently,
anemia has been linked to decline in physical performance in the elderly
[57]. In addition, higher levels of Hb have been associated with better
early functional recovery, as a function of distance walked at discharge, in
elderly patients following total hip replacement surgery [58]. Clearly, optimization of RBC transfusion therapy remains to be precisely and clearly
defined.

Platelet transfusion

The major purpose of platelet transfusion therapy is to afford primary hemostasis, which is critical in stopping or preventing hemorrhage. Patients in need
of platelet transfusion therapy are those with a physiologically important
reduction in platelets, usually as a result of lack of production or those with a
physiologically important dysfunction in platelet function rendering them
incapable of providing primary hemostasis [59]. Platelets are not otherwise
indicated (see Case 21). Assessment of platelet dysfunction may be achieved by
use of the platelet function analyzer (PFA-100®), which offers a more standardized *in vitro* approach, compared to the bleeding time. In some disorders,
namely thrombotic thrombocytopenia purpura (TTP), heparin-induced
thrombocytopenia (HIT), posttransfusion purpura (PTP) and idiopathic
thrombocytopenia purpura (ITP), platelets may be profoundly reduced, commonly below 10 000/μl. Yet, despite profound thrombocytopenia in these
disorders, platelet transfusion therapy is medically contraindicated except in
instances of life-threatening hemorrhage (Table 2.1). In the case of TTP and
HIT it is generally acknowledged that platelet transfusion therapy results in
worsening of the thrombotic process; with PTP and ITP the presence of antibodies against high-frequency platelet antigens limits the effectiveness of
platelet transfusion therapy and results in severe reactions (PTP) or might
induce confounding alloimmunization (ITP) [60–62]. Splenic sequestration
may result in profound thrombocytopenia. Again, platelet transfusion therapy
should be reserved for instances of life-threatening hemorrhage, since

generally such transfusion will be associated with rapid platelet removal thereby limiting the effectiveness.

The first use of platelets as a therapeutic modality was by Duke in 1910 [63]. Despite the qualified success of his work, little effort was made to exploit the therapeutic value of platelets until a reliable method became available to separate platelets from whole blood and store them as a separate blood component. Then in 1954 Gardner *et al.* described a procedure for the use of plastic equipment for platelet transfusion [64]. Gaydos *et al.*, noting the important relationship between platelet count and hemorrhage in patients with acute leukemia, suggested an important role for platelet transfusion therapy in the management of hematopoietic disorders [65]. Murphy and Gardner further revolutionized the practice of platelet transfusion therapy in the 1960s and 1970s by demonstrating maintenance of platelet function during several days of storage at room temperature [66]. Although they noted concern regarding the potential risk of bacterial contamination, they did not believe this to be a problem based on sampling a small number of units. Subsequently, it has been demonstrated, that bacterial contamination of platelets represents the single greatest infectious threat from transfusion therapy [67–70]. Nonetheless, use of platelet transfusion therapy, from its inception, revolutionized the treatment of hematopoietic malignant disorders, and today is a mainstay of treatment of numerous malignant disorders requiring ablative chemotherapy (see Cases 6 and 7) as well as a variety of benign medical and especially complex surgical disorders [71,72]. Indeed, in some tertiary care centers, the number of units of platelets transfused may exceed the number of RBC units transfused, since the required dose of platelet concentrates is often 5–10 units per dose (with 1 unit acquired from each whole blood donor). This has been offset, to some degree, by an increasing reliance on collection of platelets by apheresis technology in which a unit of apheresis platelets can be collected from a single donor in about 60–90 min; the dose is equivalent to about 5–8 platelet concentrate units acquired from whole blood donations [73].

While the therapeutic use of platelets in bleeding patients with thrombocytopenia or platelet dysfunction is well accepted, the prophylactic use of platelet transfusion – to prevent hemorrhage – has been, and remains, somewhat controversial [74–87]. The 'time-honored' platelet transfusion threshold of 20 000/μl clearly is evolving to lower levels [78–80,84,86,88,89]. Several investigators have demonstrated the utility of a 5000–10 000/μl threshold for prophylactic platelet use. In particular, Gmur *et al.* [76] have provided threshold criteria for the transfusion, in nonbleeding patients, of prophylactic platelets as follows: clinically stable patients −5000/μl; patients with a temperature or history of recent hemorrhage −10 000/μl; and patients with an ongoing coagulopathy or who have an anatomic lesion likely to bleed −20 000/μl. This approach, as with that of the transfusion of RBCs, focuses primarily on clinical need but relies on the platelet count as an additional important guideline.

There is also an increased recognition that physiologic platelet function is closely dependent on the patient's RBC mass. Lack of a sufficient number of RBCs, even at levels not typically thought of as requiring RBC transfusion for clinical management of anemia, may have a profound effect on a patient's bleeding tendency even when the platelet count is normal. Thus, Valeri *et al.* demonstrated that on average, in a group of 22 men and 7 women undergoing 2 units of RBC autologous phlebotomy, the Hct decreased from 41% to 35%, the platelets decreased from 220 000/μl to 200 000/μl and the bleeding time increased from < 5 min to nearly 8 min. In contrast, when plateletpheresis was performed lowering the platelet count from 238 000/μl to 163 000/μl while maintaining the Hct at 40%, there was essentially no change in the bleeding time of approximately 4 min. Thus, a novel use of RBC transfusion therapy – representing a largely unrecognized positive benefit – might be to improve hemostasis by improving platelet function. While the exact mechanisms of how RBCs promote hemostasis, even in thrombocytopenic patients, is not yet clearly defined, an Hct level of > 34% has been shown to be adequate to reduce both the bleeding time and nonsurgical blood loss without the need for transfusion of platelets or fresh frozen plasma (FFP) in patients undergoing cardiopulmonary bypass [90].

Again, as in the case of RBC transfusion therapy, there is a tendency to monitor for overtransfusion of platelet therapy with less attention to auditing for the potential undertransfusion of platelet therapy [53].

Plasma component therapy
Fresh frozen plasma (FFP)

FFP is the fluid portion of whole blood and is prepared from whole blood collection or by apheresis collection. FFP is composed of over 90% water, 6–8% protein, lipids and carbohydrates, and all of the coagulation proteins including the labile coagulation factors, V and VIII, which without freezing will degrade over time. One international unit (IU) of each coagulation factor is present in each milliliter of undiluted plasma. Indications for plasma transfusion include the coagulopathy of liver disease, reversal of warfarin and replacement fluid for therapeutic plasma exchange, in TTP (see Case 11), for rare congenital factor deficiencies for which concentrates are not available (see Case 10), and in massive transfusion [91]. The patient's weight, indication for use and half-life of the deficient factor determine the dose of FFP. Generally, for adults 10–15 ml of FFP per kilogram of body weight is given. For replacement of isolated coagulation factor deficiencies, plasma dosing also considers the half-life of the deficient factor with those factors with shorter half-lives requiring more frequent doses. FFP *should not* be used when a coagulopathy might be corrected more effectively with specific therapy (i.e. vitamin K, CRYO, factor concentrate), nor should it be used solely as a volume expander. In patients with liver disease the risk of both bleeding and thrombosis may be increased [92,93]. The risk of bleeding may be increased because of decreased production of clotting factors, decreased production of antiplasmin, abnormal or decreased fibrinogen production, thrombocytopenia and increased levels of tissue plasminogen activator (TPA). The risk of thrombosis may be increased because of increased production of factor VIII and von Willebrand's factor (vWF), and decreased levels of antithrombin, protein C, protein S and plasminogen. If a patient with liver disease requires surgery or is actively bleeding, 10–15 ml of FFP per kilogram of body weight may be given, and this dose may need to be repeated every 6–12 h to achieve adequate hemostasis. Factor VII has a half-life of 6 h; consequently, a patient may require FFP every 6 h to normalize to the International Normalized Ratio (INR) or to stop bleeding.

FFP is used to reverse the effect of warfarin on the vitamin K–dependent clotting factors (factors II, VII, IX and X) when immediate reversal is required and/or further anticoagulation is anticipated. Plasma should never be used to reverse the effect of heparin (Table 2.1) since such therapy may exacerbate the effect of the heparin (antithrombin).

Hemophilia A, hemophilia B and von Willebrand's disease (vWD) account for 80–85% of all inherited bleeding disorders with deficiencies of factors I, II, V, VII, X, XI, XII and XIII accounting for the remainder. FFP may be used to replace isolated coagulation factor deficiencies (factors II, VII, X, XI and XIII). Acquired factor deficiencies are seen in conditions ranging from autoimmune disorders to malignancy and may present with a wide clinical spectrum in the severity of bleeding. Diagnosis depends on demonstration of decreased factor activity. Treatment of these rare clotting factor deficiencies consists of using the most purified blood product available that contains the missing factor and may involve the use of purified concentrates, CRYO, FFP, recombinant factor VIIA and factor XIII. FFP is used in the setting of massive blood transfusion or major blood loss to replace depleted clotting factors that are typically not present in RBC units [94]. Generally in the setting of massive transfusion, the dose of FFP is at least 10–15 ml of FFP per kilogram of body weight; the dose may need to be repeated more than once and may vary with the clinical situation.

Cryoprecipitate

CRYO contains fibronectin, fibrinogen, vWF, factor XIII and factor VIIIC. Each unit of CRYO should contain at least 80 IU factor VIIIC units and at least 150 mg of fibrinogen in approximately 15 ml of plasma. CRYO is indicated for a variety of conditions depending on the plasma protein being replaced [95–99]. The appropriate dosage depends on the indication or condition being treated. CRYO is indicated for replacement of plasma fibrinogen in cases of congenital afibrinogemia (see Case 8), dysfibrinogemia and hypofibrinogenemia, both congenital and acquired. CRYO contains vWF but is second-line therapy for vWD and should be used *only* if virus-inactivated factor VIII concentrates are not available for management of patients with vWD (Table 2.1). Factor XIII (FXIII) is a heterotetramer consisting of A subunits (XIIIA) and B subunits (XIIIB). FXIII catalyzes intermolecular crosslinking between fibrin monomers, which increase the strength of the forming fibrin clot. Thus a deficiency of FXIII results in a defective cross-linking pattern, and a resultant weakened fibrin clot with hemostatic abnormalities [100,101]. Congenital FXIII deficiency (see Case 9) is a severe autosomal recessive bleeding disorder associated with a characteristic pattern of neonatal hemorrhage and a lifelong bleeding diathesis with intracranial hemorrhage and, in females, spontaneous miscarriage. CRYO is indicated for treatment of factor XIII deficiency. However, for patients who can tolerate the volume of an FFP transfusion, FFP is the preferred vehicle to deliver factor XIII to deficient patients, since there is twice as much factor XIII per unit of FFP as per unit of CRYO. CRYO is used to treat the coagulopathy associated with uremia. The precise mechanism leading to the benefit is unknown.

Clinical vignettes

Clinically appropriate transfusion therapy
Red blood cells
Case 1

Transfusion in an elderly woman with a gastrointestinal (GI) bleed
A 76-year-old female presented to the emergency room with a 7-day history of passing dark, tarry stools, dizziness and dyspnea. Her laboratory values were: normal prothrombin time [(PT) – 10.8 s], normal activated partial thromboplastin time [(APTT) – 25 s] and Hb 4.1 g/dl. She received 4 units of RBC; her follow-up laboratory values were Hb 11.0 g/dl and Hct 31.6%, and her clinical signs and symptoms abated.

Case 2

Transfusion in a young adult with profound anemia associated with new onset acute myelogenous leukemia (AML)
A 22-year-old college student visited her dentist over several weeks for dental pain attributed to her wisdom teeth. The teeth were extracted, but following the extraction there was marked swelling of the oral mucosa and poor healing. 2 weeks after the extraction the patient developed profound dizziness, severe headache, shortness of breath and fatigue. She visited her private physician, and a complete blood count (CBC) revealed Hct 11.1%, platelets 80 000/μl and white blood cells (WBCs) 120 000 with 75% blasts. 2 units of RBC were administered immediately, followed by 3 more units of RBC, after which there was complete relief of symptoms. The patient was referred for further medical management.

Case 3

Transfusion in a 12-year-old child with excessive vaginal bleeding
A 12-year-old girl was brought to an emergency room with the chief complaint of excessive and continuous vaginal bleeding for more than 48 h. Her family history revealed that an uncle had recurrent epistaxis. A pregnancy

test was negative. Her Hb was 6.9 g/dl and plasma fibrinogen level was 158 mg/dl. Based on additional laboratory testing, a combination of vWD and dysfibrinogenemia was suspected. The patient was transfused with both RBCs and CRYO, following which there was cessation of the hemorrhage.

Case 4
RBC exchange in a pregnant patient with sickle cell disease
A 19-year-old 30-week-pregnant African-American female presented to the emergency room with fever and dyspnea. Her oxygen saturation (by pulse oximeter) was in the low 80s on room air, and she was transferred to the medical intensive care unit (MICU). After diagnosis of acute chest syndrome, an emergent RBC exchange was performed with 14 units of RBC. A fetal monitor was used during the exchange. Following the RBC exchange, there was abatement of the acute sickle crisis and she went on to have a successful delivery.

Case 5
RBC exchange maintenance in a young male status post stroke
A 25-year-old male with sickle cell disease suffered a stroke at age 3. Since the stroke, he has undergone 22 years of prophylactic RBC exchange to prevent a recurrent stroke. The RBC exchange transfusions were performed every 8 weeks with 10 units of RBC per exchange. He is a college graduate who is completing a graduate program to prepare for a career in teaching high school Spanish. He became infected with Hepatitis C virus (likely from one of the transfused RBC units), but is asymptomatic without any evidence of active liver disease.

Platelets
Case 6
Platelets and RBCs
A 48-year-old female with a history of multiple myeloma status post bone marrow transplant in 1996 presented 6 years later to an emergency department with neutropenic fever, dehydration and vomiting. At the time of her emergency department visit, her laboratory values were platelets 9000/µl and Hct 24%. She received 10 units of platelet concentrates and 2 units of RBC; her posttransfusion laboratory values were platelets 177 000/µl and Hct 29.4%.

Case 7
Symptomatic bleeding
A 23-year-old male with newly diagnosed Hodgkin's disease developed severe thrombocytopenia (platelets 6000/µl) followed by epistaxis. He received 10 units of platelet concentrates, following which the epistaxis resolved and his platelet count increased to 46 000/µl.

Cryoprecipitate
Case 8
Congenital afibrinogenemia
A 17-year-old male was diagnosed at birth with congenital afibrinogenemia at which time he was found to have prolonged PT and APTT, and undetectable fibrinogen. Since birth the patient has been sustained with transfusion of CRYO – approximately 6–8 units every 4–6 weeks. He has had no serious bleeding complications to date and his infectious disease testing remains negative (hepatitis B virus (HBV), hepatitis C virus (HCV) and human immunodeficiency virus (HIV)).

Case 9
Congenital factor XIII deficiency
A 21-year-old female with congenital factor XIII deficiency has been maintained since birth with monthly infusions of CRYO. She contemplates pregnancy and discusses it with her hematologist. She is successfully managed through pregnancy and delivery with transfusions of CRYO.

Plasma
Case 10
Plasma in isolated factor deficiency
A 31-year-old white male presented with newly diagnosed intractable epilepsy. A preoperative screening work-up revealed a prolonged APTT. A CT scan demonstrated a left temporal lobe lesion for which an angiogram needed to be performed prior to surgery. The cause of the prolonged APTT was determined to be due to a factor XI level of only 2%. Because of the markedly low level of factor XI and the high risk of bleeding during the angiogram and/or ensuing surgery, the patient was transfused with 6 units of FFP; his factor XI level post transfusion increased to 42%. An angiogram showed a right parietal lobe arteriovenous malformation in addition to the left temporal lesion. Prior to resection of the left temporal lobe lesion (pathology: grade 1 glioma) he underwent plasmapheresis with 12 units of FFP to increase his factor XI to approximately 50%. Postoperatively the patient received 4–6 units of FFP daily to maintain the factor Xl level in the 40–50% range. One week following the temporal tumor resection, he underwent gamma knife therapy for treatment of the arteriovenous malformation. Infusions of FFP are planned to maintain the factor Xl level in the 20–30% range for about 1 month postoperatively.

Case 11
Plasma in TTP
A 26-year-old obese African-American female presented in 1997 with thrombocytopenia, microangiopathic hemolytic anemia and acute mental status changes. She was immediately started on emergent therapeutic plasma exchange (TPE) for a diagnosis of TTP. She underwent a total of 200 TPEs over the course of 4 years and received over that period a total of 4000 units

of FFP. Her tests for hepatitis B and C and HIV remain negative emphasizing the safety of the blood supply.

Errors of omission with transfusion therapy

Case 12

Failure to receive transfusion therapy in a timely manner – surgical patient

A 50-year-old female with Hb 6.3 g/dl and Hct 20.5% was admitted for dialysis catheter revision. Because of multiple antibodies she was crossmatch compatible only with frozen deglycerolyzed RBCs (FDRCs). During surgery, extensive and uncontrolled bleeding occurred; the 4 available units of FDRC were used and additional units were ordered. The operating room was told that no compatible blood was immediately available. If needed, group O uncrossmatched, partially matched or least incompatible blood could be sent. Because the blood bank received no further communication, a laboratory physician went to the operating room to assess the situation. In the operating room, the patient lay with ongoing blood loss and an evolving flat electrocardiogram (ECG) tracing without the administration of blood transfusion therapy. 2 units of group O uncrossmatched RBC were ordered and delivered by the pathologist to the operating room, STAT. These were hung and within 5 min the ECG reverted to a normal sinus rhythm. 2 additional units, partially matched, were also administered and additional FDRC units were ordered. Postoperative values were Hb 7.2 g/dl and Hct 23.7%. Unfortunately, the patient expired on the second postoperative day.

Case 13

Failure to receive transfusion therapy in a timely manner – medical patient

A 47-year-old male with a past history of mixed Hodgkin's and non-Hodgkin's lymphoma presented with a 3-week history of left-sided weakness. The patient had a past history of a right cerebrovascular accident (CVA) and had a previous right carotid endarterectomy. Physical examination on admission showed findings characteristic of a right CVA. Initial laboratory studies revealed Hb 3.7 g/dl, Hct 12.8%, reticulocyte count 19.8%, bilirubin – total 2.8 mg/dl, direct 0.8 mg/dl, direct antiglobulin test (DAT) IgG 1+, C3d w+, and numerous spherocytes on the peripheral blood smear. The peripheral blood smear morphology and blood bank serology were interpreted as characteristic of a warm autoimmune hemolytic anemia. Upon questioning a medical resident regarding the apparent delay in transfusion therapy, a laboratory physician was told that the clinical team was awaiting the availability of crossmatch compatible blood. Because of the evolving central nervous system symptoms and profound anemia, the laboratory physician suggested immediate transfusion therapy with 'least incompatible' blood. Following a total of 5 units of 'least incompatible' RBCs, the Hct increased to 21.5% and the central nervous system symptoms abated.

Case 14

Failure to receive transfusion therapy in a timely manner – medical patient

A 47-year-old group O Rh positive male with Coombs' positive autoimmune hemolytic anemia was started on steroids and transferred to a tertiary care facility. There was no history of coronary artery or cerebrovascular disease. Hct levels, 12 h apart, prior to the hospital transfer were 30.4% and 17.6%. On arrival, 3 days after clinical presentation, the Hct was 12.3%. The patient appeared alert and clinically stable with 'satisfactory' oxygen extractions, and transfusion was not initiated, despite florid hemolysis, pending completion of a serological evaluation by the laboratory. The patient became bradycardic and hypotensive, following which he required intubation and pressors. Despite the immediate transfusion of 3 units of uncrossmatched group-specific blood, he expired. Final characterization of the patient's serum antibody revealed a panreactive warm autoantibody without evidence of alloimmunization.

Case 15

Failure to receive transfusion therapy in a timely manner – medical patient

An 81-year-old female was sent from her nursing home to a tertiary care facility with disorientation, dehydration, emesis and an elevated glucose level. 5 days earlier the patient been treated at the same tertiary care facility for a right distal femoral fracture. Upon her arrival in the emergency room at 9 AM her Hb was 4.1 g/dl and Hct 12.6%. Her vital signs were BP 87/59, pulse 96, respirations 20 and temperature 37.4°C. She was noted to be awake but disoriented, responding to verbal commands. About 12 h following her admission she was noted to have trouble breathing, became unresponsive, and no pulse oximetry or BP was obtainable. An ECG showed a rate of 30–40 with wide complexes. A note in the chart indicated the following: 'and, they don't have the blood ready'. Further investigation revealed an apparent communication breakdown between the clinical and laboratory services regarding the urgency for transfusion. The blood bank, unaware of this patient's severe anemia and deteriorating status, had identified several new antibodies including anti-Fya, Kell and M. Initially, the clinical service did not indicate any particular urgency regarding the need for transfusion. Ultimately, the Transfusion Service medical director was apprised of the circumstances and urged immediate transfusion therapy, with or without the availability of fully matched blood. The patient was then aggressively managed with fluid replacement with several units of compatible blood. Despite this, the patient had a massive acute myocardial infarction and expired the day following her admission. It is likely that severe anemia (associated with blood loss from a recent orthopedic procedure) with delay in RBC transfusion administration contributed to a massive myocardial infarction and resultant death in this case.

Case 16

Failure to receive transfusion therapy in a timely manner – medical patient

A 45-year-old group O Rh positive white male came to the emergency room with bleeding esophageal varices. The patient was reported to be clinically unstable with Hb 5.0 g/dl and Hct 15.8% and ongoing hemorrhage. Because of the patient's prior history of anti-E the emergency room was afraid to use group O negative blood (the latter was immediately available in the emergency room refrigerator). Fortunately, based on the above and similar cases, the laboratory physician covering the hospital blood bank was proactively contacted by the blood bank staff and advised of these circumstances. In order to avoid further delay in transfusion therapy, the laboratory physician intervened and advised immediate use of group O Rh negative blood for this patient. The emergency room staff was advised that in this case the clinical risk in delaying transfusion was likely to prove more harmful than the slight risk for possible accelerated hemolysis in this patient. 2 units of group O Rh negative uncrossmatched blood (one later shown to be positive for the E antigen) were administered without difficulty. The patient stabilized and was admitted to the MICU. There was no clinical or laboratory evidence of accelerated hemolysis from the single E-positive unit administered (despite the presence of anti-E). About 6 months later the patient returned to the MICU with a history of massive upper GI bleeding and Hb 3.0 g/dl, Hct 10.6, platelet count 87 000/μl. Once again, a type and screen revealed the presence of antibody activity. The clinician, stating that the patient appears clinically stable, refused transfusion until compatible blood could be made available. The patient received his first RBC transfusion nearly 13 h following admission. He received 6 units of RBC over 2 days with his Hb and Hct increasing to 10.3 g/dl and 30.8 respectively.

Case 17

Underdosing of CRYO

A 56-year-old male presented to the emergency room with acute hepatic failure. He had a history of alcohol and cocaine abuse and weighed 110 kg. His fibrinogen level was noted to be < 50 mg/dl. An order for 6 units of CRYO was placed with the blood bank. The blood bank contacted a laboratory physician who was covering the Transfusion Service in order to verify the requested CRYO dose. The laboratory physician determined that the ordered dose of CRYO was insufficient based on the patient's fibrinogen level, Hct and patient weight; the correct dose of CRYO was actually 48 units. The ordering clinician was contacted and the order was changed to provide an adequate dose.

Comment: Calculating the proper dose of a blood component is analogous to calculating the proper dose of a medication. One must consider the patient's size (and body weight). Larger patients require larger amounts of both drugs and blood components; smaller patients (see below) require smaller amounts. In the above case the administration of 6 units of CRYO was clearly underdosing, where each unit raises the fibrinogen by approximately 10 mg/dl per 70 kg, which would have been grossly insufficient to raise the fibrinogen level to a hemostatic level in this patient.

Errors of commission with transfusion therapy

Case 18

Overdosing of platelets

A 7-year-old boy with neuroblastoma was undergoing chemotherapy and radiation treatment and was persistently thrombocytopenic with platelet counts ranging from 6000 to 10 000/μl. He weighed 24 kg and received daily platelet transfusion therapy (three platelet concentrates). During one of the patient's platelet transfusion episodes, an intern ordered 3 single-donor platelets, apheresis units (rather than three platelet concentrates) for the child – a dose approximately six times greater than appropriate; fortunately the blood bank caught the ordering error and an appropriate dose was issued to the patient.

Case 19

Overdosing of platelets

A 26-week gestational age, 556 g infant with APGARS of 2 and 6 was admitted to the neonatal intensive care unit (NICU) immediately after birth. On day 1 the neonate went to the operating room for an exploratory laparotomy for a gastric perforation. The preoperative platelet count was 82 000/μl. In the operating room a total of 49 cc of platelets and 12 cc of crystalloid was transfused for an estimated blood loss of approximately 10 cc. Peri- and postoperatively, the infant did poorly with a platelet count of 2.342×10^6/μl; an emergency whole blood exchange transfusion reduced the platelet count to 1.095×10^6/μl. However, a hepatic vein thrombosis was noted on day 7. The infant expired 2 weeks after birth. This patient received an approximately 20-fold platelet overdose with possible or at least perceived clinical consequences.

Case 20

Transfusion therapy without defined clinical need – RBCs

An 87-year-old female with organic brain syndrome resides at a nursing home. She was noted to be slightly more lethargic than usual. Laboratory testing revealed an Hct of 35%. There was no evidence of clinical bleeding and no acute cardiac symptoms. The clinician requested that she be transported to a local hospital and receive as an outpatient 2 units of RBCs over a total of 8 h. Shortly after completion of the second unit, the patient developed dyspnea. Over the course of the next several hours she developed congestive heart failure and acute pulmonary edema. The patient expired the following day.

Case 21
Transfusion therapy without defined clinical need – platelets
A 58-year-old male is admitted to the hospital for biopsy of a brain mass. Past medical history is significant for insulin-requiring diabetes mellitus. On admission, the laboratory values reveal Hb 16.8g/dl, Hct 47%, platelet count 237 000/μl, PT 11.2 s, INR 1.09, PTT 25 s. There is no evidence of active bleeding and he is on no aspirin-containing medication. The clinician orders 10 units of platelets, later reduced to 5 units, as a precautionary measure despite no obvious indications. A platelet function assay (PFA) to objectively assess platelet function – and therefore the necessity for platelet transfusion – was not ordered.

Case 22
Transfusion therapy without defined clinical need – laboratory error
An 18-year-old female weighing 45 kg receives as an outpatient routine dialysis for lupus-induced nephritis. She also has lupus-induced myelosuppression and is on erythropoietin and Neupogen. Her Hct levels normally range from 24% to 28%. Her laboratory values during a dialysis treatment one day were reported as Hb 4.3 g/dl and Hct 13.1%. 2 days prior to this the Hct was reported as 25.1%. The patient had no evidence of bleeding and clinically appeared to be in her normal state of health. Because of this laboratory result, the patient was transfused with 1 unit of RBC, and then sent home. Her next Hct reading, 2 days later, was 29.2%. It is likely that an error in blood sampling, possibly a sample diluted with dialysis fluid, was submitted to the laboratory for testing; and, instead of repeating the result on a new, separate sample, the patient was simply and likely inappropriately transfused.

Clerical errors
Case 23
Wrong blood in tube
A 77-year-old male presented with urinary retention and a creatinine of 15.8 mg/dl. He underwent a suprapubic prostatectomy after which he developed postoperative hematuria and anemia (Hct 24%). RBC transfusion therapy was ordered. A type and screen revealed that he was blood group A Rh positive. His blood type was 'confirmed' by repeat testing of the same sample, by a different medical technologist in the blood bank. There was no prior typing result for this patient on file in the blood bank. Based on the type and screen results of this single blood sample, the patient received 5 units of group A Rh (D) positive and 1 unit of group O Rh (D) negative RBC over the next 3 days postoperatively. Nonetheless, the patient's Hct failed to increase, remaining at 24.3%. Since he required further transfusion therapy more than 3 days after procurement of the initial type and screen sample, a new sample was submitted for further crossmatching and RBC transfusion therapy. The type and screen this time showed the patient to be group B Rh positive. The group B status of this second sample was confirmed by repeat

testing. In addition, a third sample was drawn, which also typed as group B. Two group B Rh positive RBC units were transfused, and this time the patient's Hct rose to 28.2% the day following transfusion and 30.6% 4 days later. He made an otherwise uneventful recovery. An investigation was initiated. In retrospect, the ongoing postoperative 'hematuria' was attributed to hemolysis, as was the 1.5°C increase in temperature postoperatively. Neither the 'hematuria' nor the fever was reported to the blood bank as a possible transfusion reaction since both findings were attributed to the patient's postoperative condition. A root cause analysis in this case revealed that the phlebotomist who collected the sample for the initial type and screen had mislabeled the patient's initial sample tube, which led to the wrong blood being in the tube. Realizing at the time that a mislabeling had occurred, she drew a new, correctly labeled sample – but failed to retrieve the mislabeled sample from the blood bank. The blood bank, in receipt of two samples labeled identically, assumed the second sample was a duplicate and set it aside. Subsequently, this 'duplicate' sample was retrieved and confirmed as group B Rh positive. The incorrect sample, typing as group A Rh positive, was confirmed to be from a patient in an adjacent room. The patient in the adjacent room did not require RBC transfusion.

Case 24
Operating room administration error
A 68-year old male presenting with heart failure is scheduled to undergo a repeat heart valve replacement. In an adjacent operating room another cardiac procedure is in progress. For the valve surgery case 4 RBC units are sent in an igloo in anticipation of immediate need. They are placed in the corridor between these two rooms rather than in the specific room for the intended patient. When blood is needed for the valve surgery case, it is erroneously obtained from the nearby refrigerator rather than the 'misplaced' igloo. The name and hospital number of the wrong blood were 'verified' by the nurse and perfusionist prior to use and the blood placed in the bypass machine. Only when the blood was nearly all infused was it noted that the patient's name and the name on the unit did not match. The blood bank was contacted. Luckily, both patients were group A Rh positive. The root cause investigation revealed that the specially prepared igloo was actually in the hallway between the operating rooms rather than in the room designated for the specific heart valve patient. The operating room staff has been retrained regarding the use of blood from igloos.

Inadvertent adverse clincial outcomes
Case 25
Volume overload in plasmapheresis
An 81-year-old female with a 15-year history of diabetes complicated by retinopathy and atherosclerotic heart disease called her primary care physician complaining of weakness, dizziness and early satiety. Physical

examination revealed splenomegaly. Laboratory testing revealed Hct 23%, WBC 29 000/μl with 77% lymphocytes with lymphoplasmacytoid cells and rouleaux formation on the peripheral blood smear. The total protein was elevated with IgM 5455 (normal range 33–232) and serum viscosity 3.97 (normal range 1.40–1.80). A diagnosis of Waldenström's macroglobulinemia was made and plasmapheresis was initiated. At the completion of the plasmapheresis, during which about 200 cc of whole blood were rinsed back from the plasmapheresis bowl over a 20-min time frame, the patient had a respiratory arrest and expired 2 days later. This was reported to the Food and Drug Administration (FDA) as a potential transfusion-associated fatality associated with volume overload.

Case 26
Volume overload in platelet transfusion
A 58-year-old female who had undergone an allogeneic stem cell transplant for acute myelogenous leukemia 2 months ago entered a tertiary care facility with a fungal infection of the lungs, acute renal failure and a history of hypertension. Because of suspicion of ongoing pulmonary hemorrhage and thrombocytopenia (platelet count −21 000/μl), transfusion therapy with 2 single-donor apheresis units was ordered. Prior to transfusion the vital signs were as follows: temperature 36.7°C, pulse 96, respirations 20 and BP 172/80. The patient then received 2 apheresis platelet units, with a total volume of 720 ml of platelet-rich plasma over 1 h 15 min. Following the completion of the transfusion, the patient became acutely short of breath and complained of back pain. Her vital signs following the reaction were as follows: temperature 36.6°C, pulse 150, respirations > 30 and BP 190/108. An increase in her baseline peripheral edema was noted. She was transferred to the MICU and treated with diuresis and positive pressure ventilation by mask. Her oxygen saturation, in the 80s during the acute event, improved to 97% with the above therapy. A chest X-ray (CXR) revealed scattered infiltrates consistent with pulmonary edema, which improved following the above therapy. Despite the clinical diagnosis of acute pulmonary edema by the intensive care staff, the clinical oncology service suspected a diagnosis of transfusion-related acute lung injury (TRALI) and asked the Transfusion Service to provide further therapeutic recommendations, especially since the patient was refusing to accept blood transfusion lest she have a further reaction. The Transfusion Service concluded, based on the history and signs and symptoms noted above, that the reaction was classic for volume overload rather than TRALI. The clinical oncology team together with the patient were counseled regarding the need to provide as indicated, infusion of blood components more slowly, reduced volume blood components, diuresis before, during or after transfusion therapy; and, provide close monitoring and reassurance during transfusion therapy. There has been no recurrence despite ongoing transfusion therapy.

Case 27
Transmission of infectious agents – platelet bacterial contamination
A 39-year-old male with multiple myeloma was admitted for autologous stem
cell transplant. While receiving 5 units of platelet concentrates (administered
as a 5-unit pool), he developed rigors, tachycardia, shortness of breath,
wheezing and a flushed face. Prior to the transfusion, vital signs were:
temperature 37°C, pulse 92, respirations 24 and BP 170/86. Immediately
following the transfusion, the temperature rose to 39–40°C and the BP fell
to 70/38. He was treated with intravenous (IV) fluids, steroids and dopamine.
A transfusion reaction report was initiated, and Gram Stain of the pool and
one out of five of the individual units was positive for gram-negative rods.
Cultures of the pool and implicated unit, 3 days storage age at the time of
transfusion, were positive for *Pseudomonas aeruginosa* with 1.1×10^6 CFU/ml
in the pool and 1.6×10^7 CFU/ml in the implicated unit. A blood culture
obtained shortly after the transfusion grew *P. aeruginosa*. A clinical diagnosis
of endotoxic shock was made. The patient developed multiorgan system
failure, became increasingly comatose and died 5 days following receipt of
the contaminated transfusion.

Case 28
Transfusion-related aucte lung injury
A 73-year-old male was admitted to a hospital for elective repair of an
abdominal aortic aneurysm. On the day after his admission, the aneurysm
was repaired, during which the patient received 9 units of RBC. Immediately
after the operation, the patient's condition was stable. During the next
30 min the patient received 2 units of FFP and 1 L each of normal saline
and 5% dextrose in half-normal saline. Within the next 2 h the patient
became profoundly leukopenic (predominantly neutrophils and monocytes)
with a rise in immature neutrophils. The alveolar-to-arterial oxygen (A–a O_2)
gradient rose substantially and after about 7 h severe bilateral pulmonary
infiltrates developed without change in heart size or significant elevation in
the pulmonary artery wedge pressure. The platelet count fell to 83 000/μl.
The neutropenia lasted approximately 15 h. The pulmonary infiltrates
resolved over 24 h. The A-a O_2 gradient gradually returned to baseline over
4 days. The patient was given two IV boluses of methylprednisolone, 2 g and
1 g respectively, 6 h 30 min and 12 h after the clinical onset. Subsequent
recovery was uneventful. In this case, 9 of 11 of the blood donors were
available for follow-up investigation. One of the donors, a healthy 52-year-
old female with a history of 13 pregnancies and one previous blood transfusion exhibited an anti-NA2 neutrophil-specific antibody in her plasma at a
titer of 1/8 by agglutination and 1/128 by immunofluorescence. No reactivity
was detected in the granulocyte cytotoxicity assay. The patient's neutrophils
were NA2 positive and reacted with this donor's serum in the minor cross-
matches.

Case 29
Transfusion-associated graft versus host disease (GVHD)
A male baby was admitted to a tertiary care facility with multisystem deteri-oration including pancytopenia, coagulopathy and skin rash. The 4-week-old baby, weighing 5 lb 9 oz, was born at another hospital to a G_3P_3 mother at $35\frac{1}{2}$ weeks gestation, following an uneventful pregnancy. At birth, the baby's platelet count was 7000/μl and petechiae were noted. A diagnosis of isoim-mune neonatal thrombocytopenia was made. Initially, random-donor plate-let concentrates were administered to the baby, with no clinical response. Subsequently, maternal platelets were harvested and transfused at another hospital, but these platelets were neither irradiated nor leukocyte-reduced. The platelet count normalized and the baby was discharged. Three weeks later, the baby was readmitted to a second hospital with a temperature of 38°C. A work-up for septicemia was negative, and following 3 days of anti-biotic therapy, the baby was discharged. The platelet count on discharge was 202 000/μl. Three days later, the baby was again admitted to the hospital, this time with a bulging fontanelle, generalized edema, lethargy, petechiae and a single generalized seizure. A diffuse bright red skin rash was present and a skin biopsy was suggestive of GVHD. The baby was transferred again to the tertiary care facility. Upon admission, a prominent diffuse bright red rash was once again noted. The baby was started on high-dose steroids and cyclosporine for the presumed diagnosis of GVHD. He underwent rapid clinical deterioration with multisystem failure including profound pancyto-penia and expired 6 days following his final hospital admission. The cause of death was attributed to GVHD presumably associated with transfusion of maternal platelets in the neonatal period.

Case 30
Hemolysis – delayed hemolytic transfusion reaction
A 46-year-old multiparous African-American female was admitted to a tertiary care facility for an abdominal hysterectomy. On admission her Hct was 36%. She was noted to be blood group O Rh positive with a negative screen for unexpected red cell antibodies. Her surgery was complicated by excessive bleeding necessitating the transfusion of 4 units of RBCs. Her Hct at discharge was 33%. Four days following discharge, she noted brown urine and increasing frequency of urination. Scleral icterus was noted and she was readmitted to the hospital. On readmission her Hct was 24.7%, falling to 18% with rehydration. A DAT and antibody screen on readmission were both positive due to anti-Jk^b and anti-E. Her plasma was noted to be red in color. Retrospective investigation revealed that 3 of the 4 units transfused 10 days previously were positive for Jk^b and 2 units were positive for E. Other laboratory work revealed total bilirubin 5.4 (direct 0.5), SGOT (AST) 117, LDH 1325, U/A 2+ blood/Hb with rare RBCs. This case was interpreted as a delayed hemolytic transfusion reaction manifest-ing with predominantly intravascular hemolysis. When she initially presented, the clinicians were more concerned about the possibility of posttransfusion

hepatitis than of a transfusion reaction. The patient was managed with hydration. She received 2 additional RBC transfusions negative for the corresponding antibodies. She was discharged 5 days later with a Hct of 28%.

Case 31
Hemolysis – hemolytic transfusion reaction syndrome
A 25-year-old African-American female with a history of sickle β thalassemia presented to an outside hospital with anemia, fever and left upper quadrant pain, and was transferred to a tertiary care facility for further management. Her baseline Hct normally ranged from 30% to 36%, however her Hct was only 18.9% on admission. She was found to have a left subphrenic abscess. Fluid drainage revealed polymicrobial growth and she was treated with vancomycin, ciprofloxacin and Flagyl. She was known to have multiple alloantibodies (anti-hr^B, anti-E and anti-D related to partial D IIIa type) and autoantibody reactivity. Despite the incompatibility, the initial plan was transfusion to raise the Hct so that the abscess could be surgically drained. Her Hct stabilized between 30.1% and 36.4% over the next 8 days during which she received 6 units of RBC – 2 compatible and 4 'least' incompatible. On day 9 her Hct fell to 25% and on day 10 to 21%. For the next 3 days she received 4 units of 'least' incompatible blood. Her Hct continued to decrease from 21% to 16.5%. Meanwhile, the total and direct bilirubin increased to 32 mg/dl and 22 mg/dl respectively. The blood urea nitrogen (BUN) and creatinine were 67 and 3.8 respectively. On day 13 her Hct had decreased to 13%. She received IVIG, Epogen and steroids. She also received 3 more incompatible RBC transfusions. During this period, her Hct further decreased to 11.8%. She was placed on oxygen therapy. A single unit of compatible blood, located by the New York Blood Center was shipped – she received this unit in increments of one-half each over 4 h for the onset of chest pain. Bone marrow biopsy revealed a hypercellular bone marrow with pure red cell aplasia. Parvovirus serology was negative. On day 16 following admission, RBC transfusions were stopped despite the extremely low Hct and presence of pure red cell aplasia in the bone marrow. Within a few days, the bilirubin had decreased to 4.3 mg/dl and the Hct values improved to the course of 12.6–15.1%. Indeed, the resulting hemolysis attributed to the transfusions, increasing in severity over time, likely triggered in this patient the so-called sickle cell hemolytic transfusion reaction syndrome with its resultant red cell aplasia.

Comment: In this case, the withdrawal of transfusion therapy (where compatible blood was not readily available) in conjunction with the use of steroids, IVIG and erythropoietin, despite the profoundly low Hct, was likely lifesaving.

The risks of transfusion therapy

The safety of blood transfusion therapy represents a combination of blood component safety and blood transfusion process safety. Application of technology over the last two decades has vastly improved blood component safety [102]. However, little attention has been devoted to blood transfusion process safety [103]. Blood transfusion process safety includes all processes and procedures that ensure that a blood component is safely administered to a patient. Failure in blood component safety – leading to *product risks*, or blood transfusion process safety – leading to *process risks*, diminishes transfusion safety.

Product/component risks

Infectious disease testing of blood donations started with testing for syphilis (1940s), followed by testing for hepatitis B surface antigen (HBsAg) (1970), antibody to human immunodeficiency virus (HIV) (1985), antibody to hepatitis B core (anti-HBc) (1986), antibody to human T-cell lymphotropic virus (HTLV)-I (1988), antibody to hepatitis C virus (HCV) (1990), antibody to HIV-1/2 (1992), HIV-1 p24 antigen (1996) and antibody to HTLV-I/II (1998) [102]. These serologic tests, the implementation of nucleic acid amplification test (NAT) [104], and blood donor screening questions targeted at high-risk behavior have substantially decreased the risk for transfusion-transmitted viruses (TTVs) [105–107]. The most recent estimated frequencies in the USA per unit transfused for TTV are for HIV-1 1 in 2.1×10^6, for hepatitis B virus (HBV) 1 in 2.0×10^5, for HCV 1 in 1.9×10^6 [108] and for HTLV-I/II 1 in 2.9×10^6 (see Table 2.2) [105].

While over 99.99% of the time transfusions are safe from these viral agents [106], the public's perception of blood safety continues to be one of doubt, and its demand for a 'zero-risk blood supply' persists. Recognition of transfusion-transmitted HIV in the mid-1980s heightened sensitivity in the private, public and governmental spheres to the potential risk of transfusing infectious agents and negatively transformed the public's perception of the safety of the US blood supply [107,109,110]. The evolution and appearance of previously unknown pathogens such as new variant Creuztfeldt–Jakob disease [111], West Nile virus (WNV) and SARS raise questions for regulatory agencies and the blood industry regarding the potential impact on the blood supply from these previously unknown and/or emerging infectious agents. Table 2.2 provides current data on the frequency of the various transfusion-transmitted infectious agents.

Despite the ongoing recognition of new and emerging infectious threats and the fear this generates among donors, recipients and the blood industry, the most important infectious risk related to transfusion therapy, as illustrated in Case 27, is bacterial contamination of room temperature–stored platelets. Although the problem of bacterial contamination of blood was identified over 60 years ago, it is only in 2003 and 2004 that the College of American Pathologists and American Association of Blood Banks have promulgated standards to reduce and identify instances of bacterially contaminated platelets. While most of the focus of transfusion is on the risk of infectious disease transmission, numerous other risks as detailed in Tables 2.3 and 2.4 are also possible.

Table 2.2 Known infectious agents transmitted by blood transfusion.

Viruses	Estimated frequency in the USA (per unit transfused)
CMV	1: 300
EBV	1: 200
HAV	Rare
HBV	1: 205 000
HCV	1: 1 935 000
HDV	1: 3000
HGV	Unknown
Retroviruses	
HTLV-I/II	< 1: 2 993 000
HIV-1	< 1: 2 135 000
HIV-2	Extremely rare
Bacteria	
T. pallidum	Rare
GN enterics	Uncommon
GP organisms	1: 2000 (in platelets)
B. burgdorferi	Unknown
Parasites	**(Incidences in the USA are rare to very rare)**
Plasmodium sp.	0.25: 1 000 000
Babesia microti	< 1: 1 000 000
Trypanosoma cruzi	< 1: 1 000 000
Leishmania sp.	< 1: 20 000 000

Note: CMV, cytomegalovirus; EBV, Epstein–Barr virus; GN, Gram negative; GP, Gram positive; HAV, HBV, HCV, HDV and HGV are hepatitis A, B, C, delta and G viruses respectively; HTLV-I/II, human T-lymphotrophic viruses, types I and II; HIV, human immunodeficiency virus.

Process risks

The transfusion therapy process includes all steps and procedures that ensure that a blood component is safely administered to a patient (Figure 2.3). These steps and procedures represent a complex interplay of activities occurring within the blood bank/transfusion service laboratory, at the patient bedside and at a variety of interdepartmental interface points between the blood bank and bedside. We have dubbed this in-between terrain the 'twilight zone' to reflect the often ill-defined nature of these interface activities. While the proper application of these complex processes is critical to transfusion safety, dependency on numerous diverse human interactions makes these processes particularly prone to accidents and errors [112]. Indeed, blood administration–related errors – many of which occur outside the confines of blood bank/transfusion service laboratory (see Cases 22–24) [113] – represent a significant cause of transfusion morbidity and mortality.

Table 2.3 Immune-mediated adverse effects.

Adverse effect	Estimated frequency per unit	Comment
Acute hemolytic reaction		
Death	1: 100 000 to 1: 800 000	Fortunately, only a fraction of ABO incompatible transfusions are fatal
ABO incompatibility	1: 10 000 to 1: 20 000	
Delayed hemolytic reaction		RBC alloimmunization occurs more commonly than clinical signs and/or symptoms
Hemolytic reaction	1: 4000	
Serologic reaction	1: 1500	
Febrile transfusion reaction (nonhemolytic)	1: 200	Cytokine or WBC-induced; much more common in multitransfused recipients
Alloimmunization to RBC, WBC, or platelets	1: 100	50–100% incidence in heavily transfused populations
Allergic transfusion reactions	1: 333	1–3% in patients requiring large plasma transfusions, such as therapeutic plasma exchange
Transfusion-related acute lung injury (TRALI)	1: 5000	Due chiefly to anti-WBC antibodies in transfused plasma; the anti-WBC antibody containing plasma can be in RBCs, platelets, FFP or CRYO; this reaction is probably underreported. For more information, go to the following web site: *http://www.cbbsweb.org/enetTRALI.html*
Acute anaphylaxis	1: 20 000 to 1: 50 000	Plasma protein mediated; can be associated with anti-IgA in IgA-deficient patients or antihaptoglobin in haptoglobin-deficient patients. For more information, go to the following web site: *http://www.ncbi.nih.gov/entrez/query.fcgi?cmd=Retrieve&db=PubMed&list_uids=10666182&dopt=Abstract*
Posttransfusion purpura	Rare to very uncommon	Platelet antibody-mediated; multiparous females most susceptible
Transfusion-associated graft-versus-host disease (GVHD)	Unknown	US incidence extremely low, except in specific susceptible recipients; preventable with appropriate use of gamma irradiation of cellular components

Table 2.4 Nonimmune-mediated adverse effects.

Adverse effect	Estimated frequency per unit	Comment
Circulatory overload	1: 100 to 1: 200	Common, but underreported
Transfusion-associated sepsis	1: 10 000 to 1: 15 000 patients get sepsis from platelet transfusions;	More prevalent in platelets, due to room temperature storage, especially with platelets stored for 5 days
Bacterial contamination	1: 2000 platelet units contaminated	
Mechanically hemolyzed unit	Infrequent	Occur randomly and episodically
Thermally hemolyzed unit	Infrequent	Occur randomly and episodically
Cold-induced thrombopathy	Infrequent	Occur randomly and episodically; warming the patient and use of blood warmers is helpful
Osmotically hemolyzed unit	Infrequent	Use *only* 0.9% saline for dilution of cellular components
Electrolyte imbalances (K^+, Mg^{++}, citrate toxicity)	Uncommon	More common in massive transfusion recipients
Transfusional hemosiderosis	Uncommon	Lifelong risk high in thalassemias and SCD

The decision to transfuse assumes a proper procurement of an adequately labeled sample. In some cases a properly identified sample may be erroneously procured, leading to a false Hb or Hct level (see Case 22) [53,114–117]. While fortunately only a fraction of errors lead to erroneous transfusion [118], the risk of receipt of an ABO incompatible RBC transfusion is greater than the combined risk of all known TTV infections [119]. Surveillance data support the notion that [114–116,120,121] the weakest links in the blood transfusion process, potentially resulting in the erroneous administration of blood, are those involving misidentification. To be sure, the erroneous administration of ABO incompatible RBC units, as the result of a misidentification during the transfusion process, is the leading cause, worldwide, of acute RBC transfusion-associated mortality. The occurrence of this event has continued largely unabated over the last several decades despite increasing awareness of, and attention to, this problem. While errors in identification may occur anywhere throughout the transfusion process sequence, they most often occur outside the confines of the blood bank/Transfusion Service [113], either upstream at the time of phlebotomy (see Case 23) or downstream at the time of transfusion (see Case 24). Nursing personnel are those who have the best opportunity to interdict or prevent blood transfusion errors [122] since they are usually responsible for the final activities in the transfusion process, namely blood administration and monitoring, and at times for the initial activity, namely phlebotomy. Specimen procurement and blood

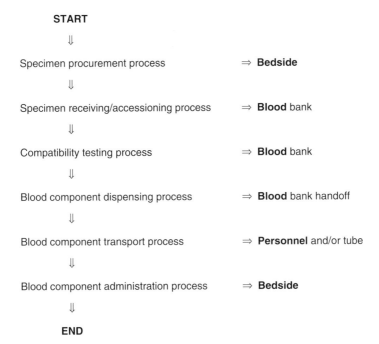

START

⇓

Specimen procurement process   ⇒ **Bedside**

⇓

Specimen receiving/accessioning process   ⇒ **Blood** bank

⇓

Compatibility testing process   ⇒ **Blood** bank

⇓

Blood component dispensing process   ⇒ **Blood** bank handoff

⇓

Blood component transport process   ⇒ **Personnel** and/or tube

⇓

Blood component administration process   ⇒ **Bedside**

⇓

END

Figure 2.3 The transfusion therapy process.

administration are particularly susceptible to errors in identification (see Cases 23 and 24). Work by Shulman and others [119,123–125] has demonstrated the importance of ongoing audits of the blood transfusion process as a means to identify and reduce errors in the blood transfusion process. Indeed, Shulman has noted that the fewest errors occur in blood component administration practices on those nursing units whose staff routinely performs self-assessment of the blood transfusion process [119]. It is hoped that improvements in automation and especially computerized bar code technology will become available in the not-too-distant future, assisting in the identification process that matches blood units to patients. However, in the absence of such technology, a particularly concerted effort must be made to optimize the blood transfusion process, as it currently exists in most hospitals. Only with increasing attention to blood component process safety can we state with a clear conscience that blood transfusion has never been safer.

Summary and conclusions: the balancing act

While many of the risks and benefits of transfusion therapy are well known and have been clearly defined, as noted throughout this chapter, there remain undefined risks and benefits, which may be unknown and evolve as our scientific knowledge base increases. Because risk, especially of the unknown, evokes fear and anxiety, there is a tendency to focus on uncertain risks rather than on unknown benefits. Further, in some instances risk and benefit are so intimately intertwined as to make it difficult to decipher which parameter – risk or benefit – is more important at any given point in time.

Each patient whose clinical condition warrants consideration of transfusion therapy should be evaluated objectively by his or her physician(s) and/ or other health care providers, and offered, when appropriate, the use of blood product transfusions. Those who refuse blood product transfusions, after appropriate counseling regarding the risks and benefits of receiving versus risks and benefits of refusal, should be afforded their rights as individuals in the USA to refuse transfusion. For the immediate future, transfusion of blood components will remain a cornerstone of medical surgical treatment. Promises of transfusion alternatives and possibly, in the future, transfusion substitutes should be tempered with a clear understanding and appreciation of their benefits, risks and cost-effectiveness. The best combination of clinical utility and cost-effectiveness should guide the application of transfusion practice.

Dr Richard Lower, a pioneer in animal transfusion studies, in describing the potential uses of human blood transfusion in a simulation of a seventeenth-century debate, commented:

As far as I can see, physicians seem to fall into one of three general groupings. There are those who approve the intervention and maintain that it could be prescribed for a wide variety of diseases. Others look on it as a useless novelty, while the last group haven't made up their minds, and claim to be waiting for more evidence one way or another.

Let us hope that at the dawn of the twenty-first century we have ample evidence to appreciate the risks and benefits of blood transfusion therapy and provide transfusion therapy in an optimal manner to improve patient care. As noted in Ecclesiastes 3:1, 'There is a time for everything, a season for every activity under heaven.' So may it be with transfusion therapy – to use this modality wisely in the appropriate context, in the appropriate amount, and at the appropriate time.

References

1 Starr D. Blood: an epic history of medicine and commerce. In: Moore P, ed. *Blood and Justice*. Chichester, UK: John Wiley & Sons, 2003.
2 Spencie L. *One Blood: The Death and Resurrection of Charles R. Drew*. Chapel Hill, North Carolina: The University of North Carolina Press, 1996.
3 Koscick RL, Yomtovian RAK. The red blood cell transfusion trigger: how low can we go? American Society of Clinical Pathologists, Check Sample 1998. *Transfusion Medicine 98-8* TM-228: 103–19.

4 Counts RB. Transfusion medicine in the surgical patient. In: Speiss BD, Counts RB, Gould SA, eds. *Perioperative Transfusion Medicine*. Balimore, MD: Williams & Wilkins, 1998: 15–43.

5 Carson JL, Duff A, Berlin JA, Lawrence VA, Poses RM, Huber EC, O'Hara DA, Noveck H, Strom BS. Perioperative blood transfusion and postoperative mortality. *JAMA* 1998; **279**: 199–205.

6 Stehling L. The red blood cell transfusion trigger: physiology and clinical studies. *Arch Path Lab Med* 1994; **118**: 429–34.

7 Tuchschmidt J, Oblitas D, Fried JC. Oxygen consumption in sepsis and septic shock. *Crit Care Med* 1991; **19**: 664–70.

8 Crosby, ET. Perioperative haemotherapy – I: indications for blood component transfusion. *Can J Anaesth* 1992; **39**: 695–707.

9 Hebert PC, Wells G, Blajchman MA, Marshall J, Martin C, Pagliarello G, Tweeddale M, Schweitzer I, Yetisir E. A multicenter, randomized, controlled clinical trial of transfusion requirements in critical care. *N Engl J Med* 1999; **340**: 409–17.

10 Hebert PC, Yetisir E, Martin C, Blajchman MA, Wells G, Marshall J, Tweeddale M, Pagliarello G, Schweitzer I. Is a low transfusion threshold safe in critically ill patients with cardiovascular diseases? *Crit Care Med* 2001; **29**: 227–34.

11 Freudenberger RS, Carson JL. Is there an optimal hemoglobin value in the cardiac intensive care unit? *Curr Opin Crit Care* 2003; **9**: 356–61.

12 Mangano DT, Hollenberg M, Fegert G, Meyer ML, London MJ, Tubau JF, Krupski WC. Perioperative myocardial ischemia in patients undergoing noncardiac surgery – I: incidence and severity during the 4-day perioperative period. The Study of Perioperative Ischemia (SPI) Research Group. *J Am Coll Cardiol* 1991; **17**: 843–50.

13 Hogue CW Jr, Goodnough LT, Monk TG. Perioperative myocardial ischemic episodes are related to hematocrit level in patients undergoing radical prostatectomy. *Transfusion* 1998; **38**: 924–31.

14 Nelson AH, Fleisher LA, Rosenbaum SH. Relationship between postoperative anemia and cardiac morbidity in high-risk vascular patients in the intensive care unit. *Crit Care Med* 1993; **21**: 860–6.

15 American Society of Anesthesiologists Task Force on Blood Component Therapy. Practice Guidelines for Blood Component Therapy. *Anesthesiology* 1996; **84**: 732–47.

16 Welch HG, Meehan KR, Goodnough LT. Prudent strategies for elective red blood cell transfusion. *Ann Intern Med* 1992; **116**: 393–402.

17 Carson JL, Duff A, Poses RM, Berlin JA, Spence RK, Trout R, Noveck H, Strom BL. Effect of anaemia and cardiovascular disease on surgical mortality and morbidity. *Lancet* 1996; **348**: 1055–60.

18 Reinecke H, Trey T, Wellman J, Heidrich J, Fobker M, Wichter T, Walter M, Breithardt G, Schaefer RM. Haemoglobin-related mortality in patients undergoing percutaneous coronary interventions. *Eur Heart J* 2003; **24**: 2142–50.

19 Szachniewicz J, Petruk-Kowalcyzk J, Majda J, Kaczmarek A, Reczuch I, Kalra PR, Piepoli MF, Anker SD, Banasiak W, Ponikowski P. Anaemia is an independent predictor of poor outcome in patients with chronic heart failure. *Int J Cardiol* 2003; **90**: 303–8.

20 Spiess BD, Ley C, Body SC *et al*. Hematocrit value on intensive care unit entry influences the frequency of Q-wave myocardial infarction after coronary artery bypass grafting. The Institutions of the Multicenter Study of perioperative Ischemia (McSPI) Research Group. *J Thorac Cardiovasc Surg* 1998; **116**: 460–7.

21 Blair SD, Janvrin SB, McCollum CN *et al*. Effect of early blood transfusion on gastrointestinal hemorrhage. *Br J Surg* 1986; **73**: 783–5.

22 Bracey AW, Radovancevic R, Riggs SA *et al*. Lowering the hemoglobin threshold for transfusion in coronary artery bypass procedures: effect on patient outcome. *Transfusion* 1999; **39**: 1070–7.

23 Bush RL, Pevec WC, Holcroft JWA. Prospective, randomized trial limiting perioperative red blood cell transfusions in vascular patients. *Am J Surg* 1997; **174**: 143–8.

24 Carson JL, Terrin ML, Barton FB *et al*. A pilot randomized trial comparing symptomatic vs. hemoglobin-level-driven red blood cell transfusions following hip fracture. *Transfusion* 1998; **38**: 522–9.

25 Furtune JB, Feustel PJ, Saifi J *et al*. Influence of hematocrit on cardiopulmonary function after acute hemorrhage. *J Trauma* 1987; **27**: 243–9.

26 Hebert PC, Wells G, Marshall J *et al*. Transfusion requirements in critical care: a pilot study. Canadian Critical Care Trials Group (published erratum appears in *JAMA* 1995; **274**: 944). *JAMA* 1995; **273**: 1439–44.

27 Johnson RG, Thurer RL, Kruskall MS *et al*. Comparison of two transfusion strategies after elective operations for myocardial revascularization. *J Thorac Cardiovasc Surg* 1992; **104**: 307–14.

28 Weiskopf RB. Do we know when to transfuse red cell to treat anemia? *Transfusion* 1998; **38**: 517–21.

29 McLellan SA, McClelland DB, Walsh TS. Anaemia and red blood cell transfusion in the critically ill patient. *Blood Rev* 2003; **17**: 195–208.

30 Petrides M. Red cell transfusion "trigger": a review. *South Med J* 2003; **96**: 664–7.

31 Crosby E. Re-evaluating the transfusion trigger: how low is safe? *Am J Ther* 2002; **9**: 411–16.

32 Carson JL, Hill S, Carless P, Hebert P, Henry D. Transfusion triggers: a systematic review of the literature. *Transfus Med Rev* 2002; **16**: 187–99.

33 Carson JL, Chen AY. In search of the transfusion trigger. *Clin Orthop* 1998; **357**: 30–5.

34 Pearlman ES. When to transfuse blood in sickle cell disease? Lessons learned from Jehovah's Witnesses. *Ann Clin Lab Sci* 1994; **24**: 396–400.

35 Hill SR, Carless PA, Henry DA, Carson JL, Hebert PC, McClelland DB, Henderson KM. Transfusion thresholds and other strategies for guiding allogeneic red blood cell transfusion. *Coch Database Sys Rev* 2002; **2**: CD002042.

36 Lundsgaard-Hansen P. Safe hemoglobin or hematocrit levels in surgical patients. *World J Surg* 1996; **20**: 1182–8.

37 Engelfriet CP, Reesink HW, McCullough J, Hebert PC, McIntyre LA, Carson JL, Ferreira G, Thurer RL, Brock H, Boyce N, Jones J, Wulf H, Lukasewitz P, Kretschmer V, Walsh TS, McClelland B. Perioperative triggers for red cell transfusions. *Vox Sang* 2002; **82**: 215–26.

38 Viele MK. What can we learn about the need for transfusion from patients who refuse blood? The experience with Jehovah's Witnesses. *Transfusion* 1994; **34**: 396–401.

39 Carson JL, Poses RM, Spence RK, Bonavita G. Severity of anaemia and operative mortality and morbidity. *Lancet* 1988; **1**: 727–9.

40 Spence RK, Carson JA, Poses R, McCoy S, Pello M, Alexander J, Popovich J, Norcross E, Camishion RC. Elective surgery without transfusion: influence of preoperative hemoglobin level and blood loss on mortality. *Am J Surg* 1990; **159**: 320–4.

41 Carson JL, Armas-Loughran B. Blood transfusion: less is more? *Crit Care Med* 2003; **31**: 2409–10.

42 Fitzgerald RD, Martin CM, Dietz GE. Transfusing red blood cells stored in citrate phosphate dextrose adenine-1 for 28 days fails to improve tissue oxygenation in rats. *Crit Care Med* 1997; **25**: 726–32.

43 Marik PE, Sibbald WJ, Burton AC. Effect of stored-blood transfusion on oxygen delivery in patients with sepsis. *JAMA* 1993; **269**: 3024–9.

44 Zallen G, Offner PJ, Moore EE, Blackwell J, Ciesla DJ, Gabriel J, Denny C, Silliman CC. Age of transfused blood is an independent risk factor for postinjury multiple organ failure. *Am J Surg* 1999; **178**: 570–2.

45 Purdy FR, Tweeddale MG, Merrick PM. Association of mortality with age of blood transfused in septic ICU patients. *Can J Anaesth* 1997; **44**: 1256–61.

46 Mynster T, Nielsen HJ. The impact of storage time of transfused blood on post-operative infectious complications in rectal cancer surgery. Danish RANX05 Color-ectal Cancer Study. *Scand J Gastroenterol* 2000; **35**: 212–17.

47 McMahon TJ, Moon RE, Luschinger BP, Carraway MS, Stone AE, Stolp BW, Gow AJ, Pawloski JR, Watke P, Singel DJ, Piantadosi, Stamler JS. Nitric oxide in the human respiratory cycle. *Nat Med* 2002; **8**: 711–17.

48 Lane P, Gross S. Hemoglobin as a chariot for NO bioactivity. *Nat Med* 2002; **8**: 657–8.

49 Mair B, Agosti SJ, Foulis PR, Hamilton RA, Benson K. Monitoring for under-transfusion. *Transfusion* 1996; **36**: 533–5.

50 Lenfant C. Transfusion practice should be audited for both undertransfusion and overtransfusion. *Transfusion* 1992; **32**: 873–4.

51 Sazama K. Is undertransfusion occurring? *Transfusion* 2001; **41**: 577–8.

52 Pinkerton PH, Tasev T, Coovadia AS. Changes in red-cell transfusion practice in a tertiary care hospital during the 1990s: a 7-year study. *Transfus Med* 1998; **8**: 179–84.

53 Saxena S, Wehrli G, Makarewicz K, Sartorelli J, Shulman IA. Monitoring for underutilization of RBC components and platelets. *Transfusion* 2001; **41**: 587–90.

54 Gorman DF, Teanby DN, Sinha MP, Wotherspoon J, Boot DA, Molokhia A. Pre-ventable deaths among major trauma patients in Mersey Region, North Wales and the Isle of Man. *Injury* 1996; **27**: 189–92.

55 Yee H, Mra R, Nyunt KM. Cardiac abnormalities in the thalassaemia syndromes. *SE Asian J Trop Med Pub Health* 1984; **15**: 414–21.

56 Carson JL, Noveck H, Berlin JA, Gould SA. Mortality and morbidity in patients with very low postoperative Hb levels who decline blood transfusion. *Transfusion* 2002; **42**: 812–18.

57 Penninx BWJH, Guralnik JM, Onder G, Ferrucci L, Wallace R, Pahor M. Anemia and decline in physical performance among older persons. *Am J Med* 2003; **115**: 104–10.

58 Lawrence VA, Silverstein JH, Cornell JE, Pederson T, Noveck H, Carson JL. Higher Hb level is associated with better early functional recovery after hip fracture repair. *Transfusion* 2003; **43**: 1717–22.

59 National Institutes of Health Consensus Conference. Platelet transfusion therapy. *JAMA* 1987; **257**: 1777–80.

60 Drews RE. Critical issues in hematology: anemia, thrombocytopenia, coagulopa-thy, and blood product transfusions in critically ill patients. *Clin Chest Med* 2003; **24**: 607–22.

61 McCarthy LJ, Danielson FM, Miraglia C *et al*. Platelet transfusion and thrombotic thrombocytopenic purpura. *Transfusion* 2003; **43**: 829.

62 De la Rubia J, Plume G, Arriaga F *et al*. Platelet transfusion and thrombotic thrombocytopenic purpura. *Transfusion* 2002; **42**: 1384–5.

63 Duke WW. The relation of blood platelets to hemorrhagic disease. *JAMA* 1910; **60**: 1185–92.

64 Gardner FH, Howell D, Hirsch EO. Platelet transfusions utilizing plastic equipment. *J Lab Clin Med* 1954; **43**: 196–207.

65 Gaydos LA, Freireich EJ, Mantel N. The quantitative relation between platelet count and hemorrhage in patients with acute leukemia. *N Engl J Med* 1962; **266**: 905–9.

66 Murphy S, Gardner FH. Effect of storage temperature on maintenance of platelet viability: deleterious effect of refrigerated storage. *N Engl J Med* 1969; **280**: 1094–8.

67 Goodnough LT, Shander A, Brecher ME. Transfusion medicine: looking to the future. *Lancet* 2003; **361**: 161–9.

68 Dodd RY. Bacterial contamination and transfusion safety: experience in the United States. *Transfus Clin Biol* 2003; **10**: 6–9.

69 Blajchman MA. Incidence and significance of the bacterial contamination of blood components. *Dev Biol* 2002; **108**: 59–67.

70 Yomtovian R. Bacterial contamination of blood: lessons from the past road map for the future. *Transfusion* 2004; **44**: 450–60.

71 McCullough J. Current issues with platelet transfusion in patients with cancer. *Semin Hematol* 2000; **37**(2 Suppl. 4): 3–10.

72 Schiffer CA, Anderson KC, Bennett CL, Bernstein S, Elting LS, Goldsmith M, Goldstein M, Hume H, McCullough JJ, McIntyre RE, Powell BL, Rainey JM, Rowley SD, Rebulla P, Troner MB, Wagnon AH. Platelet transfusion for patients with cancer: clinical practice guidelines of the American Society of Clinical Oncology. *J Clin Oncol* 2001; **19**: 1519–38.

73 Rock G, Moltzan C, Alharbi A, Giulivi A, Palmer D, Bormanis J. Automated collection of blood components: their storage and transfusion. *Transfus Med* 2003; **13**: 219–25.

74 Patten E. Controversies in transfusion medicine: prophylactic platelet transfusion revisited after 25 years – con. *Transfusion* 1992; **32**: 381–5.

75 Baer MR, Bloomfield CD. Controversies in transfusion medicine: prophylactic platelet transfusion therapy – pro. *Transfusion* 1992; **32**: 377–80.

76 Gmur J, Burger J, Schanz U, Fehr J, Schaffner A. Safety of stringent prophylactic platelet transfusion policy for patients with acute leukemia. *Lancet* 1991; **338**: 1223–6.

77 Higby DJ, Cohen E, Holland JF, Sinks L. The prophylactic treatment of thrombocytopenic leukemic patients with platelets: a double blind study. *Transfusion* 1974; **14**: 440–6.

78 Lawrence JB, Yomtovian RA, Hammons T, Masarik SR, Chongkolwatana V, Creger RJ, Manka A, Lazarus H. Lowering the prophylactic platelet transfusion threshold: a prospective analysis. *Leuk Lymph* 2001; **41**: 67–76.

79 Gil-Fernandez JJ, Alegre A, Fernandez-Villalta MJ, Pinilla I, Garcia VG, Martinez C, Tomas JF, Arranz R, Figuera A, Camara R, Fernandez-Ranada JM. Clinical results of a stringent policy on prophylactic platelet transfusion: non-randomized comparative analysis in 190 bone marrow transplant patients from a single institution. *Bone Marr Transpl* 1996; **18**: 931–5.

80 Wandt H, Frank M, Ehninger G, Schneider C, Brack N, Daoud A, Fackler-Schwalbe I, Fischer J, Gackle R, Geer T, Harms P, Loffler B, Ohl S, Otremba B, Raab M, Schonrock-Nabulsi P, Strobel G, Winter R, Link H. Safety and cost effectiveness of a $10 \times 10(9)/L$ trigger for prophylactic platelet transfusions compared with the traditional $20 \times 10(9)/L$ trigger: a prospective comparative trial in 105 patients with acute myeloid leukemia. *Blood* 1998; **91**: 3601–6.

81 Sagmeister M, Oec L, Gmur J. A restrictive platelet transfusion policy allowing long-term support of outpatients with severe aplastic anemia. *Blood* 1999; **93**: 3124–6.

82 Murphy MF, Murphy W, Wheatley K, Goldstone AH. Survey of the use of platelet transfusions in centres participating in MRC leukaemia trials. *Br J Haematol* 1998; **102**: 875–6.

83 Finazzi G. Prophylactic platelet transfusion in acute leukemia: which threshold should be used. *Haematologica* 1998; **83**: 961–2.

84 Heckman KD, Weiner GJ, Davis CS, Strauss RG, Jones MP, Burns CP. Randomized study of prophylactic platelet transfusion threshold during induction therapy for adult acute leukemia: 10,000/microL versus 20,000/microL. *J Clin Oncol* 1997; **15**: 1143–9.

85 Rebulla P, Finazzi G, Marangoni F *et al*. The threshold for prophylactic platelet transfusions in adults with acute myeloid leukemia. *N Engl J Med* 1997; **337**: 1870–5.

86 Navarro JT, Hernandez JA, Ribera JM, Sancho JM, Oriol A, Pujol M, Milla F, Feliu E. Prophylactic platelet transfusion threshold during therapy for adult acute myeloid leukemia: 10,000/microL versus 20,000/microL. *Haematologica* 1998; **83**: 998–1000.

87 Tinmouth AT, Freedman J. Prophylactic platelet transfusions: which dose is the best dose? A review of the literature. *Transfus Med Rev* 2003; **17**: 181–93.

88 Zumberg MS, del Rosario ML, Nejame CF, Pollock BH, Garzarella L, Kao KJ, Lottenberg R, Wingard JR. A prospective randomized trial of prophylactic platelet transfusion and bleeding incidence in hematopoietic stem cell transplant recipients: 10,000/microL versus 20,000/microL trigger. *Biol Blood Marr Transpl* 2002; **8**: 569–76.

89 Callow CR, Swindell R, Randall W, Chopra R. The frequency of bleeding complications in patients with haematological malignancy following the introduction of a stringent prophylactic platelet transfusion policy. *Br J Haematol* 2002; **118**: 677–82.

90 Valeri CR, Cassidy G, Pivacek LE, Ragno G, Lieberthal W, Crowley JP, Khuri SF, Loscalzo J. Anemia-induced increase in the bleeding time: implications for treatment of nonsurgical blood loss. *Transfusion* 2001; **41**: 977–83.

91 National Institutes of Health Consensus Conference. Fresh-frozen plasma: indications and risks. *JAMA* 1985; **253**: 551–3.

92 Kaul V, Munoz SJ. Coagulopathy of liver disease. *Curr Treat Options Gastroenterol* 2000; **3**: 433–8.

93 Amitrano L, Guardascione MA, Brancaccio V *et al*. Coagulation disorders in liver disease. *Semin Liver Dis* 2002; **22**: 83–96.

94 Downes KA, Sarode R. Massive blood transfusion. *Ind J Pediatr* 2001; **68**: 145–9.

95 Bianco C. Choice of human plasma preparations for transfusion. *Transfus Med Rev* 1999; **13**: 84–8.

96 Di Paola J, Nugent D, Young G. Current therapy for rare factor deficiencies. *Haemophilia* 2001;Suppl. 1: 16–22.

97 Thompson HW, Touris S, Giambartolomei S, Nuss R. Treatment of congenital afibrinogenemia with cryoprecipitate collected through a plasmapheresis program using dedicated donors. *J Clin Apheresis* 1998; **13**: 143–5.

98 Janson PA, Jubelirer SJ, Weinstein MJ *et al.* Treatment of the bleeding tendency in uremia with cryoprecipitate. *N Engl J Med* 1980; **303**: 1318–22.

99 Poon MC. Cryoprecipitate: uses and alternatives. *Transfus Med Rev* 1993; **7**: 180–92.

100 Duckert F. Documentation of the plasma factor XIII deficiency in man. *Ann NY Acad Sci* 1972; **202**: 190–9.

101 Lak M, Peyvandi F, Ali Sharifian A, Karimi K, Mannucci PM. Pattern of symptoms in 93 Iranian patients with severe factor XIII deficiency. *J Thromb Haemost* 2003; **1**: 1852–3.

102 Downes KA, Yomtovian R. Advances in pre-transfusion infectious disease testing: assuring the safety of transfusion therapy. *Clin Lab Med* 2002; **22**: 475–90.

103 Dzik WH, Corwin H, Goodnough LT, Higgins M, Kaplan H, Murphy M, Ness P, Shulman IA, Yomtovian R. Patient safety and blood transfusions: new solutions. *Transfus Med Rev* 2003; **17**: 169–80.

104 Nucleic Acid Amplification Testing of Blood Donors for Transfusion Transmitted Infectious Disease. Report of the Interorganizational Task Force on Nucleic Acid Amplification Testing of Blood Donors. *Transfusion* 2000; **40**: 143–59.

105 Busch MP. HIV, HBV and HCV: new developments related to transfusion safety. *Vox Sang* 2000; **78**(Suppl. 2): 253–6.

106 Busch MP. Closing the windows on viral transmission by blood transfusion. In: Stramer SL, ed. *Blood Safety in the New Millennium*. Bethesda, MD: American Association of Blood Banks, 2001: 33–54.

107 Sazama K. Interactions between science, government, and media on selection and testing of donors. *Vox Sang* 1998; **74**(Suppl. 2): 503–6.

108 Dodd RY, Notari EP IV, Stramer SL. Current prevalence and incidence of infectious disease markers and estimated window-period risk in the American Red Cross blood donor population. *Transfusion* 2002; **42**: 975–9.

109 AuBuchon JP, Birkmeyer JD, Busch MP. Safety of the blood supply in the United States: opportunities and controversies. *Ann Int Med* 1997; **127**: 904–9.

110 Busch M, Chamberland M, Epstein J *et al.* Oversight and monitoring of blood safety in the United States. *Vox Sang* 1999; **77**: 67–76.

111 Heye N, Hensen S, Muller N. Creutzfeldt–Jakob disease and blood transfusion. *Lancet* 1994; **33**: 693–7.

112 Joint Commission on Accreditation of Health Care Organizations, Sentinel Event Alert, Issue Ten. Blood transfusion errors: preventing future occurrences, August 30, 1999.

113 Sharma RR, Kumar S, Agnihotri SK. Sources of preventable errors related to transfusion. *Vox Sang* 2001; **81**: 37–41.

114 Sazama K. Death from transfusion: sources of error. In: *Best Practices for Reducing Transfusion Errors*. OBRR/CBER/FDA Workshop; Bethesda, MD, February 14, 2002.

115 Linden J. Transfusion errors. In: *Best Practices for Reducing Transfusion Errors*. OBRR/CBER/FDA Workshop; Bethesda, MD, February 14, 2002.

116 Williamson LM, Lowe S, Love EM, Cohen H, Soldan K, McClelland DBL, Skacel P, Barbara JAJ. Serious hazards of transfusion (SHOT) initiative: analysis of the first two annual reports. *BMJ* 1999; **319**: 16–19.

117 Andreu G, Morel P, Forestier F, Debeir J, Rebibo D, Janvier G, Herve P. Hemovigilance network in France: organization and analysis of immediate transfusion incident reports from 1994 to 1998. *Transfusion* 2002; **42**: 1356–64.

118 Callum JL, Kaplan HS, Merkley LL, Pinkerton PH, Fastman BR, Romans RA, Coovadia AS, Reis MD. Reporting of near-miss events for transfusion medicine: improving transfusion safety. *Transfusion* 2001; **41**: 1204–11.

119 Shulman IA, Saxena S, Ramer L. Assessing blood administering practices. *Arch Pathol Lab Med* 1999; **123**: 595–8.

120 Sazama K. Reports of 355 transfusion-associated deaths: 1976 through 1985. *Transfusion* 1990; **30**: 583–90.

121 Linden JV, Wagner K, Voytovich AE, Sheehan J. Transfusion errors in New York State: an analysis of 10 years' experience. *Transfusion* 2000; **40**: 1207–13.

122 Bradbury M, Cruickshank JP. Blood transfusion: crucial steps in maintaining safe practice. *Br J Nurs* 2000; **9**: 134–8.

123 Shulman IA, Lohr K, Derdiarian AK, Pickaric JM. Monitoring transfusionist practices: a strategy for improving safety. *Transfusion* 1994; **34**: 11–15.

124 Shulman IA, Jones, FS. Practical aspects of the self-assessment of the issue and administration of blood: a review of two hospitals' experiences. *Am J Clin Pathol* 1997; **107**(Suppl. 1): S17–S22.

125 Motschman TL, Moore SB. Error detection and reduction in blood banking. *Clin Lab Med* 1996; **16**: 961–73.

CHAPTER 3

Preoperative Management and Preparation for Transfusion-Free Surgery

Lawrence T Goodnough

Introduction

Bloodless medicine refers to emerging clinical strategies for medical care without allogeneic blood transfusion, and is a well-defined area in blood management. The Circular of Information distributed with blood and blood products recommends that all physicians be familiar with the alternatives that are a part of bloodless medicine. The Circular states that 'red cell–containing components should not be used to treat anemias that can be corrected with specific medications' [1]. The purpose of this chapter is to present an overview of this approach in the preoperative assessment and management of the surgical patient.

Preoperative assessment

Thorough preoperative planning is essential to reducing or avoiding peri-operative allogeneic transfusion. Preoperative assessment requires accurate history taking and physical examination. Attention should be paid to any personal or family history of bleeding disorders. In patients requesting transfusion-free care who require major cardiac and orthopedic surgical procedures, aggressive preoperative work-ups have yielded excellent results [2,3]. Table 3.1 summarizes presurgical assessment and planning.

Patients with low hemoglobin (Hb) levels prior to surgery are at higher risk of receiving allogeneic transfusion. To minimize this risk, patients should have their red cell mass increased preoperatively. The use of recombinant human erythropoietin (EPO) and/or iron therapy has been effective for this purpose.

A simple measure to conserve the patient's own blood consists of restricted diagnostic phlebotomy (reducing the number of tests and the volume of blood withdrawn) [4]. Another measure is careful management of anticoagulation, including discontinuation or substitution of agents that could

Table 3.1 Preoperative assessment and planning

Methodical history taking, physical examination, supplemented by judicious laboratory tests

Identify appropriate combinations of strategies for prevention and treatment of anemia and/or bleeding

Optimize preoperative hemoglobin level with erythropoietin, iron, folate, vitamin B12

Avoid pharmacologic coagulopathies

Manage anticoagulation

Restrict diagnostic phlebotomy

adversely affect clotting in the perioperative period (e.g. acetylsalicylic acid (ASA) and medication containing aspirin, nonsteroidal anti-inflammatory drug (NSAIDs), antiplatelet agents, anticoagulants).

Physicians are obligated to inform their patients of preoperative autologous donation (PAD) as an alternative to allogeneic transfusion [5,6]. However, it is not without significant cost or inconvenience. For every 2 units donated, on average only 1 unit gets transfused [7]. The patient may not entirely avoid exposure to allogeneic blood, since approximately 50% of patients who donate blood prior to surgery are anemic on the day of surgery [8]. PAD is also associated with higher rates of clerical errors than allogeneic blood and is not without infectious risks. Increased costs, inconvenience to patient and possible clerical errors are some of the reasons for the recent decline in enthusiasm for PAD [5,9]. Nonetheless, it is important to consider the patient's peace of mind and informed choice. PAD is not acceptable to patients who are Jehovah's Witnesses.

Optimizing red cell mass

Little is known about current utilization in the USA of technologies or techniques to reduce allogeneic blood transfusion. The results of a survey sent to 1000 US hospitals in 1997 that reported using such technologies (autologous blood procurement and/or pharmaceutical therapy in patients undergoing surgery) are illustrated in Figure 3.1 [10]. As many as 43% of respondents stated that EPO therapy was available, although only 11% stated that EPO was routinely (2%) or sometimes (9%) prescribed. The remainder stated that EPO was never (57%) or almost never (32%) used. Despite approval for perisurgical use of EPO therapy in the USA in 1996, acceptance for its utilization as an alternative to blood transfusion has been slow, probably due to high costs and poor cost-effectiveness (more than $7 million per quality-adjusted life year (QALY) saved [11]).

A review recently summarized knowledge gained regarding the relationship between EPO, iron and erythropoiesis in patients undergoing PAD (as a model for blood loss anemia), with or without EPO therapy [12]. A summary

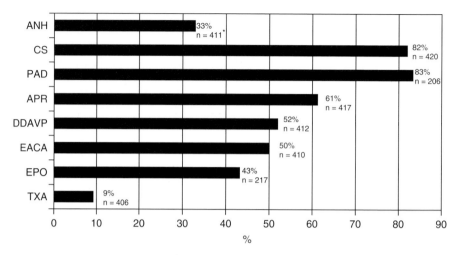

Figure 3.1 Percentage of hospitals using technologies to reduce allogeneic blood transfusion. Techniques: acute normovolemic hemodilution (ANH); cell salvage (CS); preoperative autologous donation (PAD). Pharmaceuticals: aprotinin (APR); desmopressin (DDAVP); epsilon-aminocaproic acid (EACA); recombinant human erythropoietin (EPO); tranexamic acid (TXA). *Different denominators are the result of different sources of data (e.g. anaesthesiologist vs. surgery). (*Source*: Hutchinson *et al.* [10] with permission.)

of selected, prospective controlled trials of patients undergoing PAD discussed in the review is presented in Table 3.1. Endogenous EPO-mediated erythropoiesis in response to PAD under standard conditions of 1 blood unit donated weekly, in this setting, generates 397–568 ml RBC, or the equivalent of 2–3 units of blood. Exogenous EPO therapy in patients undergoing PAD generates 358–1102 ml, or the equivalent of 2–5 units of blood (Table 3.2). With enhanced erythropoiesis during exogenous EPO therapy, iron-restricted erythropoiesis occurs even in patients with measurable storage iron (Figure 3.2). The superior erythropoietic response in a patient with hemochromatosis further suggests that iron-restricted erythropoiesis occurs in patients receiving EPO therapy (Table 3.2), even with oral iron supplementation.

Erythropoietin therapy and erythropoietic response

An analysis of the relationship between EPO dose and the response in red blood cell (RBC) production has demonstrated a good correlation (Figure 3.3), and can be used to determine the appropriate EPO dose to generate the desired increase in red cell mass [13]. EPO-stimulated erythropoiesis is independent of age and gender [14], and the variability in response among patients is in part due to iron-restricted erythropoiesis [15]. There is no evidence that surgery or EPO therapy affects the endogenous EPO response to anemia, or the erythropoietic response to EPO [16].

Table 3.2 Endogenous erythropoietin-mediated erythropoiesis (data expressed as means).

Patients (n)	Blood removed (donated)				Blood produced		
	Requested/ donated units	RBC (ml)	Baseline RBC (ml)		RBC (ml)	Expansion (%)	Iron therapy
Standard phlebotomy							
108	522	2.7	522		1884	351	19	PO
22	590	2.8	590		1936	220	11	None
45	621	2.9	621		1991	331	17	PO
41	603	2.9	603		1918	315	16	PO + IV
Aggressive phlebotomy							
30	540	3.0	540		2075	397	19	None
30	558	3.1	558		2024	473	23	PO
30	522	2.9	522		2057	436	21	IV
24	683	4.1	683		2157	568	26	PO
23	757	4.6	757		2257	440	19	PO

Note: PO, oral; IV, intravenous.
Source: Goodnough *et al.* [12].

RBC expansion is seen with an increase in reticulocyte count by day 3 of treatment in nonanemic patients treated with EPO who are iron-replete [17]. As illustrated in Figure 3.4, the equivalent of 1 blood unit is produced by day 7 and the equivalent of 5 blood units produced over 28 days [18]. If 3–5 blood units are necessary in order to minimize allogeneic blood exposure in patients undergoing complex procedures such as orthopedic joint replacement surgery, the preoperative interval necessary for EPO-stimulated erythropoiesis can be estimated to be 3–4 weeks.

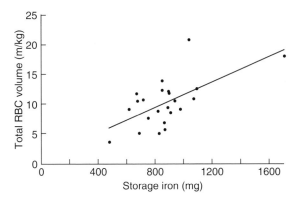

Figure 3.2 Relationship between initial storage iron (mg) and red blood cell volume expansion (ml/kg) in patients undergoing aggressive phlebotomy, with erythropoietin therapy. Linear regression analysis demonstrates a significant correlation ($r = 0.6$; $P = 0.02$). (*Source*: Goodnough and Marcus [15] with permission.)

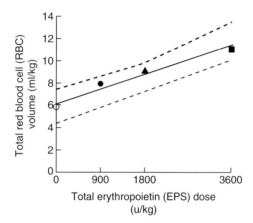

Figure 3.3 The dose-response relationship between total (cumulative) amount of erythropoietin (EPO) administered (units/kg body weight for six treatments over 3 weeks) and the red blood cell (RBC) volume increases (ml/kg body weight) during the preoperative interval for patients treated intravenously with placebo – 150 u/kg, 300 u/kg, and 600 u/kg. Doses of EPO are given in total (cumulative) units/kg body weight for all six treatments combined over a period of 3 weeks; increases in red cell volume are given in ml/kg body weight. The dotted lines indicate the 95% confidence interval. (*Source*: Goodnough LT, *et al.* [13].)

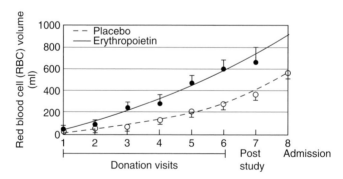

Figure 3.4 Red blood cell (RBC) production during autologous blood donation in 23 placebo-treated (○) and 21 erythropoietin-treated (●) patients. Data points represent calculated RBC production (ml) at donation visits 1 through 6, the post-study visit, and hospital admission. RBC production is indicated by a polynomial regression curve for each treatment group (*n* = 44 at each point). The rate of RBC production can be derived for any preoperative interval. The mean cumulative interval since donation visit 1 is 3.5 days to visit 2; 7.2 days to visit 3; 10.6 days to visit 4; 14.2 days to visit 5; 17.6 days to visit 6; 20.9 days to visit 7 (post-study visit); and 26.3 days to visit 8 (hospital admission). (*Source*: Goodnough LT, *et al.* [18].)

Normal individuals have been shown to have difficulty providing sufficient iron to support rates of erythropoiesis that are greater than three times basal [19]. A recent study confirmed that the maximum erythropoietic response in the acute setting, seen in EPO-treated patients with measurable storage iron, is approximately four times basal marrow RBC production [15]. Previous investigators have shown that conditions associated with enhanced plasma iron and transferrin saturation produce a greater marrow response, such as in patients with hemochromatosis [20] or in patients supplemented with intravenous (IV) iron administration [21].

In hemochromatosis, marrow response has been estimated to increase by six- to eightfold over baseline RBC production with aggressive phlebotomy [20]. The term 'relative iron deficiency' has thus been termed by Finch [22] to occur in individuals when the iron stores are normal but the increased erythron iron requirements exceed the available supply of iron.

Iron supplementation with at least 100 mg elemental iron per day taken with food can cover the increased iron needs from the endogenous EPO response in autologous blood donors [12]. However, a randomized trial of EPO therapy found that the optimal erythropoietic response was in patients who received IV iron supplementation [23]. Another study found that for iron-replete patients there is a significant relationship between storage iron and marrow response in patients receiving EPO therapy [15]. These results suggest that both storage iron and iron supplementation are important for maintaining sufficient plasma transferrin saturation for optimal erythropoiesis in the setting of EPO therapy.

Iron therapy

In circumstances with significant ongoing iron losses, oral iron does not provide enough iron to correct the iron-deficient erythropoiesis, and IV iron therapy should be considered. Renal dialysis patients have such blood losses, and the role of IV iron therapy has been best defined in clinical trials achieving target hematocrit (Hct) levels in this setting. Addressing iron deficiency with IV iron therapy allows correction of anemia along with utilization of lower EPO dosage [24]. Another role for IV iron therapy is in the arena of bloodless medicine and bloodless surgery programs for patients who refuse blood transfusions on the basis of religious beliefs. Common clinical settings here include pregnancy [25] and patients with dysfunctional uterine bleeding who are scheduled for hysterectomy [26].

IV iron therapy has been closely scrutinized for risks and adverse events. Imferon (iron dextran BP) is an iron preparation previously associated with a 0.6% risk of life-threatening anaphylactoid reactions and 1.7% risk of severe, delayed reactions that were serum sickness–like and characterized by fever, arthralgias and myalgias [27]. An increased incidence of delayed reactions of up to 30% and severe reactions of 5.3% was subsequently described [28]; this product was eventually withdrawn from use.

InFed (iron dextran USP) is currently approved for parenteral (intramuscular (IM) or IV) use, with widespread use as IV administration in renal dialysis patients. Clinical studies have shown that InFed administered IV during the dialysis procedure was associated with clinically significant adverse reactions in 4.7% patients, of which 0.7% were serious or life-threatening, and another 1.75% were characterized as anaphylactoid reactions [29]. The prevalence of these reactions does not appear to differ among patients receiving low-dose (100 mg) or higher-dose (250–500 mg) infusions [30]. A recent review reported 196 allergic/anaphylaxis cases with the use of iron dextran in the USA between 1976 and 1996, of which 31 (15.8%) were fatal [31].

Safety aspects of parenteral iron in patients with end-stage renal disease for iron dextran, ferric gluconate and iron saccharate have been scrutinized [32]. Iron saccharate is a preparation available in Europe but not in the USA, in which allergic reactions are very rare. Possible adverse effects include a metallic taste, arthralgia, chest pain or brochospasm [32–34]. Ferric gluconate (Ferrlecit) was approved for use in the USA in February 1999 as an IV iron preparation in renal dialysis patients. Dosage of Ferrlecit is limited to 125 mg over a 1-h infusion at each administration [35]. The rate of allergic reactions (3.3 episodes per million doses) appears lower than iron dextran (8.7 episodes per million doses) and the safety profile of iron gluconate is substantially better; among 74 adverse events reported as severe with its use from 1976 to 1996, there were no deaths [31].

Adverse events that have been reported associated with ferric gluconate include hypotension, rash, chest or abdominal pain, with an incidence of less than 5% [36]. Another potential adverse effect of IV iron therapy is a clinical syndrome of acute iron toxicity (nausea, facial reddening and hypotension), which has been attributed to oversaturation (> 100%) of transferrin. This has been described with rapid infusion of ferric gluconate (62.5–125 mg within 30 min) in a study of 20 dialysis patients [37]. However, a recent report disputed the existence of this effect (i.e. oversaturation of transferrin) by demonstrating that two laboratory assays for measurement of serum iron yield misleading results for transferrin saturation if performed within 24 h after infusion [38]. Serious reactions including one hypotensive event were reported in only 3 (1.3%) of 226 patients undergoing renal dialysis while treated with ferric gluconate in one European study [39].

Previous studies [40] have indicated that the increased erythropoietic effect (4.5–5.5 times basal) of IV iron dextran (with an estimated half-life of 60 h) is transient and lasts 7–10 days, after which the iron is sequestered in the reticuloendothelial system, and erythropoiesis returns to 2.5–3.5 times normal [41]. IV iron therapy is therefore recommended to be administered at intervals of 1–2 weeks. A dose-response relationship of EPO and erythropoiesis that is affected favorably by IV iron, even in iron-replete individuals, has important implications for EPO dosage [11], especially if the cost of therapy is taken into account. IV iron may potentiate the erythropoietic response in the setting of EPO therapy by improving iron-restricted erythropoiesis induced by EPO therapy.

Current safety issues

Thrombotic events were described in an initial uncontrolled trial of epoietin alfa therapy in patients undergoing dialysis [42]. The observation of thrombotic events with epoietin alfa administration in this setting required a subsequent randomized placebo-controlled trial. Diastolic blood pressures showed a mild but significant elevation in epoietin alfa–treated patients maintained at 'higher' levels of Hb (115–130 g/dl) compared with 'lower' (95–110 g/dl) levels or placebo-treated patients; venous access clotting was similarly increased [43]. Studies of epoietin alfa therapy in the setting of uremia suggested that effects on platelet number, platelet aggregation, blood coagulation and/or fibrinolysis could influence the risk of thrombosis during epoietin alfa therapy in patients who are uremic [44–46]. The shortening of the bleeding time in these patients treated with epoietin alfa, however, is related to increased Hct [47,48]; any thrombotic effect may, in part, be related to acute increases in Hct affecting blood rheology in patients at risk [49].

Subsequently, a randomized trial was conducted in hemodialysis patients with clinical evidence of congestive heart failure or ischemic heart disease to study the risks and benefits of normalizing Hct (to achieve and maintain an Hct of 42%) compared to maintenance of Hct at 30% [50]. The primary end point was length of time to death or a first nonfatal myocardial infarction. The study was halted after 29 months with 183 deaths and 19 first nonfatal myocardial infarctions in the normal Hct cohort compared to 150 and 14, respectively, in the low Hct group; while the differences were not statistically significant, they were sufficient to preclude any possibility that the study would reveal a benefit for the normal Hct cohort. Of note, the mortality rates decreased with increasing Hct in both groups.

Thrombotic events have not been associated with epoietin alfa therapy in carefully controlled trials of patients scheduled for surgery. The safety of epoietin alfa therapy in patients undergoing noncardiac surgery has been demonstrated by the equal distribution of concomitant adverse events between patients treated with epoietin alfa or placebo in over 1000 surgical patients participating in clinical trials. The overall prevalence of thrombotic events in 10 (2.8%) of 365 evaluable patients in three clinical trials [51–53] undergoing preoperative autologous blood donation, with or without epoietin alfa therapy, is similar to rates of thrombotic complications reported in patients undergoing orthopedic surgery. The occurrence of myocardial infarction in the setting of autologous blood donation ABD has also been described in patients undergoing radical prostatectomy [54]. Careful studies of hemostasis, fibrinolysis and rheology in autologous blood donors have failed to identify (pro)thrombotic changes [55,56]. In view of the thrombotic events reported during the preoperative blood donation interval in both (placebo and epoietin alfa) patient cohorts, volume replacement in patients undergoing aggressive (twice weekly) phlebotomy in any patient known to have cardiovascular risks seems prudent.

An unresolved question is the safety of epoietin alfa therapy in patients undergoing cardiac surgery, and its role in this setting. In a European trial

Table 3.3 Erythropoiesis during blood loss and erythropoietin therapy (data are expressed as means)

Patients (n/sex)	Total EPO dose (U/kg)	Units	Blood removed			Blood produced		
			RBC (ml)	Baseline RBC (m)	RBC (ml)	Expansion (%)	Iron therapy	
10/F	900 SQ	3.4	435	1285	358	28	IV	
24	900 IV	5.2	864	1949	621	32	PO	
10/F	1800 SQ	4.3	526	1293	474	37	IV	
26	1800 IV	5.5	917	2032	644	32	PO	
11/F	3600 IV	4.9	809	1796	701	39	PO	
12/M	3600 IV	5.9	1097	2296	1102	48	PO	
23	3600 IV	5.4	970	2049	911	45	PO	
18	3600 IV	5.6	972	2019	856	42	PO	
1/M	4200 IV	8	1600	2241	1764	79	Hemochromatosis	

Source: Goodnough *et al.* [12].

[57], the investigators found no differences in mortality, thrombotic events or serious adverse events in their 76 patients between the epoietin beta–treated and placebo cohorts, nor any differences in hemostatic parameters in their patients during the 14-day preoperative interval in which increased Hct levels (from $42 \pm 3\%$ to $48 \pm 3\%$) were demonstrated (Table 3.3) [56]. In fact, the investigators in the European trial were able to demonstrate that epoietin beta–treated patients had an improved extractable oxygen perioperatively, when compared with placebo-treated patients, which was also associated with a lower incidence of lactic acidosis in the epoietin beta–treated patients [58]. A US study [59] also observed no differences in adverse events between epoietin alfa– and placebo-treated patients, and concluded that epoietin alfa therapy was well tolerated (Table 3.4). However, these findings indicated that an uneven distribution of these events between the placebo- and the epoietin alfa–treated groups could not be ruled out to any degree of certainty. For

Table 3.4 Serious adverse events in two clinical trials of cardiac surgical patients treated with erythropoietin or placebo.

Parameter	European trial*		US trial[†]	
	Placebo	EPO	Placebo	EPO
Number of patients	38	38	56	126
Thrombosis or other serious adverse event	5	2	17	35
Mortality	4	4	0	7

Source: Sowade *et al.* [58].
[†]*Source*: D'Ambra *et al.* [59].

example, even if the true mortality rate was 0% in the placebo group and 6% in the combined epoietin groups, there is only 23% probability (power of 0.229) that the resulting data would produce a statistically significant p value of < 0.05 [60].

What is the current role of EPO therapy in cardiac surgery, particularly in the USA, where cardiac and vascular surgeries are excluded as an indication for its use? This approach remains a valuable tool for patients with special requirements, such as Jehovah's Witness patients for whom blood transfusion is not an option [61]. Until additional safety data are forthcoming, the off-label use of EPO therapy in patients undergoing cardiac or vascular surgery cannot be recommended. Emerging data on the use of EPO therapy in noncardiac procedures, such as elderly men undergoing radical prostatectomy [62], may provide additional evidence that perioperative elevations of Hct, even in patients at risk for ischemic heart disease, are well tolerated. Potential concerns that a 'too rapid' rise in Hct may be harmful are not supported by experience in two clinical settings: patients receiving blood transfusions who have immediate and substantial increases in Hct (which is actually the desired effect), and iron-deficient patients receiving total-dose iron infusions who were reported to have 2 g/dl Hb increases within 1-week interval, with no adverse consequences [63].

Of more recent concern is the increasing identification of patients since 1998 who have developed pure red cell aplasia (PRCA) while undergoing EPO therapy (compared to a total of five cases prior to 1998) [64]. This complication has been associated with the demonstration of neutralizing antibodies to EPO [65,66]. From 1998 through 2001, 87 cases of PRCA were reported, which were antibody-mediated PRCA and where the patient was exposed to a single erythropoietic product. Data submitted to the FDA suggest important differences among brands of epoietin; almost all (84 of 87) of the reported cases in 1998–2001 involve patients receiving Eprex, which is manufactured and distributed to patients outside the USA. This product has undergone a significant manufacturing change since 1998 with the removal of human serum albumin as a stabilizer. PRCA has been reported predominantly among dialysis patients who have taken the drug subcutaneously but not intravenously. These observations have led to speculation that the immunogenicity of the recombinant product has been enhanced through possible combinations of changes in the manufacturing, handling and/or administration of the recombinant product. For this reason, the route of Eprex administration in patients with chronic renal failure has now been recommended to be IV.

Central nervous system effects

An intriguing demonstration of an effect of EPO in addition to its central role in erythropoiesis is that EPO crosses the blood–brain barrier and exerts a neuroprotective effect in animal models of experimental brain injury [67]. Similar to its regulation in the peripheral circulation, EPO within the central nervous system (CNS) is inducible by hypoxia. Systemically administered EPO therapy has been shown to function as a neuroprotective agent in animal models of focal brain ischemia, concussive brain injury, experimental autoimmune encephalitis (EAE) and kainate-induced seizures [67]. The manner in which EPO serves as a neuroprotectant is unclear. One hypothesis is that EPO could rescue cells from death through modulation of apoptosis, a role well defined in erythropoiesis and since extended to neurone-like cells *in vitro*. Important clinical implications are the potential benefit of improving cognition in the elderly and in protecting cognition in patients receiving chemotherapy, who have been demonstrated to have impaired cognitive dysfunction [68].

Darbopoietin alfa

Another important event is the development and characterization of a novel erythropoiesis-stimulating protein, darbopoietin alfa. This is a genetically engineered molecule that is biochemically distinct from recombinant human erythropoietin (epoietin alfa), containing additional carbohydrate and sialic acid moieties, which prolong its serum half-life and thus increase its *in vivo* biological activity [69]. In pharmacokinetic studies in patients with renal disease, darbopoietin alfa was shown to have a threefold longer half-life than epoietin alfa after IV administration (25.3 h vs. 8.5 h respectively). Subcutaneous (SC) administration extended the half-life of darbopoietin alfa to 48.8 h. Darbopoietin alfa is now approved in many countries worldwide for treatment of anemia associated with chronic renal failure.

Darbopoietin alfa has also undergone clinical trials in patients with cancer [70,71]. In one trial [69], the feasibility of reduced-dose frequency with darbopoietin alfa compared to epoietin alfa was demonstrated, comparing weekly darbopoietin alfa vs. thrice-weekly epoietin alfa (according to current labeling indications), and comparing every other week and even every third week darbopoietin alfa vs. weekly epoietin alfa (according to current prevailing practice in oncology). This trial [70] also demonstrated a dose-dependent relationship between darbopoietin alfa and multiple measures of efficacy, including a proportion of patients responding (defined as an increase in Hb > 2 g/dl) to darbopoietin alfa. In a worldwide (non-USA) trial of darbopoietin alfa in cancer patients not receiving chemotherapy, up to 83% of patients responded to once-weekly SC administration of darbopoietin alfa [71]. Darbopoietin alfa was well tolerated in all trials, and there has been no evidence of antibody formation in over 126 000 patients with 68 000 patient-years exposure as of December 2002. Darbopoietin alfa is now approved for treatment of anemia in patients with nonmyeloid malignancies receiving chemotherapy in the USA, European Union and Australia.

Conclusion

Although the strategies discussed can be used individually with success, they are most effective when employed preoperatively in a blood management strategy that is individualized to a specific patient. For example, a patient scheduled for an elective joint replacement surgery that typically leads to a 2-unit RBC transfusion should be assessed several weeks before surgery to look for anemia or iron deficiency. If present, these can be corrected with the use of iron and EPO therapy to increase Hct, thereby improving the patient's tolerance to anticipated blood loss.

In summary, there are therapeutic options for the preoperative management of patients without allogeneic blood transfusion. Physicians should consider blood management using these options for all patients. This philosophy will provide patients with safe and effective therapy, minimize the risks of allogeneic blood, and help preserve our decreasing blood resources for those truly in need.

References

1 Circular of information for the use of human blood and blood components. American Association of Blood Banks, America's Blood Centers, and American Red Cross. 2000.
2 Wittmann PH, Wittmann FW. Total hip replacement surgery without blood transfusion in Jehovah's Witnesses. *Br J Anaesth* 1992; **68**: 306–7.
3 Helm RE, Rosengart TK, Gomez M *et al.* Comprehensive multimodality blood conservation: 100 consecutive CABG operations without transfusion. *Ann Thorac Surg* 1998; **65**: 125–36.
4 Smoller BR, Kruskall MS. Phlebotomy for diagnostic laboratory tests in adults: pattern of use and effect on transfusion requirements. *N Engl J Med* 1986; **314**: 1233–5.
5 Brecher ME, Goodnough LT. The rise and fall of preoperative autologous blood donation. *Transfusion* 2001; **41**: 1459–62.
6 Goodnough LT, Brecher ME, Kanter MH, Aubuchon JP. Transfusion medicine Part II: blood conservation. *N Engl J Med* 1999; **340**: 525–33.
7 Goldman M, Savard R, Long A, Gelinas S, Germain M. Declining value of preoperative autologous donation. *Transfusion* 2002; **42**: 819–23.
8 Forgie M, Wells P, Laupacis A, Fergusson D. Preoperative autologous donation decreases allogeneic transfusion but increases exposure to all red cell transfusion: results of a meta analysis. International Study of Perioperative Transfusion (ISPOT) Investigators. *Arch Intern Med* 1998; **158**: 610–16.
9 Krombach J, Kampe S, Gathof BS, Kiefenbach C, Kasper SM. Human error, the persisting risk of blood transfusion: a report of five cases. *Anesth Analg* 2002; **94**: 154–6.
10 Hutchinson AB, Fergusson D, Graham ID, Laupacis A, Herrin J, Hillyer CD. Utilization of technologies to reduce allogeneic blood transfusion in the United States. *Transfus Med* 2001; **11**: 79–85.
11 Goodnough LT, Monk TG, Andriole GL. Erythropoietin therapy. *N Engl J Med* 1997; **336**: 933–8.
12 Goodnough LT, Skikne B, Brugnara C. Erythropoietin, iron, and erythropoiesis. *Blood* 2000; **96**: 823–33.
13 Goodnough LT, Verbrugge D, Marcus RE, Goldberg V. The effect of patient size and dose of recombinant human erythropoietin therapy on red blood cell expansion. *J Am Coll Surg* 1994; **179**: 171–6.

14 Goodnough LT, Price TH, Parvin CA. The endogenous erythropoietin response and the erythropoietic response to blood loss anemia: the effects of age and gender. *J Lab Clin Med* 1995; **126**: 57–64.

15 Goodnough LT, Marcus RE. Erythropoiesis in patients stimulated with erythropoietin: the relevance of storage iron. *Vox Sang* 1998; **75**: 128–33.

16 Goodnough LT, Price TH, Parvin CA *et al.* Erythropoietin response to anaemia is not altered by surgery or recombinant human erythropoietin therapy. *Br J Haematol* 1994; **87**: 695–9.

17 Goodnough LT, Brittenham G. Limitations of the erythropoietic response to serial phlebotomy: implications for autologous blood donor programs. *J Lab Clin Med* 1990; **115**: 28–35.

18 Goodnough LT, Price TH, Rudnick S. Soegiarso RW. Preoperative red blood cell production in patients undergoing aggressive autologous blood phlebotomy with and without erythropoietin therapy. *Transfusion* 1992; **32**: 441–5.

19 Coleman PH, Stevens AR, Dodge HT, Finch CA. Rate of blood regeneration after blood loss. *Arch Int Med* 1953; **92**: 341–8.

20 Crosby WH. Treatment of hemochromatosis by energetic phlebotomy: one patient's response to getting 55 liters of blood in 11 months. *Br J Haematol* 1958; **4**: 82–8.

21 Goodnough LT, Merkel K. The use of parenteral iron and recombinant human erythropoietin therapy to stimulate erythropoiesis in patients undergoing repair of hip fracture. *Int J Hematol* 1996; **1**: 163–6.

22 Finch CA. Erythropoiesis, erythropoietin, and iron. *Blood* 1982; **60**: 1241–6.

23 Auerbach M, Barker L, Bahrain H *et al.* Intravenous iron optimizes the response to recombinant human erythropoietin in cancer patients with chemotherapy-induced anemia: a multicenter, open-label, randomized trial. *JCO* 2004; **22**: 1301–7.

24 Muirhead M, Bargman J, Burgess E, Jindal KK, Levin A, Nolin L, Parfrey P. Evidence-based recommendations for the clinical use of recombinant human erythropoietin. *Am J Kid Dis* 1995; **26**: S1.

25 Kaisi M, Ngwalle EWK, Runyoro DE, Rogers J. Evaluation and tolerance of response to iron dextran (Imferon) administered by total dose infusion to pregnant women with iron deficiency anemia. *Int J Gynecol Obstet* 1988; **26**: 235.

26 Mays T, Mays T. Intravenous iron dextran therapy in the treatment of anemia occuring in surgical, gynecologic, and obstetric patients. *Surg Gyn Obstet* 1976; **143**: 381.

27 Hamstra RD, Block MH, Schocket AL. Intravenous iron dextran in clinical medicine. *JAMA* 1980; **243**: 1726.

28 Woodman J, Shaw RJ, Shipman AJ, Edwards AM. A surveillance program on a long-established product: Imferon (Iron Dextran BP). *Pharmaceut Med* 1987; **1**: 289.

29 Fishbane S, Ungureanu VD, Maeska JK *et al.* The safety of intravenous iron dextran in hemodialysis patients. *Am J Kid Dis* 1996; **28**: 529–34.

30 Auerbach M, Winchester J, Wahab A, Richards K, McGinley M, Hall F, Anderson J, Briefel G. A randomized trial of three iron dextran infusion methods for anemia in EPO-treated dialysis patients. *Am J Kid Dis* 1998; **31**: 81.

31 Faich G, Strobos J. Sodium ferric gluconate complex in sucrose: safer intravenous iron therapy than iron dextran. *Am J Kid Dis* 1999; **33**: 464.

32 Sunder-Plassmann G, Horl WH. Safety aspects of parenteral iron in patients with end-stage renal disease. *Drug Safety* 1997; **17**: 241.

33 Silverberg DS, Blum M, Peer G, Kaplan E, Iaina A. Intravenous ferric saccharate as an iron supplementation in dialysis patients. *Nephron* 1996; **72**: 413.

34 Sunder-Plassmann G, Horl WH. Importance of iron supply for erythropoietin therapy. *Nephrol Dial Transpl* 1995; **10**: 2070.

35 Nissenson AR, Lindsay RM, Swan S, Sellgman P, Strobos J. Sodium ferric gluconate complex in sucrose is safe and effective in hemodialysis patients: North American trial. *Am J Kid Dis* 1999; **33**: 471.

36 Calvar C, Mata D, Alonso C, Ramos B, Lopez de Novales E. Intravenous administration of iron gluconate during haemodialysis. *Nephrol Dial Transpl* 1997; **12**: 574.

37 Zanen AL, Adriaansen HJ, Van Bommel EFH, Posthuma R, Th. de Jong GM. "Over saturation" of transferrin after intravenous ferric glucomate (Ferrlecit) in haemodialysis patients. *Nephrol Dial Transpl* 1996; **11**: 820.

38 Seligman PA, Schleicher RB. Comparison of methods used to measure serum iron in the presence of iron gluconate or iron dextran. *Clin Chem* 1999; **45**: 898.

39 Pascual J, Teruel JL, Liano F, Sureda A, Ortuna J. Serious adverse reactions after intravenous ferric gluconate. *Nephrol Dial Transpl* 1992; **7**: 271.

40 Hillman RS, Henderson PA. Control of marrow production by the level of iron supply. *J Clin Invest* 1969; **48**: 454.

41 Henderson PA, Hillman RS. Characteristics of iron dextran utilization in man. *Blood* 1969; **34**: 357.

42 Eschbach JW, Egrie JC, Downing MR *et al.* Correction of the anemia of end-stage renal disease with recombinant human erythropoietin: results of a combined phase I and II clinical trial. *N Engl J Med* 1987; **316**: 73–8.

43 Muirhead N. Recombinant human erythropoietin (epoietin alpha) in anemic patients on hemodialysis: Canada. In: Erslev AJ, ed. *Erythropoietin.* Baltimore, MD: Johns Hopkins University Press, 1991: 241–68.

44 Kaupke CJ, Butler GC, Vaziri ND. Effect of recombinant human erythropoietin on platelet production in dialysis patients. *J Am Soc Nephrol* 1993; **10**: 1672–5.

45 Taylor JE, Henderson IS, Stewart WK *et al.* Erythropoietin and spontaneous platelet aggregation in heamodialysis patients. *Lancet* 1991; **338**: 1361–2.

46 Taylor JE, Belch JJF, McLaren M *et al.* Effect of erythropoietin therapy and blood withdrawal on blood coagulation and fibrinolysis in hemodialysis patients. *Kid Int* 1993; **44**: 182–90.

47 Gordge MP, Leaker B, Patel A *et al.* Recombinant human erythropoietin shortens the uremic bleeding time without causing intravascular haemostatic activation. *Thromb Res* 1990; **57**: 171–82.

48 Vigano G, Benigni A, Mendogni P *et al.* Recombinant human erythropoietin to correct uremic bleeding. *Am J Kid Dis* 1991; **1**: 44–9.

49 Raine AEG. Hypertension, blood viscosity, and cardiovascular morbidity in renal failure: implications for erythropoietin therapy. *Lancet* 1988; **1**: 97–100.

50 Besarab A, Bolton WK, Browne JK *et al.* The effects of normal as compared with low hematocrit values in patients with cardiac disease who are receiving hemodialysis and epoietin. *N Engl J Med* 1998; **339**: 584–90.

51 Goodnough LT, Rudick S, Price TH *et al.* Increased collection of autologous blood preoperatively with recombinant human erythropoietin therapy. *N Engl J Med* 1989; **321**: 1163–7.

52 Goodnough LT, Price TH, EPO Study Group. A phase III trial of recombinant human erythropoietin in non-anemic orthopaedic patients subjected to aggressive autologous blood phlebotomy: dose, response, toxicity, and efficacy. *Transfusion* 1994; **34**: 66–71.

53 Price TH, Goodnough LT, Vogler W *et al.* The effect of recombinant erythropoietin therapy administration on the efficacy of autologous blood donation in patients with low hematocrits. *Transfusion* 1996; **36**: 29–36.

54 Goodnough LT, Monk TG. Evolving concepts in autologous blood procurement: case reports of perisurgical anemia complicated by myocardial infarction. *Am J Med* 1996; **101 (2A)**: 33S–37S.

55 Biesma DH, Bronkhorst PJH, de Groot PG *et al.* The effect of recombinant human erythropoietin on hemostasis, fibrinolysis, and bloood rheology in autologous blood donors. *J Lab Clin Med* 1994; **124**: 42–7.

56 Sowade O, Ziemer S, Sowade B *et al.* The effect of preoperative recombinant human erythropoietin therapy on platelets and hemostasis in patients undergoing cardiac surgery. *J Lab Clin Med* 1997; **129**: 376–83.

57 Sowade O, Warnke H, Scigalla P *et al.* Avoidance of allogeneic blood transfusions by treatment with epoietin beta (recombinant human erythropoietin) in patients undergoing open heart surgery. *Blood* 1997; **89**: 411–18.

58 Sowade O, Gross J, Sowade B *et al.* Evaluation of oxygen availability with oxygen status algorithm in patients undergoing open heart surgery treated with epoietin beta. *J Lab Clin Med* 1997; **129**: 97–105.

59 D'Ambra MN, Gray RJ, Hillman R *et al.* Effect of recombinant human erythropoietin on transfusion risk in coronary bypass patients. *Ann Thorac Surg* 1997; **64**: 1686–93.

60 Goodnough LT, Despotis GJ, Parvin CA. Erythropoietin therapy in patients undergoing cardiac operations. *Ann Thorac Surg* 1997; **64**: 1579–80.

61 Goodnough LT, Spence R, Shander A. Bloodless Medicine. *Transfusion* 2003; **43**: 668–76.

62 Monk TG, Goodnough LT, Brecher ME *et al.* A prospective, randomized trial of three blood conservation strategies for radical prostatectomy. *Anesthesiology* 1999; **91**: 24–33.

63 Kaisi M, Ngwalle EWK, Runyoro DE, Rogers J. Evaluation of tolerance of and response to iron dextran administered by total dose infusion to pregnant women with iron deficiency anemia. *Int J Gynecol Obstet* 1988; **26**: 235–43.

64 Anand S, Nissenson AR. Pure red cell aplasia: an emerging epidemic in dialysis patients? *Perit Dial Int* 2003; **23**: 317–19.

65 Lasadevall N, Nataf J, Viron B *et al.* Pure red-cell aplasia and antierythropoietin antibodies in patients treated with recombinant erythropoietin. *N Engl J Med* 2002; **346**: 469–75.

66 Gershon SK, Luksenburg H, Cote TR, Braun MM. Pure red-cell aplasia and recombinant erythropoietin. *N Engl J Med* 2002; **346**: 1584–5.

67 Brines ML, Ghezzi P, Keenan S *et al.* Erythropoietin crosses the blood-brain barrier to protect against experimental brain injury. *PNAS* 2000; **97**: 10526–31.

68 Brezden CB, Phillips KA, Abdolell M. Bunston T, Tannock IF. Cognitive function in breast cancer patients receiving adjuvant chemotherapy. *J Clin Onc* 2000; **18**: 2695–701.

69 Egrie JC, Browne JK. Development and characterization of novel erythropoiesis-stimulating protein (NESP). *Br J Cancer* 2001; **84**(Suppl. 1): 3–10.

70 Glaspy J, Jadeja JS, Justice G *et al.* A dose-finding and safety study of novel erythropoiesis-stimulating protein (NESP) for the treatment of anaemia in patients receiving multicycle chemotherapy. *Br J Cancer* 2001; **84**(Suppl. 1): 17–23.

71 Smith RE, Jaiyesimi IA, Meza LA, Tchekmedylan NS, Chan D, Griffith H *et al.* Novel erythropoiesis-stimulating protein (NESP) for the treatment of anaemia of chronic disease associated with cancer. *Br J Cancer* 2001; **84**(Suppl. 1): 24–30.

CHAPTER 4

Intraoperative Strategies for Transfusion-Free Surgery

Joseph D Tobias

Introduction

When evaluating the use of blood and blood products, the predominant scenario in which such agents are administered is the perioperative period. Perioperative transfusions account for greater than half of the estimated 20 million units of blood and blood products that are administered every year in the USA. Therefore, many of the techniques to limit the need for allogeneic blood products have focused on the intraoperative period or are meant to be used intraoperatively when the greatest blood loss may occur. Of the surgical procedures recognized as being associated with significant blood loss, cardiothoracic, hepatic and major orthopedic procedures – especially those involving the hip, pelvis and spine – lead the list as having the potential for significant blood loss with estimated losses that may exceed one-half to an entire blood volume [1]. During these procedures, as blood is lost and replaced with allogeneic blood, additional blood loss may be exacerbated by the development of a coagulopathy related to the dilution of normal coagulation factors, alterations in acid–base status, hypothermia or disseminated intravascular coagulation (DIC).

Although in most circumstances the administration of blood and/or blood products including fresh frozen plasma (FFP), cryoprecipitate (CRYO) and platelet concentrates can be used to effectively correct hemoglobin (Hb) concentrations and coagulation function, there is a growing body of evidence that demonstrates the potential adverse effects of the administration of allogeneic blood products including the transmission of infectious diseases, immunosuppression, transfusion-related acute lung injury (TRALI), transfusion reactions and graft-versus-host disease (GVHD) [2–4]. There is also a growing body of evidence that demonstrates the potential deleterious effects of the immunosuppressive effects of allogeneic transfusion [5–7]. This latter effect may be particularly problematic during the perioperative period and may impact on the incidence of perioperative infections. Taylor *et al.* reviewed the potential impact of the administration of allogeneic blood products to 1717 adult intensive care unit (ICU) patients [5]. The nosocomial infection rates for the transfused versus the nontransfused groups were 15.38% and 2.92% respectively ($p < 0.005$). They also noted a dose-response curve in that for each unit of packed red blood cells (RBCs) transfused, the odds of developing a nosocomial infection increased by a factor of 1.5. There was a significant increase in mortality rates and length of hospitalization in patients who received packed RBC transfusions. Additional evidence for the potential deleterious effects of allogeneic transfusion is provided by Carson *et al.* who reviewed 9598 consecutive patients undergoing surgery for hip fracture [6]. They noted a 35% greater risk of serious bacterial infection and a 52% greater risk of pneumonia in patients receiving allogeneic blood. They calculated an increased cost of $14 000 in patients having a nosocomial infection.

Potential problems also exist with the use of FFP including the transmission of infectious diseases, volume overload, anaphylactoid reactions and alterations in serum ionized calcium, which may lead to hypotension, cardiovascular compromise and even cardiac arrest [7]. Cote *et al.* evaluated the hemodynamic changes and alterations in ionized calcium levels during the administration of FFP [7]. Their study was prompted by their retrospective review of 17 children with thermal injury undergoing burn debridement who had intraoperative cardiovascular events including hypotension and bradycardia, which was severe enough to require cardiopulmonary resuscitation (CPR) in some cases. Eight of these events occurred during the administration of FFP. The prospective study included 49 intraoperative infusions of FFP to 29 children undergoing burn debridement for thermal injury. The FFP infusions were randomized to rates of 1.0, 1.5, 2.0 and 2.5 (ml/kg/min). They noted statistically significant decreases in ionized calcium during each of the four infusion rates, the greatest decrease occurring with the most rapid infusion rate. Although they noted a significant reduction in mean arterial pressure (MAP) of $\geq 20\%$ from baseline in five patients, this did not correlate with the magnitude of the drop in ionized calcium. They concluded that clinically important decreases in MAP can occur with the administration of FFP and these changes may be prevented by the administration of exogenous calcium.

Given these and other concerns, there remains significant interest in avoiding or limiting the need for allogeneic blood products. Chapter 4 reviews several of the potential options for limiting allogeneic blood product use during orthopedic surgery. Among the techniques discussed in this chapter, many are undoubtedly effective alone; however, the goal of performing major surgical procedures without the use of allogeneic blood products can only be accomplished by combining several of these techniques.

General considerations

Effective preoperative evaluation and preparation of the patient are essential to limit allogeneic blood product use. Patients presenting for major surgery may have chronic medical conditions that affect coagulation function. In pediatric patients, many patients with scoliosis presenting for posterior spinal fusion have associated cerebral palsy and static encephalopathy, at times complicated by seizure disorders. The chronic administration of anticonvulsant agents including phenytoin and carbamazepime may adversely effect coagulation function. Additionally, in these patients or chronically ill elderly patients, nutritional issues and poor intake of vitamin K may predispose to chronic low levels of vitamin K–dependent coagulation factors resulting in chronic coagulation dysfunction. Preoperative screening of coagulation function and simple measures such as the administration of vitamin K (oral or intramuscular (IM)) may alleviate such problems.

Other associated medications may also affect platelet function. Patients with chronic orthopedic problems and pain frequently use nonsteroidal anti-inflammatory drugs (NSAIDs) that may affect platelet function. Although acetylsalicylic acid (ASA) irreversibly inhibits cyclo-oxygenase and platelet function for the life of the platelet, NSAIDs result in reversible inhibition of platelet function, which is dependent on the plasma concentration and hence the half-life of the NSAID. Discontinuation of most NSAIDs for 2–5 days prior to surgery will result in return of normal platelet function.

Intraoperative issues can also impact on blood loss including choice of anesthetic technique (see below for a full discussion of controlled hypotension), fluid therapy, temperature control and patient positioning. Although control of intraoperative blood pressure and use of controlled hypotension are significant factors in intraoperative blood loss, other aspects of the anesthetic technique may also impact on the need for allogeneic blood transfusions. Gall *et al.* evaluated the perioperative effects of intrathecal morphine, administered in the lumbar intrathecal space prior to the start of surgery, in 30 children (9–19 years of age) undergoing posterior spinal fusion for idiopathic scoliosis [8]. In addition to improved analgesia, they also noted decreased blood loss with intrathecal morphine. Estimated blood loss (ml/kg) in patients receiving 0, 2 and 5 μg/kg of intrathecal morphine was 41 ± 23, 34 ± 19 and 14 ± 10 ($p < 0.05$ vs. other two groups) respectively in the three groups.

Maintenance of normothermia is also of paramount importance in controlling blood loss in orthopedic surgery. Prospective trials have shown a decrease in blood loss, requirements for allogeneic blood products, postoperative infections and hospital stay with the maintenance of normothermia [9,10]. Hypothermia below 34°C is a risk factor for the development of coagulopathy in trauma patients [11] while even mild hypothermia has been shown to increase blood loss during hip arthroplasty [10,12]. Widman *et al.* demonstrated the thermogenic effect of the infusion of an amino acid solution during hip arthroplasty in adults during spinal anesthesia [13]. In those patients receiving the amino acid solution, the pre-anesthesia temperature increased by $0.4 \pm 0.2°C$ while it was unchanged in the control group. At the completion of the surgical procedure, temperature decreased by $0.4 \pm 0.3°C$ in patients receiving the amino acid infusion and by $0.9 \pm 0.4°C$ in control patients. Blood loss was 702 ± 344 ml in controls and 516 ± 272 ml ($p < 0.05$) in study patients. Although this technique is intriguing, it is also somewhat cumbersome and costly. In most anesthetic suites, maintenance of normothermia is provided by a combination of warming the room until the patient is anesthetized, positioned and draped, plus the use of forced air-warming blankets and blood/fluid warmers to warm intravenous (IV) fluids. These techniques generally effectively maintain normothermia without the need for other modalities.

The choice of intraoperative fluid administration may affect coagulation function, thereby impacting on blood loss. During ANH (see below), blood including RBCs, coagulation factors and platelets is removed and replaced with crystalloids and/or colloids. Although it might be assumed that coagulation would be adversely impacted due to the dilution of coagulation factors and platelets, the opposite effect occurs. Due to the dilution of proteins with anticoagulatory effects such as antithrombin III, a 25–30% hemodilution with replacement by isotonic crystalloids results in an augmentation of coagulation function [14].

Colloids used for volume expansion and blood replacement may adversely affect coagulation function. Albumin and gelatins are generally considered to have no effect on, or to improve, coagulation function [15]. However, a limited number of other studies have suggested a decrease in factor VIII/von Willebrand factor (vWF) complex beyond what would be expected for the degree of hemodilution provided, as well as reduced quality of the clot formed with the administration of gelatins [16,17]. Future studies are needed to define the clinical significance of this effect. Medium– or high–molecular weight hydroxyethyl starches (HES), because of their effects on vWF, can adversely affect coagulation function, in particular platelet function, through a decrease in the factor VIII/vWF concentration, when administered in doses exceeding 20–25 ml/kg [18]. The effect of the HES on coagulation function varies with the molecular weight and the degree of substitution (number of hydroxyethyl groups per glucose molecule).

An additional factor that may impact, depending on the surgical procedure, is patient positioning. The latter becomes particularly important with prone positioning. In such cases, padding under the chest and hips prevents pressure on the abdomen. Inadvertent pressure on the abdomen can increase intraabdominal pressure and impede venous return, thereby increasing venous pressure. This may increase venous bleeding from the venous system around the vertebral column.

Isovolemic hemodilution and autologous blood donation

Acute isovolemic hemodilution

There are three means of obtaining autologous blood for transfusion: ANH, preoperative autologous donation (PAD) and perioperative salvage of shed blood. ANH involves phlebotomy and blood collection with replacement of the removed blood with either crystalloid or colloid to maintain normal intravascular volume. The technique can be carried out immediately prior to or immediately following the induction of anesthesia at the start of the surgical procedure. Hemodilution decreases the hematocrit (Hct) of blood shed during surgery, thereby limiting the mass of RBCs lost, and provides autologous blood with active coagulation factors and platelets for reinfusion at the completion of the case. The degree of hemodilution is defined by the final Hct. Moderate hemodilution is defined as a final Hct between 25% and 30%; severe hemodilution, which is not routinely employed, is defined as a Hct between 10% and 20%.

Technique of isovolemic hemodilution

Isovolemic hemodilution should be considered in adult patients in whom a 1000–2000 ml blood loss is anticipated [19]. In children, hemodilution may be considered if the blood loss is expected to be greater than 50% of the estimated blood volume. Despite the relative safety of this technique, there may be specific contraindications to its use (Table 4.1). The initial Hct should be ≥36%; however, values as low as 24% may be acceptable. Any type of ongoing disturbance in coagulation function is one contraindication to ANH, as replacement of blood with asanguineous fluid further dilutes coagulation factors and platelets. Renal insufficiency or failure is also a relative contraindication since diuresis of the fluids after the reinfusion of blood may be impaired. Other relative contraindications include severe pulmonary disease, cirrhosis, severe hypertension, significant cerebrovascular disease or any concurrent illness, which may not allow the patient to tolerate the lower Hct or may preclude the increase in cardiac output (CO) to compensate for it. In the absence of comorbid features, age should not be considered a contraindication except for the fact that the techniques are not indicated in infants less than 6 months of age. An increase in oxygen delivery cannot be provided by increasing stroke volume and the presence of fetal Hb with a leftward shift of the oxyhemoglobin dissociation curve impairs oxygen release at the tissue level [20].

Hemodilution can be performed in an awake or anesthetized patient immediately preceding surgery. The quantity of blood to be withdrawn can be

Table 4.1 Relative contraindications to ANH

Coagulation defect
Renal failure
Severe pulmonary disease
Severed hypertension
Underlying cardiac disease
Significant cerebrovascular disease
Infant less than 6 months of age

calculated, using the patient's current blood volume (BV), initial Hct (H_1) and the final desired Hct (H_E). The volume of blood to be withdrawn is $BV \times (H_1 - H_E)/H_{AV}$ where H_{AV} is the average of H_1 and H_E. Blood is collected in standard blood bank collection bags containing an anticoagulant (usually citrate phosphate dextrose). It is imperative to measure the amount of blood withdrawn so that adequate volume resuscitation may be performed. This can be calculated by weighing the bag to determine the volume of blood removed. The procedure can be accomplished with two large-bore IV catheters or a central line and a large-bore IV. In either case, one catheter is used for infusion of replacement fluid while the other is used for blood removal. Colloid or crystalloid may be used for volume replacement (see below). Placement of an intraarterial catheter may be convenient to continuously monitor MAP as well as for intraoperative monitoring. Heart rate should be continuously monitored to assess the adequacy of volume replacement. A central venous or pulmonary artery catheter, while not necessary in all patients, may be indicated to assess volume status and oxygen delivery depending on the patient's underlying status. Once the blood is collected, it may be kept at room temperature for up to 4–6 h. If the blood is not to be reinfused within 6 h, it should be refrigerated and used within 24 h. Refrigeration will decrease or inactivate platelet function and eliminate one of the benefits of the fresh autologous blood. It is preferable to reinfuse the blood after surgical blood loss has been controlled. The order of units to be reinfused is opposite the order in which they were removed such that the last unit salvaged is the first unit reinfused. The first unit salvaged is given last because it will have the highest Hct and concentration of clotting factors and platelets.

As with resuscitation measures in general, there is controversy as to whether volume replacement for ANH should include crystalloids or colloids. Crystalloid is administered in a 3:1 volume ratio relative to the amount of whole blood removed. Only isotonic fluids should be used such as normal saline, lactated Ringer's or Plasmalyte™. The advantages of crystalloid are that it can be easily diuresed and is inexpensive. However, because the entire volume does not remain in the intravascular space, a 3:1 replacement ratio should be used. With crystalloids, colloid oncotic pressure (COP) will not be maintained, and tissue edema may result with a compromise of oxygen delivery (see below).

Korosue *et al.* [21] studied the effects of hemodilution with crystalloid (lactated Ringer's) or colloid (low–molecular weight dextran) in dogs subjected to focal cerebral ischemia and found improved neurologic outcome with the colloid solution. They attributed this to a reduction of COP by the crystalloid solution and concluded that a decrease in COP would lead to edema formation in the area of focal ischemia. However, since lactated Ringer's is not an isotonic fluid, it reduces osmolarity, which may also augment edema formation in ischemic brain. Therefore, the same outcome may not occur with true isotonic fluids such as normal saline. While different investigators have advocated one fluid over another for specific reasons, some of which are supported by laboratory or animal investigations, no clear-cut benefit on postoperative outcome has been demonstrated with any particular crystalloid or with colloid as opposed to crystalloid.

Colloids are infused as a 1:1 replacement for blood. Thus less volume is required while COP is maintained, because most colloids have a half-life longer than 4 h and may not be rapidly diuresed from the body [22]. Therefore, there is at least the theoretical risk of hypervolemia and fluid overload if the salvaged blood is reinfused rapidly during a time when there is no ongoing blood loss. Therefore, the use of short-acting colloids such as pentastarch or dextran 40 has been encouraged. These agents have half-lives of less than 4 h and are rapidly excreted. No differences regarding volume expansion have been demonstrated between albumin, gelatin, dextran and HES.

Both albumin and high–molecular weight HES have half-lives greater than 24 h. Albumin is prepared from pooled human plasma in a process that eliminates the risk of disease transmission. The chances of adverse effects are minimal, but it is expensive. Hetastarch, a high–molecular weight polysaccharide of the HES family, can have an adverse effect on hemostasis when infused in volumes greater than 20–25 ml/kg [23]. Pentastarch, an HES with a lower molecular weight than hetastarch, has less effect on hemostasis [24]. Dextran 70 and 40 have also been used for volume replacement. Dextran 70 is a water-soluble glucose polymer synthesized by bacteria from sucrose, whereas dextran 40, which has a lower molecular weight than dextran 70, is formed by chemical treatment of dextran 70 [22]. Because of the renal threshold for filtration of dextran, less dextran 70 will be filtered by the glomeruli, thereby accounting for its longer half-life. The half-life of dextran 40 is 2–4 h compared with 6–12 h of dextran 70. Both are enzymatically degraded to glucose and may result in hyperglycemia, especially in patients with altered glucose homeostasis. The maximum recommended dose of dextran 70 is 20 ml/kg for the first 24 h, followed by 10 ml/kg/day for a maximum of 5 days. Dextran 70 decreases factor VIII levels, platelet adhesiveness and aggregation, and fibrinogen levels [22]. Both of the dextran solutions induce rouleau formation and can interfere with subsequent crossmatching of blood. Allergic or true anaphylactic reactions can occur with either product, but dextran 70 has greater antigenic potential than dextran 40. The incidence of allergic reactions with dextran 70 is approximately 1 in 3300 [25]. Dextran 1, a hapten, which combines with the dextran antibody without causing an immune reaction, has been used as a pretreatment to reduce the incidence of allergic reactions [25].

Physiologic consequences

Although the purpose of hemodilution is a decrease in the Hct with a corresponding decrease in the loss of red cell mass during intraoperative bleeding in addition to the salvage of autologous blood with active platelets and coagulation factors for infusion at a later time, there are several physiologic consequences of the technique. Any alteration in the relation between the red cell mass and the plasma volume will alter microcirculatory flow and blood viscosity. Blood viscosity is influenced by shear rates and Hct. The ratio of shear stress (force required to move a fluid) to shear rate (rate at which a fluid flows) defines viscosity. For example, fluids with a higher viscosity require a higher shear stress (force) to move. Most fluids are Newtonian in that they have a constant viscosity regardless of the velocity of the flow. Therefore, a change in force causes a proportional change in flow rate. Blood is not a Newtonian fluid because changes in flow rate will produce a change in viscosity and therefore not a linear increase in flow velocity.

Viscosity also changes disproportionately to changes in Hct. A change in Hct is followed by an exponential increase or decrease in blood viscosity. The shear rate determines the rate of change. The lower the shear rate, the greater is the rate of change in viscosity. Viscosity is shear-dependent down to an Hct of 25–30%. As a result of these factors, hemodilution has the most significant effect at moderate hemodilution to an Hct of 25–30%. Hemodilution to lower Hct does not result in a further reduction of viscosity or shear rate and therefore does not help in increasing flow to and through the microcirculation.

The initial effect of isovolemic hemodilution with a reduction in the Hct is a reduction of the arterial oxygen content of the blood. Compensatory mechanisms to maintain adequate oxygen delivery include increased CO, increased oxygen extraction at the tissue level, and a rightward shift of the oxyhemoglobin dissociation curve. Increased CO is due primarily to an increase in stroke volume without significant changes in heart rate. An increase in heart rate during ANH should be considered a sign of hypovolemia or inadequate anesthesia. The primary factor responsible for the increased stroke volume is increased venous return due to reduced whole-blood viscosity and improved microcirculatory flow [26,27]. The increased venous return is reflected by an elevation of left ventricular (LV) end-diastolic pressure [28]. The reduced viscosity of the blood also results in a reduction of the systemic vascular resistance, thereby reducing afterload and improving LV ejection [29,30]. Myocardial contractility increases, most likely because of activation of cardiac sympathetic fibers [26]. Bowens *et al.* [31] demonstrated, in anesthetized dogs, that the increase in CO, due to isovolemic hemodilution, remains stable over a prolonged period of time without adverse hemodynamic consequences. The increase in CO does not require an intact autonomic system as it occurs even in dogs following either cardiac denervation or ß-adrenergic blockage [26,32].

As arterial oxygen content and delivery decline, the oxygen extraction ratio increases. In the resting state, peripheral oxygen extraction does not increase until the Hct decreases to less than 20–25% [32,33]. This relationship holds true provided that hypovolemia does not occur. In the presence of hypovolemia, the arteriovenous oxygen difference will widen even at an Hct greater than 20–25%. Although a decrease in the mixed venous oxygen generally occurs at an Hct of 15–20%, more severe degrees of hemodilution may be tolerated in the presence of normal cardiovascular reserve. Van Woerkins *et al.* [27] demonstrated a constant mixed venous PO_2 and oxygen saturation in dogs down to a mean Hct of $9.3 \pm 0.3\%$ with an exchange of 50 ml/kg of blood. In this animal model, CO doubled resulting in increased flow to all organs except the liver and adrenals. The greatest increase in flow occurred to the heart and brain. The increased flow rates and CO maintained oxygen delivery down to an Hct of 9%.

In a cohort of eight pediatric patients with a mean age of 12 years, Fontana *et al.* demonstrated no adverse effects with hemodilution to a mean Hb of 3.0 g/dl [34]. Mixed venous oxygen saturation decreased from $90.8 \pm 5.4\%$ to $72.3 \pm 7.8\%$ while oxygen extraction increased from $17.3 \pm 6.2\%$ to $44.4 \pm 5.9\%$. No adverse effects were noted despite the extreme degree of hemodilution.

The compensatory mechanisms to maintain oxygen delivery during hemodilution may not be possible in patients with underlying cardiorespiratory dysfunction. The absolute value of Hct (lowest tolerable Hct) at which a decrease in the mixed venous oxygen tension occurs will also be influenced by the use of anesthetic agents and neuromuscular blocking agents. Although these agents decrease peripheral oxygen consumption, they also may blunt the compensatory cardiovascular mechanisms. Van der Linden *et al.* demonstrated that there was a marked blunting of the CO response during hemodilution when animals were anesthetized with high-dose halothane (2 MAC) or ketamine compared to low-dose regimens (1 MAC halothane) [35].

A decrease in oxygen affinity, demonstrated by a rightward shift of the oxyhemoglobin dissociation curve, is an additional compensatory mechanism that maintains tissue oxygen delivery during hemodilution. This mechanism, which facilitates oxygen release from Hb, does not become operative until the Hct reaches 20% [36]. The mechanism responsible for the shift is an increase in 2,3-diphosphoglycerate (2,3-DPG) in erythrocytes. Sunder-Plassman *et al.* [37] found a decrease in oxygen affinity in dogs during hemodilution to a mean Hct of 10% and demonstrated a linear relation between Hb oxygen affinity and 2,3-DPG levels. The effect reaches maximum values within 90 min after hemodilution.

Van Woerkin *et al.* [27] demonstrated an additional compensatory mechanism, the redistribution of regional blood flow. The redistribution of flow is dependent on the metabolic demands of the various tissue beds. They noted increased flow to all organs except the liver and adrenal glands, with the heart and brain receiving the most delivery. When considering the coronary bed, the increased flow is disproportionately greater when compared with the increase in CO. In dogs, Holtz *et al.* [14] demonstrated a 220% increase in CO while coronary blood flow increased by 650%. This disparity results from a greater reduction in coronary vascular resistance than in flow.

The changes in myocardial oxygen consumption are dependent on the level of hemodilution. Jan and Chien [39] demonstrated that myocardial oxygen consumption and coronary sinus oxygen saturation remained constant from an Hct of 60% down to 20%. When the Hct declined below 20%, myocardial oxygen consumption declined and coronary sinus oxygen saturation began to increase. The authors inferred from these data that there was myocardial ischemia with impairment of oxygen extraction at an Hct of less than 20%. Conflicting data were published by Van Woerkins *et al.* [27] who found that myocardial oxygen consumption increased down to an Hct of 9% in anesthetized pigs. Because coronary blood flow and oxygen delivery increased, the myocardial oxygen extraction ratio remained constant. They concluded that increased myocardial blood flow was responsible for an increase in oxygen delivery, which met the metabolic demands of the myocardium.

The distribution of coronary blood flow during isovolemic hemodilution has also been a subject of controversy. Messmer [40] demonstrated a distribution of flow away from the endocardium during hemodilution to a Hct of 15%. Similar results have been reported by Buckberg and Brazier [41]. Crystal [42] observed that coronary blood flow remained unchanged between the endocardium and epicardium with hemodilution to an Hct of 7%. Although the data are conflicting, if there is a redistribution of flow away from the endocardium, it could theoretically expose the patient to ischemia despite the global increase in myocardial blood flow and apparent preservation of myocardial oxygen delivery.

Despite laboratory evidence demonstrating the preservation of coronary blood flow and myocardial oxygen delivery, alterations in flow may be observed in certain pathophysiologic states. Simple tachycardia with the resultant reduced perfusion time and increased oxygen consumption may result in ischemia. The presence of coronary artery stenosis when combined with isovolemic hemodilution may also lead to myocardial ischemia. Geha and Baue [43] examined this issue in dogs with hemodilution to an Hct of 20% followed by graded coronary occlusion. When the left anterior descending (LAD) artery was 50% occluded, there was no decrease in myocardial function, no evidence of ischemia, and an increase in coronary blood flow. However, with a 67% stenosis, there was impaired flow with ischemia. Tachycardia did not occur, although there was a 7% increase in heart rate with hemodilution to an Hct of 20%.

Spahn *et al.* [44] examined LV function with combined LAD occlusion (decrease by 95% of the vessel's cross-sectional area) and hemodilution in dogs. They found that only a marginal decrease in function occurred with hemodilution down to an Hct of $24.4 \pm 0.1\%$. They concluded that while LV function may be preserved under mild and moderate hemodilution, the critical level of isovolemic hemodilution in the presence of a critical stenosis of a coronary vessel is between an Hct of 15% and 25%. Other factors that might compromise coronary blood flow include decreased MAP and LV hypertrophy (LVH). Therefore, the minimal safe Hct in patients with compromised cardiac function is defined as the Hct at which coronary blood flow can no longer increase sufficiently to meet myocardial demand. The authors concluded that identification of this level clinically may be difficult. While hemodilution appears safe in patients with normal myocardial function, problems may arise in the presence of compromised cardiovascular function or alterations in coronary anatomy, especially if combined with tachycardia, decreased perfusion pressure or decreases in the Hct to less than 20%.

As with animal studies, human studies demonstrate differences in myocardial blood flow with hemodilution dependent on the anatomy of the coronary circulation. Kim et al. [45] demonstrated no difference in coronary sinus oxygen saturation at an Hct of 23% versus 34% following cardiopulmonary bypass (CPB) in patients with normal LV function. In a similar patient population, Weisel et al. [46] found that myocardial function may be compromised at an Hct of 20% or less. Given these data and those previously outlined from animal studies, it is logical to suggest that extremes of hemodilution should be avoided in patients with compromised cardiovascular status (abnormal LV function, clinically significant coronary artery disease).

Isovolemic hemodilution also leads to a redistribution of flow to other organ beds including the cerebral circulation with cerebral blood flow being inversely proportional to the degree of hemodilution or the Hct. Todd et al. [47] evaluated the effects of hemodilution with 6% hetastarch in Sprague-Dawley rats. Both cerebral blood flow and cerebral blood volume increased inversely with the reduction in Hct. They also noted that although the increases paralleled each other, there was not a consistent relationship between these two parameters. Therefore, arteriolar vasodilation is not the only factor responsible for the observed increase in cerebral blood flow. Other suggested mechanisms include capillary recruitment, nitric oxide release or an increase in postarteriolar volume [48].

Less information is available concerning the effects of hemodilution outside the cardiovascular system and central nervous system (CNS). Reduced viscosity, as a result of a reduction in erythrocyte and fibrinogen content, results in improved microcirculatory flow in various organs with a more even distribution of tissue PO_2. Sunder-Plassman et al. [37] demonstrated this phenomenon by continuously measuring tissue PO_2 in the liver, kidneys, pancreas, small intestine and skeletal muscle during isovolemic hemodilution to an Hct of 20%. They observed a more homogenous distribution of flow as evidenced by an equilibration of the tissue PO_2 throughout the tissue beds. They concluded that microcirculatory flow improved oxygenation to the peripheral tissues with an equal increase in all organ beds. At an Hct of 15%, a less homogenous redistribution of flow has been noted. Fan et al. [49] demonstrated that, despite a significant increase in CO, greater increases in coronary and cerebral blood flow occurred compared with smaller increases in renal and hepatic blood flow. Renal oxygen extraction has been shown to remain constant despite reductions in oxygen delivery and flow redistribution to the inner renal cortex [50]. Hepatic and gastrointestinal (GI) blood flow are preserved [51]. Utley et al. [52] using a canine model with an Hct of

$25 \pm 2\%$ and nonpulsatile CPB noted no deleterious effects on end-organ perfusion including the GI system.

Clinical applications of isovolemic hemodilution

Various studies have demonstrated the efficacy of ANH as a means of limiting the need for perioperative homologous blood transfusions. Laks *et al.* [30] reported their experience with ANH in four patients during hip arthroplasty. CO increased, while both the oxygen delivery and the arteriovenous oxygen difference decreased with no change in tissue oxygen consumption. No evidence of metabolic acidosis was noted. Additional studies have evaluated ANH during scoliosis surgery in the pediatric population [54,55]. Haberkern and Dangel [54] combined hemodilution to an Hct of 20–25% with mild hypothermia and controlled hypotension. They reported a 75% decrease in the need for homologous blood. No adverse effects were noted.

ANH has also been used for patients of the Jehovah's Witness faith when undergoing cardiac surgery. Because of the continuity of flow maintained between the patient and the CPB circuit, many patients consider this an acceptable technique. Stein *et al.* [56] reported their experience with ANH during cardiac surgery for children of Jehovah's Witnesses. The patients ranged in age from $1\frac{1}{2}$ to 17 years and in weight from 9.1 to 63 kg. Asanguineous priming of the CPB circuit was used combined with moderate to deep hypothermia. There was a decrease of the Hct to a mean of 17.9%. One death occurred related to persistent pulmonary hypertension. No adverse sequelae related to the technique were noted, although no direct measurement of regional blood flow/oxygen delivery was performed. Although the Hct was as low as 10% during CPB, the authors recommended maintaining a value of 20% when discontinuing CPB to maintain myocardial oxygen delivery and function. Following rewarming, prior to separation from CPB, ultrafiltration can be instituted to remove excess crystalloid and raise the Hct.

The literature holds no definitive answer regarding the minimal safe Hct for hemodilution. The degree of hemodilution should be based on the patient's ability to compensate hemodynamically to maintain tissue perfusion and oxygen delivery. Patients with myocardial dysfunction may not have sufficient cardiac reserve to tolerate a reduction of the Hct to 20%. The presence of valvular disease, poor ventricular function and coronary artery disease must be evaluated to determine the lowest tolerable Hct. Neonates and infants are generally not good candidates for ANH as they are incapable of increasing stroke volume to compensate for the decreased oxygen content of the blood, and the presence of fetal Hb shifts the oxyhemoglobin dissociation curve to the left, thereby further impeding oxygen delivery to the tissues.

In patients without cardiac disease, tissue oxygenation is well maintained at an Hct of 20% provided that eurolemia is maintained and the fractional concentration of oxygen is increased. An additional factor that helps maintain the oxygen supply to oxygen demand ratio is a decrease in peripheral oxygen use due to anesthetic and neuromuscular blocking agents. The prevention of factors that increase oxygen consumption, such as pain, shivering and fever, is also important. This must be continued into the postoperative period if there is persistent anemia. Robertie and Gravlee [33] have published guidelines for transfusion thresholds based on the available clinical and basic science research. These recommendations are based on assumptions concerning Hct and CO that are needed to maintain adequate oxygen content and delivery. In patients who are ASA class I, an Hb of 6 g/dl (or an Hct of 18%) may be acceptable during ANH. This level may even be tolerated postoperatively, as long as the course remains uncomplicated. ASA class II and many class III patients will tolerate hemodilution to 24%; however, patients with coronary artery disease, myocardial dysfunction or increased metabolic demands (fever, pain, agitation) may require higher Hct. Patients who are unable to increase CO and regional blood flow (those with congenital, valvular or ischemic cardiac disease) may require a minimum Hct as high as 30% [57,58]. Regardless of the patient's status, intraoperative monitoring for coronary ischemia and decreased end-organ perfusion is required. In many patients, this can be done noninvasively with electrocardiogram (ECG) monitoring, observation of heart rate, monitoring of urine output and intermittent assessment of acid–base status. When more extreme degrees of ANH are used or when the patient has associated comorbid features, invasive hemodynamic monitoring should be considered.

ANH may also be used as an alternative to preoperative autologous donation. In a prospective trial of adult patients undergoing radical retropubic prostatectomy, ANH was shown to be equally as effective as preoperative autologous donation in avoiding allogeneic blood products and maintaining postoperative Hb values while avoiding the costs of preoperative autologous donation, which were three times that of ANH [59]. Future uses of ANH may include its combination with erythropoietin (EPO) therapy as a means of increasing the preoperative Hct and augmenting the amount of blood that can be removed as well as its combination with artificial oxygen carriers or blood substitutes, a technique known as 'augmented ANH'.

Preoperative autologous donation

Although the potential for the preoperative donation of autologous blood was first suggested by Fantus in 1937 when he founded the first blood bank in the USA [60], it was not until the 1980s that autologous transfusion programs gained widespread clinical use during the heightened awareness of the risks of infectious disease transmission with allogeneic blood products. Preoperative donation of autologous blood can reduce the exposure to allogeneic blood, provides blood for patients with rare phenotypes, reduces blood shortages, avoids transfusion-induced immunosuppression and may be an option for patients who refuse transfusions based on religious beliefs [61,62].

The criteria for autologous donation are less stringent than those for allogeneic donors [63,64]. Patients with absolute contraindications to allogeneic

donation such as known malignancies and infections like human immunodeficiency virus (HIV) or hepatitis may participate. Although earlier programs
had age restrictions, many institutions now allow autologous donation in
children younger than 2 years and adults older than 80 years [65,66]. There
are no limitations in regard to a patient's weight. Patients who weigh 50 kg or
more may donate a standard unit of blood (approximately 450–500 ml),
whereas patients weighing less than 50 kg may donate proportionately smaller volumes [67,68].

The technique of blood collection is the same as for allogeneic donation
except that the blood is generally kept as whole blood and not separated into
its components. A patient's Hct is checked prior to each donation to ensure
that it is greater than 33%. Patients are placed on iron supplementation with
the initiation of donation. Donations may be made every 3 days, but the usual
practice is to donate 1 unit per week. The last unit should be donated at least
3 days prior to surgery and preferably up to 1 week to allow the Hct to
increase and plasma proteins to normalize intravascular volume prior to the
surgical procedure. Blood is collected in bags with standard anticoagulants
(CPD-A or citrate-phosphate-dextrose-adenine) for blood storage, having
shelf lives of 35–42 days.

Although it has been reported that complications requiring hospitalization
were 12 times more frequent after autologous than after allogeneic donation
[69], the autologous and allogeneic donors differed in age and first-time donor
status. First-time donors have been shown to have a higher rate of adverse
reactions and were more common in the autologous group. Autologous
predonation has relatively few contraindications (Table 4.2). The presence
of bacteremia is an absolute contraindication due to the obvious concerns
of reinfection during transfusion. Severe or unstable angina necessitating
hospitalization, severe aortic stenosis, anemia, severe pulmonary diseases,
hemodynamic instability or limited cardiac reserve due to other lesions
have been suggested as contraindications to preoperative donation [70].
However, these contraindications have been challenged by several authors.

Mann *et al.* [62] reported adverse effects in 4% of preoperative donation
among 342 'high-risk' patients, an incidence similar to that among healthy
patients. All adverse effects were attributed to transient hypotension, which

Table 4.2 Relative contraindications
to preoperative autologous donation.

Bacteremia
Agina
Underlying cardiovascular disease
Aortic stenosis
Pulmonary disease
Anemia

resulted in either light-headedness or temporary loss of consciousness. No episodes of clinically apparent myocardial ischemia were reported. Owings *et al.* [64] retrospectively reviewed the records of 291 consecutive patients scheduled for elective cardiac surgery of whom 36.8% donated between 1 and 6 units of blood preoperatively. The incidence of adverse reactions related to autologous donation was less than 1%. Goldfinger *et al.* [71] examined autologous transfusions in patients with end-stage cardiac or pulmonary disease who were awaiting organ transplantation. Of 48 heart transplant candidates, 65% were able to donate 1–8 units of blood. The exposure to homologous blood products decreased from 88% in the nondonors to 54% in the donors. Of the 24 lung transplant candidates, 63% predonated and had a homologous blood exposure rate of 45% versus 100% for those who were ineligible for donation. No serious complications were noted.

These studies demonstrated the possibility of autologous donation even in the so-called 'high-risk' groups and its efficacy in reducing the need for homologous transfusion. Age should not be considered a barrier to autologous predonation. Goodnough *et al.* [72] reported that autologous blood accounted for 95% of the transfusion requirements in 1672 patients undergoing elective spinal surgery, 60% of whom were older than 60 years. Autologous donation has also been used in pregnant women without adverse effects on either the mother or the fetus [73,74]. Autologous blood donation has been used in patients diagnosed with placenta previa. Autologous donation should be limited to the second trimester to avoid spontaneous abortions (in the first trimester) and preterm labor (in the third trimester).

The limiting factor in autologous predonation is frequently anemia despite iron supplementation [75]. This has been attributed to inadequate EPO levels. To facilitate predonation, Goodnough *et al.* [76] prospectively evaluated the efficacy of EPO in 47 patients. The patients were randomized to receive either placebo or EPO (600 units/kg) twice a week. Patients who had received EPO were able to donate 5.4 units compared to 4.1 units in the placebo group. The investigators suggested that EPO may be a useful adjunct in autologous predonation (see below for a full discussion of the perioperative applications of EPO in avoiding allogeneic transfusions).

A major issue with predonation of autologous blood is the cost and inconvenience to the patient with the need for repeated visits to the donation center. These issues gain greater importance given the reports that a significant percentage of predonated autologous blood is discarded. The percentage of autologous units that are discarded averages between 30% and 50% with reports of up to 73% of units being discarded [77,78]. The issue of 'crossing over' or using blood that was meant for autologous transfusion for general use remains controversial. In such circumstances, the allogeneic donation criteria must be applied if the blood is to be used. Despite the differences in the criteria for autologous and allogeneic donation, up to 30% of autologous blood could be used.

Autologous blood should not be given merely because it is available. The same criteria used for the transfusion of homologous blood are generally recommended when transfusing autologous blood. Because of the risks of incorrect identification and possible bacterial contamination, it is prudent to avoid transfusion unless indicated.

Intraoperative blood salvage

The intraoperative collection and reinfusion of shed blood was first used in the nineteenth century [79]. Initially used in cardiac surgery, the technique is now used in over 350 000 cases every year during trauma, vascular, orthopedic and gynecologic surgery, as well as liver transplantation. There are several devices available from different manufacturers for both intraoperative and postoperative blood salvage [80]. The blood can either be unprocessed (anticoagulated and reinfused) or processed (anticoagulated, washed with saline and then reinfused).

Semicontinuous flow devices are the most commonly used tool for intraoperative collection of shed blood. They are also the most complex to use as they involve the processing of the salvaged blood. The disposable equipment consists of a blood aspirator and anticoagulation assembly, a reservoir with filter, a centrifuge bowl, a waste bag and tubing. The double-liner aspiration set includes an anticoagulation line so that either heparin or citrate can be combined with the aspirated blood at a controlled rate. The anticoagulated blood is collected into a disposable reservoir containing a filter. The filtered blood is then pumped into a bowl, centrifuged at approximately 4000 rpm, washed with saline and pumped into a reinfusion bag. There are different sized bowls for pediatric and adult patients so that even small quantities of blood can be processed for infants and children. Most of the white blood cells (WBCs), platelets, clotting factors, free plasma Hb and anticoagulant should be removed in the washing process and eliminated in the waste bag. The entire process takes approximately 3–10 min. The RBC suspension has a Hct of approximately 45–60%.

The second type of device used for intraoperative salvage, otherwise known as the canister collection technique, includes a rigid canister with a sterile, disposable liner. Blood is aspirated from the wound and anticoagulated in a similar manner to that of semicontinuous flow devices. The blood is collected in a rigid plastic reservoir containing a disposable liner. The blood can either be washed (processed) prior to infusion or reinfused without washing (unprocessed). Functioning platelets and coagulation factors are present if the blood is left unwashed; however, there is an increased risk of adverse effects due to cellular debris, free Hb and fragmented blood components (see below).

The third type of collection is a single-use, self-contained rigid plastic reservoir that provides unprocessed blood for reinfusion. Citrate, the anticoagulant, is placed in the container in a fixed quantity prior to use. Once the container is full, it is reinfused. This apparatus can also be used for postoperative blood collection and reinfusion. The surgical drains are connected to the canister and every 4 h the blood is reinfused and a new canister attached to the surgical drains. Coagulation factors and platelets are present in the blood.

The indications for intraoperative blood salvage include anticipated loss of greater than 20% of the patient's blood volume or a surgical procedure in which more than 10% of the patients require allogeneic transfusions. Conventional salvage devices have bowls with a capacity of 125 ml and wash the blood in increments of approximately 300 ml, thus mandating that this amount of blood is lost before any of the shed blood can be returned to the patient, thereby rendering these machines ineffective in smaller patients. However, new methods using smaller bowls down to 50–60 ml allow for use of this technology with blood loss of only 100 ml. Alternatively, newer devices that allow for the continuous washing and return of shed blood are now available. These devices allow for the immediate processing of shed blood and therefore may be used even with blood loss of less than 100 ml, thereby making them effective even in neonates and infants. Despite the small volumes, the washed blood maintains a consistent quality and Hct.

Intraoperative blood salvage is most cost-effective when large volumes of blood are harvested, such as in liver transplantation and major vascular surgery [81,82]. For the semicontinuous devices that allow processing of blood, the cost includes both the disposable and nondisposable items. Disposable items (tubing, bowl, separator, reservoir, suction assembly tubing and anticoagulant) cost approximately $200–500 plus the initial cost of the device, which is $20 000–40 000. Despite this, salvaged blood still tends to be less expensive than allogeneic blood. Gardner *et al.* estimated the cost for 285 ml of blood to be $83 for salvaged blood compared to $143 for allogeneic blood [81]. These figures do not consider the potential increased cost related to adverse effects of allogeneic blood product use.

Reported contraindications to the intraoperative blood salvage are usually related to the contamination of the collected blood with infectious or noninfectious agents (Table 4.3). Salvage of blood during cancer surgery is controversial. Although there is concern regarding dissemination of tumor cells since washing does not remove the malignant cells, there have been reports regarding the use of intraoperative blood salvage in patients undergoing surgery for urologic malignant disease without adverse effects [83]. No

Table 4.3 Absolute contraindication for intraoperative cell salvage.

Bacterial contamination of the surgical site
Presence of amniotic fluid
Presence of local hemostatic agents
Cancer surgery (?)

difference in prognosis or outcome has been demonstrated in oncologic surgery patients in whom salvaged blood was used compared to those in whom it was not used. Other suggested modalities in oncologic surgery to treat salvaged blood prior to reinfusion include the use of leukocyte-depletion filters to remove, or irradiation to inactivate, cancer cells.

Intraoperative blood salvage should not be used if there is a risk of bacterial contamination from bowel contents or an infected wound. Aspiration of protamine or other hemostatic agents, e.g. thrombin, is not recommended because of the risk of initiating systemic coagulation [84]. Wound irrigants, debris and amniotic fluid should not be salvaged since these agents may also initiate intravascular coagulation [85]. The reinfusion of salvaged blood from an ectopic pregnancy is considered acceptable.

Other complications related to blood salvage include air and fat embolism, hemolysis with hemoglobinuria, pulmonary dysfunction, renal dysfunction, coagulopathy, electrolyte disturbances and sepsis [85–88] (Table 4.4). Air embolism is uncommon except with improper use of the devices. Reports of fatal air embolism have reported that the blood was reinfused under pressure [89]. Avoidance of pressurized retransfusion and de-airing of the infusion bag should eliminate this complication.

Hemolysis may occur if the suction level is too high or if the aspiration method causes excessive mixing of air with blood. Free Hb may be released during salvage and washing because of erythrocyte damage. Free Hb levels exceeding 100–150 mg/dl may lead to hemoglobinuria and acute renal failure, as the binding capacity of haptoglobin is saturated and free Hb is filtered in the renal tubules. Although there are reports of free hemoglobin levels of 350 mg/dl in salvaged blood and mild creatinine elevations [90], acute renal failure has not been reported. If adequate diuresis is maintained, Hb can be excreted without adverse effects on renal function. Simple bedside monitoring for free Hb in the urine is relatively quick and easy, as the urine will be positive for blood by dipstick yet no RBCs will be seen under microscopic examination. Diuresis should be maintained until the urine is free of Hb.

Reinfusion of fragmented cellular components and debris may lead to activation of the eicosanoid or kininogen system with systemic vasodilation and hemodynamic compromise. The fragments may also act as microemboli and contribute to pulmonary dysfunction [91]. Although pulmonary injury

Table 4.4 Complications of cell salvage.

Infection
Disseminated intravascular coagulopathy
Hemolysis
Pulmonary dysfunction
Air/fat embolism

has been induced in an animal model, such problems have not been reported in humans during reinfusion of salvaged blood [91,92]. Nevertheless, the blood should be reinfused through a 40-μm filter to remove this debris.

Coagulopathy is one of the most common adverse effects associated with intraoperative blood salvage. The incidence and severity of the coagulopathy increases with the volume of blood that is reinfused. Coagulopathy may be related to one of several factors including qualitative or quantitative platelet defects, dilution of coagulation factors or the initiation of DIC. Several coagulation factors including factors I, V, VIII and X are decreased in salvaged blood [93]. Murray *et al.* [85] reported two cases in which DIC occurred following the reinfusion of salvaged blood. They theorized that the intracellular contents of the cellular components of blood initiated the coagulation cascade resulting in DIC. Both patients had hemoglobinuria, which supported their hypothesis that damaged cellular elements were responsible for initiating DIC.

While dilution of platelets and coagulation factors is the most common cause of coagulopathy, residual anticoagulants may also interfere with the coagulation cascade. Improper washing and centrifuge techniques may lead to the infusion of excessive amounts of heparin or citrate. Monitoring of coagulation function (prothrombin time/partial thromboplastin time, activated clotting time or thromboelastogram) may be indicated when large volumes of salvaged blood are used or when clinical bleeding is noted.

Aside from coagulation disturbances, excessive quantities of citrate may lead to disturbances of calcium homeostasis. Hypocalcemia is uncommon except with massive blood loss (greater than 3000–4000 ml) or liver failure. With hepatic insufficiency, citrate metabolism may be slowed, leading to the excessive binding of calcium. Additional metabolic consequences may also occur with intraoperative blood salvage. Washing with saline and removal of bicarbonate can lead to a dilutional metabolic acidosis as well as the dilution of other electrolytes with hypomagnesemia and hypocalcemia [94]. Electrolyte and acid–base disturbances may be limited by using a balanced electrolyte solution instead of saline to wash the RBCs prior to reinfusion [95]. Periodic monitoring of serum electrolytes and acid–base status is necessary when large volumes of blood are salvaged.

Mechanical problems with the cell saver devices or human error may impart some degree of risk to health care providers. If the tubing from the cell saver to the reservoir bag is inadvertently clamped, high pressure in the tubing will cause it to disconnect and spray blood throughout the operating room. Such problems mandate that personnel involved in the use of cell saver devices be educated and familiar with the equipment prior to operating these devices. Some institutions use the perfusionist staff to operate the devices. Although this ensures a certain level of education and competency with such devices, the cost of such personnel may make the cost of the technology prohibitive.

Pharmacologic agents for blood conservation

DDAVP

DDAVP or deamino-8-D-arginine vasopressin is a synthetic analogue of vaso-pressin initially used in the treatment of diabetes insipidus [96]. DDAVP is produced by the deamination of the hemicysteine at position 1 of the natural hormone, thereby protecting the molecule from peptidase degradation. A second modification, D-arginine substitution for L-arginine at position 8, decreases the cardiovascular effects of the molecule [97]. These alterations result in a more potent and prolonged antidiuretic activity with effects at the V_2 vasopressin receptor and limited activity at the V_1 vasopressin receptor. As a result, there are no effects on the smooth muscle of the uterus or the GI tract. The *in vivo* half-life is 55–60 min.

DDAVP promotes hemostasis by augmenting the release of factor VIII and vWF from endothelial cells [98,99]. Factor VIII, a glycoprotein, accelerates the activation of factor X by activated factor IX. Hemostatic functions of vWF include increasing platelet adherence to vascular subendothelium, formation of molecular bridges between platelets to increase aggregation, protection of factor VIII in plasma from proteolytic enzymes and stimulation of factor VIII synthesis.

DDAVP is not effective in patients with severe forms of hemophilia or vWF, as these patients have impaired production of either factor VIII or vWF and therefore cannot release these compounds in response to DDAVP. Even in the normal host, tachyphylaxis may occur in response to DDAVP because of depletion of vWF stores.

The recommended dose of DDAVP is 0.15–0.3 μg/kg administered IV over 15–20 min the morning of surgery. Levels of factor VIII and vWF increase to three to five times those of baseline. Administration over 20–30 min avoids systemic hypotension since the agent can cause systemic vasodilation. DDAVP may also be given subcutaneously or intranasally with plasma levels achieved within 1 h [100,101]. Both these routes produce plasma concentrations of factor VIII and vWF that are equivalent to those seen with IV administration.

Untoward effects of DDAVP include decreased free water clearance from antidiuretic hormone activity, hypotension and the potential for an increased incidence of perioperative thrombotic events. Hyponatremia is uncommon following a single dose and is generally seen only when excessive free water is administered perioperatively. Hypotension results from endothelial cell re-lease of prostacyclin when DDAVP is administered rapidly. This can be avoided by slow administration (15 min or longer). Although there are an-ecdotal reports of thrombotic complications, prospective studies in adults undergoing coronary artery bypass grafting have indicated no difference in the perioperative myocardial infarction rates between patients who received DDAVP and control groups [102,103].

DDAVP has been used as adjuvant therapy in the treatment of vWD and hemophilia A, as well as for the correction of platelet dysfunction associated with uremia, cirrhosis and aspirin therapy [104,105]. It has also been suggested as a potential agent to decrease blood loss in major surgical procedures in patients with normal platelet function. As the studies listed below will demonstrate, the results regarding the use of DDAVP to decrease perioperative blood loss have been conflicting.

Kobrinsky *et al.* [106] evaluated the efficacy of the preoperative administration of DDAVP in adult patients with normal preoperative hemostatic function who were undergoing spinal fusion. They found that DDAVP reduced blood loss by 32.5% and reduced the need for erythrocyte transfusion by 25.6%. Salzman *et al.* [102] administered DDAVP or placebo to 70 cardiac surgery patients following reversal of heparin with protamine. Blood loss in the DDAVP group was approximately half that of the placebo group. However, more recent prospective, randomized trials in spinal surgery have demonstrated no benefit of the preoperative administration of DDAVP [107,108], while Seear *et al.* [109] demonstrated no difference in blood loss in children undergoing cardiac surgery with the use of DDAVP. In the Seear study, there was also no difference in either the bleeding time or coagulation studies when comparing DDAVP to placebo, and the investigators concluded that DDAVP was ineffective in improving hemostasis. A meta-analysis of studies in cardiac surgery patients demonstrated no effect of DDAVP during routine cardiac surgery; however, there was a significant reduction in blood loss during high-risk surgery including repeat surgery or patients with a history of recent aspirin intake [110].

Epsilon-aminocaproic acid and tranexamic acid

Epsilon-aminocaproic acid (EACA) and tranexamic acid (TXA) are γ-aminocarboxylic acid analogues of lysine. During normal coagulation function, plasminogen is converted to plasmin, which inhibits fibrin formation. EACA and TXA bind to the lysine moiety that binds plasminogen to fibrinogen, thus displacing it from the fibrinogen surface and inhibiting fibrinolysis. EACA and TXA also prevent plasmin degradation of platelet glycoprotein 1b receptors, thus preserving platelet function. These agents along with aprotinin have found greatest applications in surgeries associated with activation of the fibrinolytic systems including cardiac, hepatic and prostate surgeries. A recent meta-analysis of the available trials of the antifibrinolytic agents including EACA, TXA and aprotinin demonstrated a decrease in the exposure to allogeneic blood products in patients receiving these agents, as well as a decrease in the incidence of postoperative bleeding and the need for surgical reexploration following cardiac surgery in adult patients [111].

Dosing regimens vary somewhat depending on the study evaluated. Although oral preparations of EACA and TXA are available, for perioperative use these agents are generally administered intravenously. EACA is administered as an IV loading dose of 100–150 mg/kg followed by an infusion of 10–15 mg/kg/h. Within 4–6 h of administration 90% of EACA is excreted in the urine. TXA is seven to ten times more potent than EACA and may be used at lower doses (loading dose of 10 mg/kg followed by an infusion of 1 mg/kg/h). After approximately 24 h 90% of TXA is excreted in the urine.

Beneficial effects on blood loss and the need for allogeneic transfusions have been demonstrated in the orthopedic surgical population. Florentino-Pineda *et al.* evaluated the efficacy of EACA (100 mg/kg followed by 10 mg/kg/h) in 28 adolescents undergoing postoperative spinal fusion [112]. The anesthetic technique including the use of controlled hypotension was consistent between the two groups. Patients receiving EACA had decreased intraoperative blood loss (988 ± 411 ml vs. 1405 ± 670 ml, $p = 0.024$) and decreased transfusion requirements (1.2 ± 1.1 units vs. 2.2 ± 1.3 units, $p = 0.003$). Similar findings were reported by Neilipovitz *et al.* in their study of 40 adolescents undergoing posterior spinal fusion [113]. Patients who received TXA (10 mg/kg followed by 1 mg/kg/h) had decreased total blood transfused (cell saver plus allogeneic packed RBCs) of 1253 ± 884 ml versus 1784 ± 733 ml ($p = 0.045$). However, the amount of allogeneic blood transfused was not statistically significant between the two groups (874 ± 790 ml vs. 1254 ± 542 ml, $p = 0.08$). Three randomized controlled trials in adults undergoing orthopedic surgical procedures demonstrated a significant decrease in transfusion requirements in patients receiving TXA [114–116]. Similar effects have been demonstrated in hepatic transplantation [117], prostatectomy [118] and cardiac surgery [119,120]. Although several studies demonstrate decreased blood loss and transfusion requirements with the antifibrinolytic agents, these results are not universal. Other investigators have demonstrated no benefit of using TXA or EACA in cardiac surgery [121] and orthopedic surgery in oncology patients [122].

Adverse effects of EACA and TXA may be related either to their effects on coagulation or the route of excretion. Since these agents are cleared by the kidneys, thrombosis of the kidneys, ureters or lower urinary tract may occur if urologic bleeding is present. Both EACA and TA may be associated with nausea, vomiting, diarrhea and hypotension with rapid IV administration. Of primary concern with any agent that inhibits the fibrinolytic system is the potential to increase the incidence of postoperative thrombotic events such as deep venous thrombosis, stroke or myocardial infarction. Ovrum *et al.* [110] reported five cases of postoperative myocardial infarction in patients receiving TXA during cardiac bypass. However, the majority of the other prospective, randomized trials have demonstrated no increased incidence of such problems when comparing the EACA or TXA group to placebo patients.

Aprotinin

Although its mechanism of action is different from EACA and TXA, aprotinin is considered with these other agents under the broad heading of antifibrinolytics. Aprotinin is a naturally occurring serine protease inhibitor, first isolated from bovine lung in 1930. Aprotinin's effects on coagulation function are at least twofold. It inhibits the enzymatic formation of several serine protease enzymes including trypsin and plasma kallikrein, which convert plasminogen to plasmin. An additional mechanism of action is the preservation of platelet adhesion by protecting membrane-bound glycoprotein receptors (vWF receptor) from degradation by plasmin.

Aprotinin is administered intravenously and undergoes rapid redistribution into the extracellular fluid, followed by accumulation in renal tubular epithelium with subsequent lysosomal degradation. The dose is expressed as kallikrein-inhibitory units (KIUs). Various dosing regimens have been used in the literature. In adults, the dosing regimens are generally divided into high-dose (6 million units), intermediate-dose (2–6 million units) and low-dose (less than 2 million units) regimens. Given its rapid renal accumulation and degradation, a continuous infusion is needed to maintain adequate plasma concentrations.

To date, the majority of experience with aprotinin remains in patients undergoing cardiovascular surgical procedures. A large meta-analysis of 45 trials with a total of 5805 patients clearly demonstrated a reduction in blood loss and need for allogeneic transfusions [110,123]. Odds ratio for the need for allogeneic transfusions were significantly reduced with all three dosing regimens (high, intermediate and low) at 0.31 (range 0.25–0.39, $p < 0.0001$), 0.35 (range 0.22–0.58, $p < 0.0001$) and 0.49 (range 0.33–0.73, $p < 0.006$) respectively.

Royston [124] evaluated high-dose aprotinin in patients undergoing orthotopic heart or heart-lung transplantation. There was decreased blood loss and a decreased transfusion requirement (RBCs and platelets) in patients receiving aprotinin when compared with those receiving placebo. Blood loss was reduced by a factor of three in those patients with previous thoractomies undergoing heart-lung transplantation. An additional beneficial effect noted in the aprotinin patients included improved pulmonary gas exchange.

Several studies have also demonstrated the efficacy of aprotinin in orthopedic surgery procedures [125–127]. Capdevila et al. [125] evaluated the effects of aprotinin in patients undergoing surgery of the hip, femur or pelvis for infectious or malignant diseases. Aprotinin was administered as a bolus of 1 million KIU followed by 500 000 KIU/h during the procedure. Patients who received aprotinin when compared to placebo had decreased intraoperative blood loss (median of 1783 ml vs. 5305 ml, $p < 0.05$) and decreased need for allogeneic blood (median of 3 units vs. 7 units, $p < 0.05$). Additionally, patients who received aprotinin had higher postoperative platelet counts.

Urban et al. [126] prospectively evaluated the efficacy of aprotinin versus placebo and EACA in adult patients undergoing reconstructive procedures of the spine (anteroposterior spinal fusion) in 60 patients. EACA dosing included a 5-g loading dose followed by 15 mg/kg/h while aprotinin dosing included 1 million KIU followed by 0.25 million KIU/h. Intraoperative and total blood loss in the control, EACA and aprotinin groups were 3556/5181 ml, 2929/4056 ml and 2685/3628 ml ($p < 0.05$) respectively. Units of packed RBCs transfused in the three groups were 6 ± 2, 5 ± 2 and 4 ± 1.

Units of FFP and platelets transfused were 9/3, 3/1 and 0/0 respectively. An additional interesting finding was a decreased incidence of respiratory complications in patients who received aprotinin. The incidence of respiratory complications was 9 of 18 in the control group, 4 of 17 with EACA and 1 of 20 with aprotinin. This may be related to the potent antiinflammatory effects of aprotinin from its inhibitory action on the kallikrein-kininogen system, an effect not seen with EACA or TXA.

As with the other antifibrinolytic agents, the reports are not uniformly positive regarding the effects of aprotinin on perioperative blood loss. Boldt *et al.* [128] reported no beneficial influence of aprotinin on blood loss or transfusion requirements in children undergoing cardiac surgery. They grouped patients according to weight (greater than or less than 10 kg) and found that children weighing more than 10 kg had the greatest postoperative blood losses. Although the authors suggested that the doses of aprotinin used may have been insufficient, they were actually greater than the doses used in adult studies when based on KIU/kg.

Potential adverse effects of aprotinin include allergic reactions, increased incidence of thrombotic events and renal toxicity. Anaphylactoid reactions have been reported and are more frequent in patients previously exposed to aprotinin. With previous exposure, the incidence of anaphylaxis is low with an incidence of less than 0.1% provided that the previous exposure has been more than 6–12 months earlier. As with EACA and TXA, although there are anecdotal reports of thrombotic complications associated with the use of aprotinin, no increased incidence of these problems have been noted in prospective, randomized trials [110,111].

Reports of aprotinin's effect on renal function have been controversial. Renal toxicity is postulated to result from aprotinin's strong affinity for renal tissue and subsequent accumulation in proximal tubular epithelial cells and/or its inhibition of serine proteases (kallikrein-kininogen system). Histopathologic examination of renal tissue following high-dose aprotinin administration reveals obstructed proximal convoluted tubules and swollen tubular epithelial cells.

Additional adverse effects include a decrease in renal plasma flow, glomerular filtration rate and electrolyte excretion. These effects are thought to be the result of the inhibition of intrarenal kallikrein activation and decreased prostaglandin synthesis. The kallikrein-kininogen system leads to renal afferent arteriolar dilatation, thereby regulating renal adaptation to hemodynamic, water and electrolyte alterations. It has also been suggested that aprotinin may have a protective effect on renal function by reducing excretion of enzymes that induce renal injury and enhance glomerular filtration in models of renal ischemia.

High-dose aprotinin has been shown to enhance the anticoagulant effects of heparin during CPB and prolong activated clotting time (ACT) measured with celite. *In vitro* analysis of the effect has demonstrated that the increase in ACT results from the use of celite as the surface activator. An ACT system using kaolin as the surface activator may more accurately reflect heparin-induced anticoagulation. Therefore, if the ACT is used to evaluate heparin effect, kaolin tubes should be used. If only the celite ACT is available, the recommendation is to keep the ACT longer than the usual 400 s to more than 750 s. Aprotinin acts like activated antithrombin III to reduce the rate of coagulation of the intrinsic system. Aprotinin thereby prolongs the activated partial thromboplastin time (APTT), demonstrated by an abnormal thromboplastin time or an abnormal thromboelastogram (prolonged time, decreased alpha angle). Although the administration of FFP will correct the laboratory parameters, the abnormality is likely an artifact produced by aprotinin and does not correlate with clinical bleeding.

Recombinant factor VIIa

Factor VII plays a key role in both the extrinsic and the intrinsic coagulation cascade. Factor VII is activated after contact with tissue factor that is exposed at the site of tissue injury. Activated factor VII can then directly activate factor IX of the intrinsic cascade. Activated factor IX with activated factor XIII can then activate factor X. Alternatively through the extrinsic cascade, activated factor VII can directly activate factor X. Activated factor X can then enter the common cascade leading to the conversion of prothrombin to thrombin and subsequent fibrin formation.

Recombinant DNA technology provides the means for the production of pharmacologic quantities of various coagulation factors including factor VII. In 1988, a patient with hemophilia and inhibitors against factor VIII who was undergoing knee surgery was the first patient to be treated with recombinant factor VIIa (rFVIIa). To date, the majority of experience in both the adult and pediatric population with the use of rFVIIa has been in the treatment of patients with hemophilia who have developed autoantibodies against factor VIII (inhibitors), thereby making subsequent infusions of factor VIII ineffective. In this scenario, rFVIIa has been shown to effectively control bleeding.

Following its efficacy in the hemophilia population, there has been an increasing body of clinical experience with rFVIIa in the nonhemophiliac population with coagulation disturbances of various etiologies. In many of these cases, although anecdotal, rFVIIa has been used to control life-threatening hemorrhage when other modalities including the administration of platelets, CRYO and FFP have failed [129–131]. Scenarios have included several patients in the perioperative period including patients undergoing cardiovascular, thoracic, hepatic, intraabdominal and orthopedic procedures [132–134]. Tobias reported the intraoperative use of rFVIIa as rescue therapy in two pediatric patients who had persistent intraoperative bleeding issues when FFP (20–30 ml/kg) failed to correct coagulation function [135]. In both patients, rFVIIa subjectively controlled surgical bleeding. Friederich et al. [136] evaluated the effects of rFVII given prior to retropubic prostatectomy in patients with normal preoperative coagulation function. Patients were randomized to receive placebo, rFVIIa (20 µg/kg) or rFVIIa (40 µg/kg) prior to surgical incision. Median perioperative blood loss was 2688 ml, 1235 ml and 1089 ml respectively ($p = 0.001$) in the three groups. Of the 12 placebo patients, 7 required allogeneic RBC transfusions compared to no patients who received 40 µg/kg of rFVIIa. The authors also noted a decreased surgical time (180 min in control patients vs. 126 min and 120 min in the two rFVIIa groups, $p = 0.014$).

To date, there are limited data on which to base a recommendation for the widespread, prophylactic use of rFVIIa in patients with normal coagulation function. Additional prospective, randomized trials are needed to evaluate the efficacy of this agent in diminishing perioperative blood loss. However, rFVIIa may be effective when there is ongoing life-threatening bleeding and the coagulopathy has not responded to standard therapy (FFP, platelets, CRYO); time is not available to wait for blood typing, thawing and administration of FFP; there are concerns regarding the potential hemodynamic effects of FFP; or religious issues preclude the use of blood products. Recombinant FVIIa can be quickly reconstituted from powder with a small volume of sterile water and administered intravenously over 2–3 min.

Although clinical experience is somewhat limited, adverse effects with rFVIIa have been few with only a small number of thrombotic complications [137,138]. In the majority of these cases, the patients had several other risk factors for perioperative thromboembolic complications. As rFVIIa requires tissue factor for activation, and tissue factor is released only with vascular damage, the risk of excessive thrombogenesis should be limited [139]. However, as there are limited data in patients with normal coagulation function, future trials are needed to define the adverse effect profile of this agent and its role in the perioperative setting. Since rFVIIa does not correct other factor deficiencies, the coagulopathy may recur once the rFVIIa is cleared. Therefore, other therapies may be needed to correct other coagulation function. These additional therapies may include repeat dosing of rFVIIa, or administration of FFP or vitamin K.

Human recombinant erythropoietin

EPO is a glycoprotein, produced by the kidney in response to tissue hypoxia. It stimulates erythropoiesis by the bone marrow leading to dose-dependent increases in reticulocyte count, Hb and Hct. Recombinant technology allows the production of the hormone in a form that is indistinguishable from the endogenous hormone. Following IV administration, it undergoes biphasic clearance and has a distribution half-life of 4.4 h. IV administration results in higher plasma levels than IM or subcutaneous (SC) administration. In the perioperative period, twice weekly SC dosing of EPO is a common means of administration. Serum iron levels must be sufficient for erythropoiesis to be augmented and therefore oral iron supplementation is frequently used with EPO therapy. In rare instances, IV iron therapy may be necessary. Although originally used in the management of chronic anemia related to renal failure or in association with cancer chemotherapy, EPO now plays a key role in bloodless surgical techniques.

EPO has been previously discussed as an adjunct in the preoperative setting to increase the efficiency of autologous predonation and to augment the Hct prior to ANH [140]. Endogenous EPO secretion in response to anemia is inadequate to augment blood volume and is considered a limiting factor in autologous donation. Additionally, given that one of the major indicators of the need for perioperative allogeneic transfusions is the baseline Hct, the third application of EPO is to merely augment the preoperative Hct even in the absence of preoperative autologous donation or the planned use of ANH.

Adverse effects are more common in patients with chronic renal insufficiency and include hypertension, hypertensive encephalopathy, seizures, myocardial infarction, cerebrovascular accident, hyperkalemia, thrombosis and malaise. These effects are uncommon in patients without renal disease. It remains unclear as to whether these adverse effects are due to the primary disease, EPO therapy or a combination of the two. This drug plays a major role in the preoperative preparation of patients for surgery, and is therefore a valuable adjunct to bloodless surgery.

Controlled hypotension

Controlled hypotension (CH; also referred to as deliberate or induced hypotension) is defined as a reduction of the systolic blood pressure to 80–90 mmHg, a reduction of MAP to 50–65 mmHg or a 30% reduction of MAP from its baseline value. The latter definition being relevant for the pediatric patient whose baseline MAP may be within the 50–65 mmHg range at baseline. Although controlled hypotension is most commonly used to limit intraoperative blood loss, an additional benefit may be improved visualization of the surgical field.

CH was first described by Cushing in 1917. In 1947, Gardner described the use of arteriotomy and the removal of 1600 ml of blood to reduce systolic blood pressure and limit intraoperative blood loss. Gilles in 1948 described the first use of regional anesthesia (subarachnoid blockade) as an alternative to phlebotomy-induced hypotension. With the introduction of short-acting ganglionic blocking agents in the 1950s and continuous vasodilator infusions in the 1960s, the popularity and feasibility of CH increased. In 1966, Eckenhoff and Rich performed the first controlled study of CH and demonstrated a 50% reduction in blood loss by lowering MAP to 55–65 mmHg [141]. Other studies have provided additional evidence of the efficacy of CH, especially during major orthopedic procedures including total hip arthroplasty and spine surgery, with reported reductions of intraoperative blood loss of up to 50% [142].

With any decrease in MAP, there is a concern of the potential for a decrease in end-organ perfusion and tissue hypoxia. The theory behind CH lies in the autoregulatory function of the arteriolar bed in end-organ tissues so that with a decrease in MAP, perfusion and blood flow are maintained. Although a full review of the literature and discussion of this matter is beyond the scope of this chapter, this issue has been addressed by several studies, which have demonstrated the maintenance of end-organ perfusion and tissue oxygenation during CH with several different pharmacologic agents [143–146].

An additional question that has been raised regarding CH is whether it is the reduction in MAP or CO that determines intraoperative blood loss. Sivarajan *et al.* [147] randomized patients to sodium nitroprusside or trimethaphan for CH. Although CO increased in patients receiving nitroprusside when compared to trimethaphan, no difference in blood loss was noted between the two groups, thereby demonstrating that it is the control of MAP and not CO that determines blood loss.

Advances in drug therapy have provided the clinician with several pharmacologic options for CH. While it is now generally accepted that it is the reduction in MAP and not CO that is the primary determinant of intraoperative blood loss, there remains some controversy as to which of the many available agents is optimal for CH. In fact, it is likely that any of a number of agents can be used. The available agents can be divided into those used by themselves (primary agents) and those used to limit the dose requirements, and therefore the adverse effects, of other agents (adjuncts or secondary agents). Primary agents include regional anesthetic techniques (spinal and epidural), inhalational anesthetic agents (halothane, isoflurane, sevoflurane), nitrovasodilators (sodium nitroprusside (SNP) and nitroglycerin), trimethaphan, prostaglandin E_1 (PGE_1) and adenosine. The calcium channel blockers and beta adrenergic antagonists have been used as both primary agents and adjuncts to other agents. The pharmacologic agents used primarily as adjuncts or secondary agents include the angiotensin-converting enzyme inhibitors (e.g. captopril, enalaprilat) and alpha$_2$ adrenergic agonists such as clonidine.

SNP is one of the most commonly used agents for CH. It is a direct-acting, nonselective peripheral vasodilator that primarily dilates vessels leading to venous pooling and decreased systemic vascular resistance. It has a rapid onset of action (approximately 30 s), a peak hypotensive effect within 2 min with a return of blood pressure to baseline values within 3 min of its discontinuation. SNP releases nitric oxide (formerly endothelial-derived relaxant factor), which activates guanylate cyclase leading to an increase in the intracellular concentration of cyclic guanosine monophosphate (cGMP). cGMP decreases the availability of intracellular calcium through one of two mechanisms: decreased release from the sarcoplasmic reticulum into smooth muscle or increased uptake by the sarcoplasmic reticulum. The net result is decreased free cytosolic calcium and vascular smooth muscle relaxation. Adverse effects include rebound hypertension, coronary steal, increased intracranial pressure, increased intrapulmonary shunt with ablation of hypoxic pulmonary vasoconstriction, platelet dysfunction and cyanide toxicity. Direct peripheral vasodilation results in baroreceptor-mediated sympathetic responses with tachycardia and increased myocardial contractility. The renin-angiotensin system and sympathetic nervous system are also activated. The result is tachycardia and increased CO, which may offset the initial drop in MAP and require the addition of a beta adrenergic antagonist to control the tachycardia. Plasma catecholamine and renin activity may remain elevated after discontinuation of SNP, resulting in rebound hypertension.

An additional potential issue with SNP is the possibility of inducing coronary ischemia through a coronary steal phenomenon. The dilatation of normal coronary arteries in nonischemic areas of the myocardium may lead to an intracoronary steal with decreased oxygen delivery to areas supplied by diseased vasculature, which is unable to vasodilate in response to SNP. Since myocardial oxygen extraction is already maximal, increased coronary blood flow from the accumulation of metabolic vasodilator substances is the primary mechanism responsible for meeting increased oxygen demands. As blood pressure decreases, coronary blood flow is maintained by vasodilatation of coronary vessels. In patients with coronary artery disease and stenosis, vasodilatation may be incomplete. Therefore, ischemia may occur with a decrease in MAP to 50–60 mmHg. The potential for ischemia may be further increased by tachycardia and a decreased diastolic blood pressure.

SNP is a direct cerebral vasodilator, which may lead to increased cerebral blood flow and cerebral blood volume. Although the clinical consequences of this are minimal in patients with normal intracranial compliance, increased intracranial pressure may occur in patients with reduced intracranial compliance. A similar effect may be seen with any of the direct acting vasodilating agents. SNP may also have deleterious effects on the pulmonary vasculature and respiratory function. Hypoxic pulmonary vasoconstriction (HPV) acts as a protective mechanism to shunt blood away from unventilated alveoli, thereby maintaining the matching of ventilation with perfusion. SNP may interfere with HPV leading to increased pulmonary shunting. These effects may be further magnified by preoperative pulmonary parenchymal disease, intraoperative positioning and positive pressure ventilation. Despite these effects, the clinical consequences are generally minimal in patients with normal preoperative respiratory function.

Platelet function may be altered during SNP administration due to inhibition of thrombasthenin, a smooth muscle-like protein leading to a defect in platelet aggregation. Hines and Barash infused SNP in 19 cardiac surgery patients to maintain a MAP of 80 mmHg prior to CPB [148]. Infusion rates greater than 3 µg/kg/min (or a total dose of 16 mg in adults) decreased platelet aggregation with a prolongation of the bleeding time. ADP-aggregation studies demonstrated a 33% reduction in aggregation. Despite the alteration in laboratory evaluation of platelet function, clinical bleeding did not occur. Therefore, the clinical consequences of this phenomenon are thought to be minimal in patients with normal platelet function. Additional concerns with SNP administration are the possibility of cyanide and thiocyanate accumulation. Cyanide is a breakdown product of SNP as each molecule of SNP contains five molecules of cyanide. During metabolism by the rhodinase enzyme system of the liver, free cyanide is release. The plasma concentrations of both cyanide and thiocyanate are proportional to the total dose of SNP. Following metabolism of SNP, cyanide may either be converted to thiocyanate by the rhodinase system, combine with methemoglobin to produce cyanomethemoglobin or bind with cytochrome oxidase. The latter may result in deleterious physiologic effects through the impairment of the electron transport system and oxidative phosphorylation. Cyanide has a high affinity for cytochrome oxidase, and if conversion to thiocyanate is slow or inadequate, cellular hypoxia and metabolic acidosis may result. Clinical signs of cyanide toxicity include an elevated mixed venous oxygen tension or a significant increase in infusion requirements over time (tachyphylaxis). The risks of toxicity can be decreased by limiting the total dose of SNP as well as the duration of the infusion. Increased cyanide levels are more common with the acute administration of more than $5-8 \mu g/kg/min$ or prolonged (more than 24 h) infusion rates greater than $2 \mu g/kg/min$. As cyanide metabolism occurs primarily in the liver, patients with altered hepatic function may be at increased risk for toxicity. Toxicity is also more common in patients with dietary deficiency of vitamin B_{12} or sulfur. The latter compound is required for the hepatic conversion of cyanide to thiosulfate. Metabolism by the rhodinase system produces thiocyanate that is then excreted by the kidneys. Thiocyanate toxicity may occur in the presence of prolonged therapy or renal failure. Symptoms of toxicity include skeletal muscle weakness, mental confusion, seizures and nausea. Symptoms generally occur with plasma concentrations greater than 10 mg/dl. Thiocyanate may also alter thyroid function, leading to hypothyroidism due to the inhibition of iodine uptake into the thyroid gland.

Nicardipine is a calcium channel blocker of the dihydropyridine class that vasodilates the systemic, cerebral and coronary vasculature with limited effects on myocardial contractility and stroke volume. Unlike SNP, nicardipine does have some intrinsic negative chronotropic effects that may limit the rebound tachycardia. Like other direct acting vasodilators, nicardipine and the other calcium channel antagonists may increase intracranial pressure. Bernard *et al.* compared the efficacy of SNP versus nicardipine in 20 patients during isoflurane anesthesia for spinal surgery [149]. An initial dose of nicardipine of 6.2 ± 0.9 mg was required to achieve a MAP of 55–60 mmHg. Infusion requirements varied from 3 mg/h to 5 mg/h to maintain a similar MAP. The decrease in MAP was associated with a decrease in pulmonary and systemic vascular resistance, increased CO and decreased arteriovenous oxygen content. Unlike SNP, no change in arterial oxygenation was seen with nicardipine suggesting that it may have minimal effects on HPV. The efficacy of nicardipine compared favorably with that of SNP. One problem that was noted with nicardipine was prolonged hypotension following discontinuation of the infusion. Hypotension persisted for a mean of 43 min with a range of 27–88 min following discontinuation of the infusion. No untoward consequences of the prolonged effect were noted. A follow-up study of Bernard *et al.* [150] compared SNP to nicardipine for controlled hypotension during hip arthroplasty in 24 patients. Similar cardiovascular changes were noted with nicardipine dose requirements of $1-3\,\mu g/kg/min$ following the initial titration dose of 4.7 ± 1.5 mg. Once again, hypotension persisted for 10–20 min following discontinuation of the infusion as opposed to the rebound hypertension that was seen following discontinuation of the SNP infusion.

Hersey *et al.* [151] compared SNP with nicardipine for CH during posterior spinal fusion in 20 pediatric patients. Patients who received nicardipine had decreased blood loss when compared with SNP (761 ± 199 ml vs. 1297.5 ± 264 ml, $p < 0.05$). Time to restore blood pressure back to baseline upon discontinuation of the infusion was significantly longer with nicardipine than with SNP (26.8 ± 4.0 min vs. 7.3 ± 1.1 min, $p < 0.001$).

Summary

Increasing evidence has demonstrated the potential adverse effects of the use of allogeneic blood products. These effects may have significant deleterious effects on patients that may impact on cost and length of hospitalization, and in specific circumstances even mortality. Many of the major surgical procedures can result in significant blood loss and the need for allogeneic blood transfusions. Intraoperative options to limit the need for allogeneic blood product administration are:

1 general considerations including optimization of preoperative coagulation function, intraoperative anesthetic technique, proper patient positioning and maintenance of normothermia;
2 autologous transfusion therapy including preoperative donation with the use of EPO and intraoperative collection using ANH;
3 intraoperative and postoperative blood salvage using cell saver devices;
4 pharmacologic manipulation of the coagulation cascade with EACA, TXA, aprotinin and potentially rFVIIa; and
5 CH.

Although many of these techniques are effective alone, the combination of several of these techniques can potentially lead us to the goal of performing major surgical procedures without the use of allogeneic blood products. Many of the techniques such as autologous donation, ANH and CH have been proven in several studies to be effective. Studies regarding the efficacy of the various pharmacologic agents may not be as compelling; however, agents such as aprotinin seem promising. Since the technology of artificial blood products (see Chapter 12 for a full discussion of these agents), which may limit the need for allogeneic transfusion, may take years yet to perfect, use of the techniques described in this chapter should be considered as part of a multidisciplinary comprehensive approach to provide bloodless surgery.

References

1 Guay J, Haig M, Lortie L *et al.* Predicting blood loss in surgery for idiopathic scoliosis. *Can J Anaesth* 1994; **41**: 775–81.

2 Goodnough LT, Bercher ME, Kanter MH *et al.* Transfusion medicine: first of two parts – blood transfusion. *N Engl J Med* 1999; **340**: 438–47.

3 Parshuram C, Doyle J, Lau W *et al.* Transfusion-associated graft versus host disease. *Pediatr Crit Care Med* 2002; **3**: 57–62.

4 Schriemer PA, Longnecker DE, Mintz PD. The possible immunosuppressive effects of perioperative blood transfusion in cancer patients. *Anesthesiology* 1988; **68**: 422–8.

5 Taylor RT, Manganaro L, O'Brien J *et al.* Impact of allogeneic packed red blood cell transfusion on nosocomial infection rates in the critically ill patient. *Crit Care Med* 2002; **30**: 2249–54.

6 Carson JL, Altman DG, Duff A *et al.* Risk of bacterial infection with allogeneic blood transfusion among patients undergoing hip fracture repair. *Transfusion* 1999; **39**: 694–700.

7 Cote CJ, Drop LJ, Hoaglin DC *et al.* Ionized hypocalcemia after fresh frozen plasma administration to thermally injured children. *Anesth Analg* 1988; **67**: 152–60.

8 Gall O, Aubineau JV, Berniere J *et al.* Analgesic effect of low-dose intrathecal morphine after spinal fusion in children. *Anesthesiology* 2001; **94**: 447–52.

9 Kurz A, Sessler DI, Lenhardt R (for the Study of Wound Infection and Temperature Control Group). Perioperative normothermia to reduce the incidence of surgical wound–associated infection and shorten hospitalization. *N Engl J Med* 1996; **334**: 1209–15.

10 Schmied H, Kurz A, Sessler D *et al.* Mild hypothermia increases blood loss and transfusion requirements during total hip arthroplasty. *Lancet* 1996; **347**: 289–92.

11 Cosgriff N, Moore EE, Sauaia A *et al.* Predicting life-threatening coagulopathy in the massively transfused trauma patient: hypothermia and acidosis revisited. *J Trauma* 1997; **42**: 857–61.

12 Winkler M, Akca O, Birkenberg B *et al.* Aggressive warming reduces blood loss during hip arthroplasty. *Anesth Analg* 2000; **91**: 978–84.

13 Widman J, Hammarqvist F, Sellden E. Amino acid infusion induces thermogenesis and reduces blood loss during hip arthroplasty under spinal anesthesia. *Anesth Analg* 2002; **95**: 1757–62.

14 Ruttmann TG, James MF, Viljoen JF. Haemodilution induces a hypercoagulable state. *Br J Anaesth* 1996; **76**: 412–14.

15 Karoutsos S, Nathan N, Lahrimi A *et al.* Thromboelastogram reveals hypercoagulability after administration of gelatin solution. *Br J Anaesth* 1999; **82**: 175–7.

16 de Jonge E, Levi M, Berends F *et al.* Impaired haemostais by intravenous administration of a gelatin-based plasma expander in human subjects. *Thromb Haemost* 1998; **79**: 286–90.

17 Mardel SN, Saunders FM, Allen H *et al.* Reduced quality of clot formation with gelatin-based plasma substitutes. *Br J Anaesth* 1998; **80**: 204–7.

18 Ruttmann TG, James MFM, Aronson I. In vivo investigation into the effects of haemodilution with hydroxyethyl starch (200/0.5) and normal saline on coagulation. *Br J Anaesth* 1998; **80**: 612–16.

19 Gross JB. Estimating allowable blood loss: corrected for dilution. *Anesthesiology* 1983; **58**: 277–80.

20 Weber TP, Hartlage AG, Aken HV, Booke M. Anaesthetic strategies to reduce perioperative blood loss in paediatric surgery. *Eur J Anaesth* 2003; **20**: 175–81.

21 Korosue K, Heros RC, Oglivy CS *et al*. Comparison of crystalloids and colloids for hemodilution in a model of focal cerebral ischemia. *J Neurosurg* 1990; **73**: 576–84.

22 Davies MJ. The role of colloids in blood conservation. *Int Anesthesiol Clin* 1990; **28**: 205–9.

23 Stump DC, Strauss RG, Henricksen RA *et al*. Effects of hydroxy-ethyl starch on blood coagulation, particularly factor VIII. *Transfusion* 1985; **25**: 349–54.

24 Strauss RG, Stansfield C, Henriksen RA, Villhauer PJ. Pentastarch may cause fewer effects on coagulation than hetastarch. *Transfusion* 1988; **25**: 257–60.

25 Renck H, Ljungstrom KG, Resberg B *et al*. Prevention of dextran-induced anaphylactic reactions by hapten inhibition. *Acta Chir Scand* 1983; **149**: 349–53.

26 Glick G, Plauth WH, Braunwald E. Role of the autonomic nervous system in the circulatory response to acutely induced anemia in unanesthetized dogs. *J Clin Invest* 1964; **43**: 2112–24.

27 Van Woerkins J, Trouborst A, Duncker DJ. Catecholamines and regional hemodynamics during isovolemic hemodilution alone and in combination with adenosine-induced controlled hypotension. *J Appl Phys* 1992; **72**: 760–9.

28 Guyton AC, Richardson TQ. Effect of hematocrit on venous return. *Circ Res* 1961; **9**: 157–65.

29 Crystal GJ, Rooney MW, Salem MR. Regional hemodynamics and oxygen supply during isovolemic hemodilution alone and in combination with adenosine-induced controlled hypotension. *Anesth Analg* 1988; **67**: 211–18.

30 Laks H, Pilon RN, Klovekorn WP *et al*. Acute normovolemic hemodilution: effects on hemodynamics, oxygen, transport, and lung water in anesthetized man. *Surg Forum* 1974; **180**: 103–9.

31 Bowens C, Spahn DR, Frasco PE *et al*. Hemodilution induces stable changes in global cardiovascular and regional myocardial function. *Anesth Analg* 1993; **76**: 1027–32.

32 Tarnow J, Eberlein HJ, Hess E *et al*. Hemodynamic interactions of hemodilution anaesthesia, propranolol pretreatment and hypovolemia – I: systemic circulation. *Basic Res Cardiol* 1979; **74**: 109–22.

33 Robertie PG, Gravlee GP. Safe limits of isovolemic hemodilution and recommendation for erythrocyte transfusion. *Int Anesthesiol Clin* 1990; **28**: 197–203.

34 Fontana JL, Welborn L, Mongan PD *et al*. Oxygen consumption and cardiovascular function in children during profound intraoperative normovolemic hemodilution. *Anesth Analg* 1995; **80**: 219–25.

35 Van der Linden P, De Hert S, Mathieu N *et al*. Tolerance to acute hemodilution: effect of anesthetic depth. *Anesthesiology* 2003; **99**: 97–104.

36 Gillies IDS. Anemia and anaesthesia. *Br J Anaesth* 1974; **46**: 589–602.

37 Sunder-Plassman L, Kessler M, Jesch F. Acute normovolemic hemodilution: changes in tissue oxygen supply and hemoglobin-oxygen affinity. *Bibl Haematol* 1975; **41**: 44–53.

38 Holtz J, Bassenge E, von Restoriff W *et al*. Transmural differences in myocardial blood flow and in coronary dilatory capacity in hemodiluted conscious dogs. *Basic Res Cardiol* 1976; **71**: 36–46.

39 Jan KM, Chien S. Effect of hematocrit variations on coronary hemodynamics and oxygen utilization. *Am J Physiol* 1977; **233**: H106–H113.

40 Messmer K. Hemodilution. *Surg Clin North Am* 1975; **55**: 659–78.

41 Buckberg G, Brazier J. Coronary blood flow and cardiac function during hemodilution. *Bibl Haematol* 1975; **41**: 173–5.

42 Crystal GJ. Coronary hemodynamic responses during acute hemodilution in canine hearts. *Am J Physiol* 1988; **254**: H525–H531.

43 Geha AS, Baue AE. Graded coronary stenosis and coronary flow during acute normovolemic anemia. *World J Surg* 1978; **2**: 645.

44 Spahn DR, Smith LR, McRae RL, Leone BJ. Effects of acute isovolemic hemodilution and anesthesia on regional function in left ventricular myocardium with compromised coronary blood flow. *Acta Anaesthesiol Scand* 1992; **36**: 628–36.

45 Kim YD, Katz NM, Ng L *et al.* Effects of hypothermia and hemodilution on oxygen metabolism and hemodynamics in patients recovering from coronary artery bypass operations. *J Thorac Cardiovasc Surg* 1989; **97**: 36–42.

46 Weisel RD, Charlesworth DC, Mickleborough LL *et al.* Limitations of blood conservation. *J Thorac Cardiovasc Surg* 1984; **88**: 26–38.

47 Todd MM, Weeks JB, Warner DS. Cerebral blood flow, blood volume and brain tissue hematocrit during isovolemic hemodilution with hetastarch in rats. *Am J Physiol* 1992; **263**: H75–H82.

48 Pohl U, Busse R. Hypoxia stimulates release of endothelial-derived relaxant factor. *Am J Physiol* 1989; **256**: H1595–H1600.

49 Fan FC, Chen RY, Schuessler GB *et al.* Effects of hematocrit variations on regional hemodynamics and oxygen transport in the dog. *Am J Physiol* 1980; **238**: H545–H552.

50 Kessler M, Messmer K. Tissue oxygenation during hemodilution. *Bibl Haematol* 1975; **41**: 16–33.

51 Biernat S, Kulig A, Lepert R *et al.* Pathomorphologic and histochemical changes in the liver during hemodilution. *Am J Surg* 1974; **128**: 24–30.

52 Utley JR, Wachtel C, Cain RB *et al.* Effects of hypothermia, hemodilution and pump oxygenation on organ water content, blood flow, oxygen delivery and renal function. *Ann Thorac Surg* 1981; **31**: 121–33.

53 Rand PW, Lacombe E. Viscosity of normal human blood under normothermic and hypothermic conditions. *J Appl Phys* 1964; **19**: 117–22.

54 Olsfanger D, Jedeikin R, Metser H *et al.* Acute normovolemic hemodilution and idiopathic scoliosis surgery: effects on homologous blood requirements. *Anesth Intens Care* 1993; **21**: 429–31.

55 Haberken M, Dangel P. Normovolemic hemodilution and intraoperative autotransfusion in children: experience with 30 cases of spinal fusion. *Eur J Pediatr Surg* 1991; **1**: 30–55.

56 Stein JI, Gombotz H, Rigoler B *et al.* Open heart surgery in children of Jehovah's Witnesses: extreme hemodilution on cardiopulmonary bypass. *Pediatr Cardiol* 1991; **12**: 170–4.

57 Spence RK, Carson JA, Poses RM *et al.* Elective surgery without transfusion: influence of preoperative hemoglobin level and blood loss on mortality. *Am J Surg* 1990; **159**: 320–4.

58 Carson JA, Spence RK, Poses RM *et al.* Severity of anemia and operative mortality and morbidity. *Lancet* 1988; **157**: 727–9.

59 Monk TG, Goodnough LT, Brecher ME *et al.* A prospective randomized comparison of three blood conservation strategies for radical prostatectomy. *Anesthesiology* 1999; **91**: 24–33.

60 Fantus B. Blood preservation. *JAMA* 1937; **109**: 128–31.

61 Stehling L. Autologous transfusion. *Int Anesthesiol Clin* 1990; **28**: 190–6.

62 Mann M, Sacks HJ, Goldfinger D. Safety of autologous blood donation prior to elective surgery for a variety of potentially "high-risk" patients. *Transfusion* 1983; **23**: 229–32.

63 Scott WJ, Rede R, Castleman B. Efficacy, complications and cost of a comprehensive blood conservation program for cardiac operations. *J Thorac Cardiovasc Surg* 1992; **103**: 1001–7.

64 Owings DV, Kruskall MS, Therier RL *et al*. Autologous blood donations prior to elective cardiac surgery: safety and effect on subsequent blood use. *JAMA* 1989; **262**: 1963–8.

65 DePelma L, Luban NLC. Autologous blood transfusion in pediatrics. *Pediatrics* 1990; **85**: 125–8.

66 Klimber IW. Autotransfusion and blood conservation in oncologic surgery. *Semin Surg Oncol* 1989; **5**: 286–92.

67 Tate DE, Friedmen RJ. Blood conservation in spinal surgery: review of current techniques. *Spine* 1992; **17**: 1450–6.

68 Silvergleid DJ. Safety and effectiveness of predeposit autologous transfusion in preteen and adolescent children. *JAMA* 1987; **257**: 3403–4.

69 Popovsky MA, Whitaker B, Arnold NL. Severe outcomes of allogeneic and autologous blood donation: frequency and characterization. *Transfusion* 1995; **35**: 734–7.

70 Haugen R, Hill G. A large-scale autologous blood program in a community hospital. *JAMA* 1987; **257**: 1211–14.

71 Goldfinger D, Capen S, Czer L *et al*. Safety and efficacy of preoperative donation of blood for autologous use by patients with end-stage heart or lung disease who are awaiting organ transplantation. *Transfusion* 1993; **33**: 336–40.

72 Goodnough LT, Marcus RE. Effect of autologous blood donation in patients undergoing elective spine surgery. *Spine* 1992; **17**: 172–5.

73 McVay PA, Hoag RW, Hoag MS *et al*. Safety and use of autologous blood donation during the third trimester of pregnancy. *Am J Obstet Gynecol* 1989; **160**: 1479–88.

74 Davis R. Banked autologous blood for caesarean section. *Anaesth Intens Care* 1979; **7**: 358–61.

75 Goodnough L, Wasmen J. Limitations to donating adequate autologous blood prior to elective surgery. *Arch Surg* 1989; **124**: 494–6.

76 Goodnough L, Rudnick S, Price TH *et al*. Increased preoperative collection of autologous blood with recombinant human erythropoietin therapy. *N Engl J Med* 1989; **321**: 1163–8.

77 Goh M, Kleer CG, Kielczewski P *et al*. Autologous blood donation prior to anatomical radical retropubic prostatectomy: is it necessary? *Urology* 1997; **49**: 569–73.

78 AuBuchon JP. Autologous transfusion and directed donations: current controversies and future directions. *Transfus Med Rev* 1989; **3**: 290–306.

79 Duncan J. On reinfusion of blood in primary and other amputations. *Br Med J* 1886; **1**: 192–7.

80 Rubens FD, Boodhwani M, Lavalee G *et al*. Perioperative red blood cell salvage. *Can J Anaesth* 2003; **50**: S31–S40.

81 Gardner A, Gibbs M, Evans C *et al*. Relative cost of autologous red cell salvage versus allogeneic red cell transfusion during abdominal aortic aneurysm repair. *Anaesth Intens Care* 2000; **28**: 646–9.

82 Solomon MD, Rutledge ML, Kane LE *et al.* Cost comparison of intraoperative autologous versus homologous transfusion. *Transfusion* 1988; **28**: 379.

83 Dale RF, Kipling RM, Smith MF *et al.* Separation of malignant cells during auto-transfusion. *Br J Surg* 1988; **75**: 581.

84 Robicseck F, Duncan GD, Born GVR *et al.* Inherent dangers of simultaneous application of microfibrillar collagen hemostat and blood saving devices. *J Thorac Cardiovasc Surg* 1986; **92**: 766–8.

85 Murray DJ, Gress K, Weinstein SL. Coagulopathy after reinfusion of autologous scavenged red blood cells. *Anesth Analg* 1992; **75**; 125–9.

86 Wheeler TJ, Tobias JD. Complications of autotransfusion with salvaged blood. *J Post Anesth Nurs* 1994; **9**: 150–2.

87 Bull MH, Bull BS, Van Arsdell GS, Smith LL. Clinical implications of procoagulant and leukoattractant formation during intraoperative blood salvage. *Arch Surg* 1988; **123**: 1073–6.

88 O'Riordan WD. Autotransfusion in the emergency department of a community hospital. *JACEP* 1977; **6**: 233–7.

89 Linden JV, Kaplan HS, Murphy MT. Fatal air embolism due to perioperative blood recovery. *Anesth Analg* 1997; **84**: 422–6.

90 Symbas PN. Extraoperative autotransfusion from hemothorax. *Surgery* 1978; **84**: 722–7.

91 Litwin MS, Relihan M, Olsen RE. Pulmonary microemboli associated with massive transfusion. *Ann Surg* 1975; **181**: 51–7.

92 Mattox KL. Autotransfusion in the emergency department. *JACEP* 1975; **4**: 218–22.

93 Horst HM, Dlugos S, Fath JJ *et al.* Coagulopathy and intraoperative blood salvage. *J Trauma* 1992; **32**: 646–53.

94 Halpern NA, Alicea M, Seabrook B *et al.* Cell saver autologous transfusion: metabolic consequences of washing blood with normal saline. *J Trauma* 1996; **41**: 407–15.

95 Halpern NA, Alicea M, Seabrook B *et al.* Isolyte S, a physiologic multielectrolyte solution, is preferable to normal saline to wash cell saver salvaged blood: conclusions from a prospective, randomized study in a canine model. *Crit Care Med* 1997; **25**: 2031–8.

96 Richardson DW, Robinson HG. Desmopressin. *Ann Intern Med* 1985; **103**: 228.

97 Mannucci PM. Desmopressin: a non-transfusional form of treatment for congenital and acquired bleeding disorders. *Blood* 1988; **72**: 1449–55.

98 Horrow JC. Desmopressin and antifibrinolytics. *Int Anesthesiol Clin* 1990; **28**: 230–5.

99 Salva KM, Kim HC, Nahum K *et al.* DDAVP in the treatment of bleeding disorders. *Pharmacotherapy* 1988; **8**: 94–9.

100 Mannucci PM, Vicenti V, Alberca I *et al.* Intravenous and subcutaneous administration of desmopressin (DDAVP) to hemophiliacs: pharmacokinetics and factor VIII responses. *Thromb Haemost* 1987; **58**: 1037–9.

101 Lethagen S, Harris AS, Sjorin E, Nilsson IM. Intranasal and intravenous administration of desmopressin: effect on FVIII/vWF, pharmacokinetics and reproducibility. *Thromb Haemost* 1987; **58**: 1033–6.

102 Salzman EW, Weinstein MJ, Weintraub RM *et al.* Treatment with desmopressin acetate to reduce blood loss after cardiac surgery. *N Engl J Med* 1986; **314**: 1402–6.

103 Czer LSC, Bateman TM, Gray RJ *et al*. Treatment of severe platelet dysfunction and hemorrhage after cardiopulmonary bypass: reduction in blood product usage with desmopressin. *J Am Coll Cardiol* 1987; **9**: 1139–47.

104 Mannucci PM, Remuzzi G, Pusineri F *et al*. Desamino-8-D-arginine vasopressin shortens the bleeding time in uremia. *N Engl J Med* 1983; **308**: 8–12.

105 Mannucci PM, Vicente V, Vianello L *et al*. Controlled trial of a desmopressin in liver cirrhosis and other conditions associated with a prolonged bleeding time. *Blood* 1986; **67**: 1148–53.

106 Kobrinsky NL, Letts RM, Patel LR *et al*. 1-Desamino-8-D-arginine vasopressin (desmopressin) decreases operative blood loss in patients having Harrington rod spinal fusion surgery. *Ann Intern Med* 1987; **107**: 446–50.

107 Theroux MC, Corddry DH, Tietz AE *et al*. A study of desmopressin and blood loss during spinal fusion for neuromuscular scoliosis: a randomized, controlled, double-blinded study. *Anesthesiology* 1997; **87**: 260–7.

108 Alanay A, Acaroglu E, Oxdemir O *et al*. Effects of deamino-8-D-arginine vasopressin on blood loss and coagulation factors in scoliosis surgery. *Spine* 1999; **9**: 877–82.

109 Seear MD, Wadsworth LD, Rogers PC. The effect of desmopressin acetate (DDAVP) on postoperative blood loss after cardiac operations in children. *J Thorac Cardiovasc Surg* 1989; **98**: 217–19.

110 Laupacis A, Fergusson D. Drugs to minimize perioperative blood loss in cardiac surgery: meta-analysis using perioperative blood transfusion as the outcome. The international study of perioperative transfusion (ISPOT) investigators. *Anesth Analg* 1997; **85**: 1258–67.

111 Levi M, Cromheecke ME, de Jonge E *et al*. Pharmacological strategies to decrease excessive blood loss in cardiac surgery: a meta-analysis of clinically relevant end-points. *Lancet* 1999; **354**: 1940–7.

112 Florentino-Pineda I, Blakemore LC, Thompson GH *et al*. The effect of epsilon-aminocaproic acid on perioperative blood loss in patients with idiopathic scoliosis undergoing posterior spinal fusion. *Spine* 2001; **26**: 1147–51.

113 Neilipovitz DT, Murto K, Hall L *et al*. A randomized trial of tranexamic acid to reduce blood transfusion for scoliosis surgery. *Anesth Analg* 2001; **93**: 82–7.

114 Hippala S, Strid L, Wennerstrand MI *et al*. Tranexamic acid reduces perioperative blood loss associated with total knee arthroplasty. *Br J Anaesth* 1995; **74**: 534–7.

115 Hippala S, Strid LJ, Wennerstrand MI *et al*. Tranexamic acid radically decreases blood loss and transfusions associated with total knee arthroplasty. *Anesth Analg* 1997; **84**: 839–44.

116 Benoni G, Fredin H. Fibrinolytic inhibition with tranexamic acid reduces blood loss and blood transfusion after knee arthroplasty: a prospective, randomized double blind study of 86 patients. *J Bone Joint Surg Br* 1996; **78**: 434–40.

117 Boylan JF, Klinck JR, Sandler AN *et al*. Tranexamic acid reduces blood loss, transfusion requirements and coagulation factor use in primary orthotopic liver transplantation. *Anesthesiology* 1996; **85**: 1043–8.

118 Sack E, Spaet TH, Gentile R *et al*. Reduction of prostatectomy bleeding by epsilon-aminocaproic acid. *N Engl J Med* 1962; **266**: 541–64.

119 DelRossi AJ, Cernaianu AC, Botros S *et al*. Prophylactic treatment of postperfusion bleeding using EACA. *Chest* 1989; **96**: 27–30.

120 Horrow JC, Hlavecek J, Strong MD *et al*. Prophylactic tranexamic acid decreases bleeding after cardiac operations. *J Thorac Cardiovasc Surg* 1990; **99**: 70–4.

121 Ovrum E, Holen EA, Abdelnoor M *et al*. Tranexamic acid is not necessary to reduce blood loss after coronary artery bypass operations. *J Thorac Cardiovasc Surg* 1993; **105**: 78–83.

122 Amar D, Grant FM, Zhang H *et al*. Antifibrinolytic therapy and perioperative blood loss in cancer patients undergoing major orthopedic surgery. *Anesthesiology* 2003; **98**: 337–42.

123 Wells PS. Safety and efficacy of methods for reducing perioperative allogeneic transfusion: a critical review. *Am J Therap* 2002; **9**: 377–88.

124 Royston D, Taylor KM, Sapsford RN, Bidstup BP. Effect of aprotinin on need for blood transfusion after repeat open-heart surgery. *Lancet* 1987; **2**: 1289–91.

125 Urban MK, Beckman J, Gordon M *et al*. The efficacy of antifibrinolytics in the reduction of blood loss during complex adult reconstructive spine surgery. *Spine* 2001; **26**: 1152–7.

126 Capdevila X, Calvet Y, Biboulet P *et al*. Aprotinin decreases blood loss and homologous transfusions in patients undergoing major orthopedic surgery. *Anesthesiology* 1998; **88**: 50–7.

127 Janssens M, Joris J, David JL *et al*. High-dose aprotinin reduces blood loss in patients undergoing total hip replacement surgery. *Anesthesiology* 1994; **80**: 23–9.

128 Bidstrup BP, Harrison J. Royston D *et al*. Aprotinin therapy in cardiac operations: a report on use in 41 cardiac centers in the United Kingdom. *Ann Thorac Surg* 1993; **55**: 971–6.

129 Kalicinski P, Kaminski A, Drewniak T *et al*. Quick correction of hemostasis in two patients with fulminant liver failure undergoing liver transplantation by recombinant activated factor VII. *Transplant Proc* 1999; **31**: 378–9.

130 Tobias JD, Berkenbosch JW. Synthetic factor VIIa concentrate to treat coagulopathy and gastrointestinal bleeding in an infant with end-stage liver disease. *Clin Pediatr* 2002; **41**: 613–16.

131 Tobias JD, Groeper K, Berkenbosch JW. Preliminary experience with the use of recombinant factor VIIa to treat coagulation disturbances in pediatric patients. *South Med J* 2003; **96**: 12–16.

132 Martinowitz U, Kenet G, Segal E *et al*. Recombinant factor VII for adjunctive hemorrhage control in trauma. *J Trauma* 2001; **51**: 431–9.

133 Hendriks HGD, Meijer K, de Wolf JT *et al*. Reduced transfusion requirements by recombinant factor VIIa in orthotopic liver transplantation. *Transplantation* 2001; **71**: 402–5.

134 Murkin JM. A novel hemostatic agent: the potential role of recombinant activated factor VII in anesthetic practice. *Can J Anaesth* 2002; **49**: S21–S26.

135 Tobias JD. Synthetic factor VIIa to treat dilutional coagulopathy during posterior spinal fusion in two children. *Anesthesiology* 2002; **96**: 1522–5.

136 Friederich PW, Henny CP, Messelink EJ *et al*. Effect of recombinant activated factor VII on perioperative blood loss in patients undergoing retropubic prostatectomy: a double-blind place-controlled randomized trial. *Lancet* 2002; **36**: 201–5.

137 Roberts HR. Recombinant factor VIIa (NovoSeven) and the safety of treatment. *Semin Hematol* 2001; **38**: 48–50.

138 Roberts HR. Clinical experience with activated factor VII: focus on safety aspects. *Blood Coag Fibrin* 1998; **9**: S115–S118.

139 Gallisti S, Cvrin G, Muntean W. Recombinant factor VIIa does not induce hypercoagulability in vitro. *Thromb Haemost* 1999; **81**: 245–9.

140 Meneghini L, Zadra N, Anloni V *et al.* Erythropoietin therapy and acute preoperative normovolemic haemodilution in infants undergoing craniosynostosis surgery. *Paediatr Anaesth* 2003; **13**: 392–6.

141 Eckenhoff JE, Rich JC. Clinical experiences with deliberate hypotension. *Anesth Analg* 1966; **45**: 21–8.

142 Sollevi A. Hypotensive anesthesia and blood loss. *Acta Anaesth Scand* 1988; **89**(Suppl.): 39–43.

143 Sperry RJ, Monk CR, Durieux ME *et al.* The influence of hemorrhage on organ perfusion during deliberate hypotension in rats. *Anesthesiology* 1992; **77**: 1171–7.

144 Seyde WC, Longnecker DE. Cerebral oxygen tension in rats during deliberate hypotension with sodium nitroprusside, 2-chloroadenosine or deep isoflurane anesthesia. *Anesthesiology* 1986; **64**: 480–5.

145 Ringaert KRA, Mutch WAC, Malo LA. Regional cerebral blood flow and response to carbon dioxide during controlled hypotension with isoflurane anesthesia in the rat. *Anesth Analg* 1988; **67**: 383–8.

146 Fukusaki M, Hara MT, Maekawa T *et al.* Effects of controlled hypotension with sevoflurane anaesthesia on hepatic function of surgical patients. *Eur J Anaesthesiol* 1999; **16**: 111–16.

147 Sivarajan M, Amory DW, Everett GB *et al.* Blood pressure, not cardiac output, determines blood loss during induced hypotension. *Anesth Analg* 1980; **59**: 203–6.

148 Hines R, Barash P. Infusion of sodium nitroprusside induces platelet dysfunction in vitro. *Anesthesiology* 1989; **70**: 611–15.

149 Bernard JM, Passuti N, Pinaud M. Long-term hypotensive technique with nicardipine and nitroprusside during isoflurane anesthesia for spinal surgery. *Anesth Analg* 1992; **72**: 179–85.

150 Bernard JM, Pinaud M, Francois T *et al.* Deliberate hypotension with nicardipine or nitroprusside during total hip arthroplasty. *Anesth Analg* 1991; **73**: 341–5.

151 Hersey SL, O'Dell NE, Lowe S *et al.* Nicardipine versus nitroprusside for controlled hypotension during spinal surgery in adolescents. *Anesth Analg* 1997; **84**: 1239–44.

CHAPTER 5

Current View of the Coagulation System

Yoogoo Kang, Paul Audu

The coagulation system serves several vital functions to provide normal physiology. It maintains fluidity of blood stream to deliver oxygen and nutrients to tissues, repairs interruption in vascular integrity, and participates in inflammatory process to control or limit the harmful effects of injury or pathologic process. In surgical clinical settings, major emphasis has been placed on clot formation to avoid excessive blood loss, and control of excessive clot formation to avoid thrombosis. In this chapter, basic principles and clinical aspects of coagulation, monitoring and management are described.

Normal hemostasis

In order for blood to freely course through the vasculature, it must stay in the liquid state. Yet, it must also maintain its ability to transform into gelatinous glue to seal any breaches in the vascular integrity to prevent exsanguinations. If this property were compromised, even minor injuries or surgical procedures would be life-threatening. An intricately balanced system therefore exists to ensure attainment of these two seemingly mutually exclusive end points.

Hemostasis refers to the process by which liquid blood is transformed first into a solid state, followed by a liquid state, and is divided into five distinctive, interactive phases:

1 *vascular phase*, in which intense vasoconstriction reduces blood flow to the injured site to minimize bleeding;
2 *platelet phase*, or primary hemostasis, in which platelets amass at the site of injury and form a mechanical seal or 'platelet plug';
3 *fibrin formation phase*, or secondary hemostasis, in which a dense interwoven meshwork of fibrin invests and reinforces the plug;
4 *insoluble fibrin formation*, which follows the soluble fibrin network formation; and
5 *fibrinolysis*, which involves clot resorbtion and recanalization.

These equally important five steps take place contemporaneously and interdependently in a concert of vascular endothelium, platelets and coagulation proteins.

Vascular phase

Trauma results in intense vasoconstriction of the injured vessel within a few seconds. The response is primarily myogenic but may be enhanced by neural elements and humoral mediators, such as thromboxane A_2, serotonin and norepinephrine produced by activated platelets. Vasoconstriction may last up to 30 min. In addition, intratissue bleeding and tissue edema increase extravascular pressure to minimize extravasation.

The next important vascular phase involves vascular endothelial cells to initiate clot formation. Endothelial cells line blood vessels and play an important role in maintaining perfusion, permeability and blood fluidity. Endothelial cells are nonthrombogenic: their surface is negatively charged to repel negatively charged platelets. They produce an inhibitor of platelet aggregation (prostaglandin I_2), thrombomodulin and heparan sulfate, which activates antithrombin III (AT-III) [1–3]. Thrombomodulin binds to thrombin to interfere with further progression of coagulation, activates protein C to inactivate factors Va and VIIIa, and releases plasminogen activator. Further, stimuli including thrombin, epinephrine and trauma stimulate synthesis of PGI_2 in the endothelial cells to inhibit platelet aggregation as a negative feedback mechanism [4]. Endothelial cells are metabolically active: they produce collagen, fibronectin, proteoglycans and von Willebrand factor (vWF), and release vWF, plasminogen activator and prostanoids. Endothelium is a barrier between the blood and vessel wall, and its permeability is maintained by the junctional adaptations. Large molecules pass across the endothelium into vessel wall through patent intercellular junctions, endocytosis and via transendothelial pores. Its fenestration is affected by serotonin and norepinephrine released by platelets.

Therefore, impaired endothelial function results in a variety of hemostatic defects. For example, insufficient quantity of protein C interferes with the feedback inhibition of coagulation mediated by the thrombin–thrombomodulin complex, resulting in systemic thrombosis [5]. Thrombotic condition also develops when the release of tissue plasminogen activator is insufficient [6]. On the other hand, an increase in endothelial fenestration leads to petechiae or idiopathic thrombocytopenic purpura (ITP) [7].

Platelet phase

Platelets are disc-shaped anucleated cellular elements, measuring 2–3 μm in diameter. Platelets have several cell surface receptors that allow interaction with, and adhesion to, diverse elements of the subendothelial matrix, and their cytoplasm is rich in mitrochondria and various granules. Their production from bone marrow megakaryocytes is regulated by thrombopoietin [8], and the average adult has 150–400 billion platelets per liter of blood. Platelets have a life span of 7–10 days, and aging cells are removed from circulation by the reticuloendothelial system. Platelets are the cornerstone of hemostasis and participate in multiple phases of coagulation [9]. They adhere to the injured vessel wall and entice other platelets, leukocytes and erythrocytes into the enlarging platelet aggregate. This primary hemostasis begins within a few seconds following injury, and platelets provide phospolipid surface on which various enzyme complexes are assembled. Additionally, platelets release growth factors that assist in wound healing and tissue repair.

Platelets normally circulate in a quiescent, 'nonsticky' state. They do not adhere to the negatively charged vascular endothelium and do not stick to one another, since these aggregates would be rapidly eliminated by the reticuloendothelial system. Vascular injury, however, removes the endothelial barrier and allows platelets to come in direct contact with highly thrombogenic subendothelium to cause adhesion (Figure 5.1). In venous blood, the adhesion is achieved by the attachment of platelet glycoprotein (GP) Ia/IIa receptors to subendothelial collagen matrix. In arterial circulation, however, the interaction between a constitutively active adhesive protein complex (GP Ib/V/IX) present on the platelet surface, and vWF of the subendothelial matrix slows down platelets before adhesion.

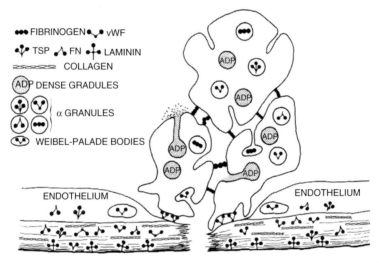

Figure 5.1. Interactions between platelets and subendothelium. Anchoring and linking platelets after vessel injury by adhesive molecule present in platelet α-granules, endothelial cells, and subendothelial extracellular matrix. vWF is shown to form multiple bonds between the platelet membrane and the subendothelium. Other components of subendothelium (collagen, thrombospondin [TSP], fibronectin [FN], and laminin) are depicted, but their role in interactions of platelets in vivo is speculative. Fibrinogen, discharged from α-granule via the surface-connecting canaliculi system, together with plasma fibrinogen provides interplatelet linkages that can also be made by vWF when fibrinogen is deficient (afibrinogenemia). ADP secreted from dense granules promotes binding of fibrinogen to platelet membrane receptors involved in interplatelet linkages. With permission from Hawiger J. Adhesive interactions of blood cells and the vessel wall. In: Colman RW, Hirsh J, Marder VJ, Salzman EW, eds. *Hemostasis and Thrombosis*. Philadelphia: Lippincott, 1987: p201.

Adhesion is a fairly slow process, and platelet plug formation is greatly amplified by platelet activation. Platelet activation is induced by binding of ligands (i.e. vWF and collagen) to platelet surface receptors, platelet adhesion per se, and agonists released during platelet degranulation (e.g. ADP, 5-HT, epinephrine, thromboxane A_2) or produced by the coagulation cascade. Platelets undergo morphological as well as functional changes on activation. Activated platelets extend cytoplasmic processes from their cell bodies and loose their surface undulation and appear smooth. They spread, flatten and increase their surface area by as much as 400% to cover an endothelial defect and also to assemble procoagulant 'factories'. During the activation process, phosphotidyl serine from the inner cell membrane migrates to outer layer to increase the amount of negatively charged phospholipid from virtually 0% to 12% [10]. Simultaneously, the binding of ligands to cell membrane receptors signals platelets to express and activate GP IIb/IIIa receptors, thus converting them from low to high affinity receptors. This process is referred to as inside-out signaling and enhances the ability of platelets to aggregate via fibrinogen bridges [11].

As platelet adhesion to the subendothelium progresses, platelets spread out on its surface and recruit additional platelets to form a mass of aggregated platelets. Platelet aggregation is an important step in hemostasis. A resting platelet has 40 000–80 000 GPIIb/IIIa receptors with a low affinity for fibrino-gen. Platelet activation not only increases the number of these receptors but also causes a conformational change, resulting in an increased affinity for fibrinogen. During this process, platelets loose a marginal band of microtu-bules to change their shape from discs to spiny spheres [12], centralize storage granules, form pseudopodia [13] and phosphorylate intracellular proteins [14]. Aggregated platelets undergo activation by forming receptor–agonist complex between surface receptors of platelets and their agonists, such as thrombin, adenosine diphosphate (ADP), epinephrine, collagen and arachi-donic acid [15].

Extracellular agonists stimulate secretory function of platelets by increasing cytoplasmic calcium level via multiple pathways. Activation of phospholipase A_2 releases free arachidonic acid to form the potent platelet aggregator, thromboxane A_2, and this in turn transports calcium from intracellular stores to cytoplasm [16,17]. Phospholipase A_2, in addition, promotes synthesis of PGD_2, an inhibitor of platelet activation, to modulate platelet actvities. ADP and platelet-activating factor (PAF), and activation of phospholipase C and protein kinase C also raise cytoplasmic calcium concentration to potentiate platelet aggregation [18].

Activation of platelets results in the release of intracellular granules, exposure of platelet receptors for plasma proteins and structural change in platelet surface membrane. Several types of granules containing a variety of chemicals are present in platelets. Dense bodies contain serotonin, adenosine triphosphate (ATP), ADP, pyrophosphate and calcium. Alpha-granules store adhesive proteins, such as fibrinogen, vWF, factor V, high–molecular weight kininogen (HMWK), fibronectin, α_1-antitrypsin, β-thromboglobulin, platelet factor 4 and platelet-derived growth factor. Lysosomes include acid hydrolases that are released during the inflammatory process [12].

Receptors for specific plasma proteins are found in the platelet membrane. Receptors for fibrinogen (GP IIb-IIIa complex) are essential in platelet aggregation and are activated by any agonists inducing platelet aggregation [19]. Therefore, lack of glycoproteins seen in patients with Glanzmann's thrombasthenia leads to significant bleeding [20]. A glycoprotein receptor for vWF (Ib) is known to be present, and interaction between glycoprotein receptors and fibronectin and thrombospondin also participate in platelet aggregation [21]. Additionally, platelets develop receptors for specific plasma coagulation factors during the course of activation. Activated factor V (Va) secreted by the platelet or circulating in the plasma serves as a binding site for factor Xa.

Cyclic 3',5'-adenosine monophosphate (cyclic AMP) is one of the most important regulatory substances that modulates activation of platelets [22]. Cyclic AMP, with the support of PGD_2 in platelets, reduces cytoplasmic free calcium to regulate platelet activation by stimulating a calcium/magnesium ATPase-dependent pump [23]. Other regulatory substances include an ADP-destroying ectoenzyme (ADPase) on the endothelial cell surface and thrombomodulin, a thrombin inhibitor.

Understanding of the platelet activation and its regulation process led to the development of new classes of antiplatelet drugs: GPIIb/IIIa receptor antagonists (abciximab and eptifibatide) and ADP receptor antagonists (clopidogrel and ticlopidine).

Coagulation phase

Clotting factors involved in the coagulation cascade are listed in Table 5.1. The liver synthesizes most coagulation protein factors, and the majority of

Table 5.1 Clotting factors.

Factor	Name
I	Fibrinogen
II	Prothrombin
III	Tissue thromboplastin (or tissue factor)
IV	Calcium
V	Proaccelerin
VII	Proconnectin
VIII	Antihemophilic factor
IX	Christmas factor
X	Stuart Prower factor
XI	Plasma thromboplastin antecedent
XII	Hageman factor
XIII	Fibrin stabilizing factor

serine proteases. Factor VIII is produced partially in the liver and partially by megakaryocytes and endothelial cells. Factors II, VII, IX and X are vitamin K-dependent factors and contain γ-glutamyl carboxyl acid (GIa) residues at the N-terminal end of the molecule [24], which require vitamin K for their synthesis by hepatocytes. The carboxyl groups of the GIa residue bind to calcium to serve as a bridge for protein binding to the phospholipid surface. Factors VII, IX and X are structurally similar with two epidermal growth factor–like domains. Prothrombin, instead, has a kringle domain (so named because it resembles a Scandinavian pastry). Coumadin, a vitamin K antagonist, inhibits factor activation and, consequently, coagulation. Factors V and VIII are not proteases but large molecular weight cofactors for the proteases. They have a structural similarity to ceruloplasmin and are referred to as labile factors owing to their short half-life. They are present in plasma in inactive forms and need to be activated by minor proteolytic cleavage.

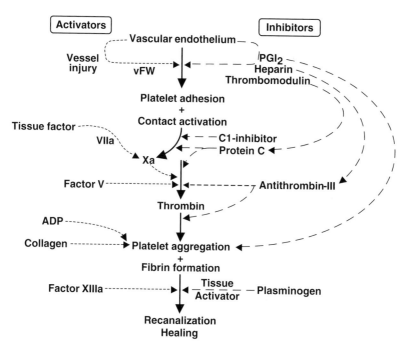

Figure 5.2. Overview of hemostasis. The process of hemostasis is illustrated by the series of cellular and coagulation factor events shown by the solid vertical arrows in the center. Activators and other procoagulants influence hemostasis as noted by the dotted arrows at left. Inhibitors of hemostasis and processes acting to degrade coagulant proteins or inhibit platelet aggregation are shown as dashed arrows at right. With permission from Colman RW, Marder VJ, Salzman EW, Hirsh J. Overview of hemostasis. In: Colman RW, Hirsh J, Marder VJ, Salzman EW, eds. *Hemostasis and Thrombosis.* Philadelphia: Lippincott, 1987: p4.

For the surface activation or intrinsic system, factor XII (Hageman factor) binds to negatively charged surfaces such as kaolin, dextran sulfate and sulfatides, and binding to these surfaces activates factor XII to XIIa by exposing its catalytic site [25,26]. Two of the major substrates of factor XIIa are prekallikrein and factor XI, both of which exist in a noncovalent molecular complex with HMWK [27]. Factor XIa activates factor IX in the presence of calcium (Figure 5.2). Factor IX is one of the vitamin K-dependent proteins, and is synthesized as prozymogens and converted to serine proteases by a limited number of proteolytic cleavages. Factor IXa, in turn, activates factor X in the presence of calcium, phospholipids and a large protein cofactor, factor VIII. Factor VIII is found in the form of a noncovalent complex with vWF [28], and accelerates the conversion of factor X to Xa by factor IXa. The absence of factors VIII and IX results in hemophilia A and hemophilia B respectively.

In addition to the intrinsic system developed within the vascular system, the extrinsic system also converts factor X to Xa with tissue factor (thromboplastin) being a cofactor. Tissue thromboplastin is a lipoprotein with a single polypeptide chain bound noncovalently to phospholipid [29]. Its cofactor activity is similar to HMWK in the contact phase, to factor VIII in the intrinsic system and to factor V in the final common pathway. Factor VII is an important next protein in the extrinsic system [30]. The coagulant activity of factor VII is potentiated by factor XIIa or factor IXa and requires tissue thromboplastin, suggesting that intrinsic and extrinsic pathways interact at several levels of the cascade.

Factor Xa formed by either the extrinsic or the intrinsic pathway converts prothrombin to thrombin. Prothrombin has functional domains for calcium binding to phospholipid, interaction with factor V, and catalytic center. Factor Xa removes the N-terminal GIa portion from prothrombin, resulting in separation of the two-chain thrombin molecule from the phospholipid surface. The interaction of factor Xa, factor V, phospholipid and calcium (prothrombinase complex) leads to an explosive activation of prothrombin on the platelet membrane. Factor V in the prothrombinase complex is secreted from α-granules and serves as a receptor for factor Xa binding to the activated platelet [31]. It is worth repeating that a negatively charged surface is involved in the initial contact system, while a phospholipid or platelet membrane provides the surface in the coagulation cascade.

Fibrin formation
The fibrin formation is the next major step in coagulation. Fibrinogen, a large glycoprotein, is present in high concentration in plasma and platelet granules, and interacts with factor XIII, fibronectin, α_2-plasmin inhibitor, plasminogen and plasminogen activator [32]. The location and concentration of these proteins determine fibrin formation, cross linking or fibrin lysis. Thrombin binds to the fibrinogen and liberates fibrinopeptides A and B [33], resulting in fibrin monomer and polymer formation. The polymer chain becomes pro-

gressively longer, and the two-stranded protofibrils interact laterally to form long, thin fibrin strands or short, broad sheets of fibrin [34]. It appears that the lateral strand association increases the tensile strength of the clot [35]. Thrombin also activates factor XIII, and factor XIIIa induces crosslinking of the fibrin polymer. In crosslinking, covalent isopeptide bonds form between lysine donors and glutamine receptors [36], with two γ-chains crosslinked rapidly to form γ-γ dimers; α-chains are crosslinked more slowly, each with two other such chains, to form a polymer network [37]. The crosslinked fibrin fiber contains approximately 100 protofibrils linked and branched together in a random fashion and is plasmin-resistant.

The fibrin mesh binds the platelets together and attaches itself to the vessel wall by binding to platelet receptor glycoproteins and by interactions with thrombospondin, fibronectin and fibrinogen released from platelet granules [38]. These proteins may serve as bridges between plasma proteins and the platelet interior, between platelets and the vessel wall, and between plasma fibrin fibers and the subendothelial matrix. Platelets play another important role: glycoprotein IIb-IIIa joins plasma fibrinogen (or α-granule fibrinogen) to intracellular actin to induce clot retraction and vasoconstriction [39].

Fibrinolysis

Fibrinolysis is the process of removing unwanted clot. Fibrinogen is broken down by plasmin into fibrin degradation products (FDPs), which are then removed from circulation by the reticuloendothelial system. The production of plasmin from its inactive precursor, plasminogen, is a closely regulated process that is accomplished by one of two activators: tissue plasminogen activator (TPA) and urokinase (uPA) [40]. uPA is produced by tissue macrophages and is present only in small concentrations in plasma. Its physiological role may be in removing fibrin from tissue. TPA is present in plasma in much larger concentrations and plays a greater role in removing intravascular clot. Thrombin is a potent stimulus for release of TPA by endothelial cells [41]. TPA has a short plasma half-life (4 min) as it is rapidly inactivated by plasminogen activator inhibitor type 1 (PAI-1) and subsequently eliminated following hepatic metabolism. However, binding to fibrinogen not only protects TPA from inactivation but also increases its affinity for plasminogen. It activates plasminogen to plasmin, which then degrades the fibrin. Bound plasmin is protected from α_2-antiplasmin, while free plasmin in the plasma is quickly inactivated [42].

Regulation of hemostasis

Excessive intravascular coagulation can cause thrombosis and tissue ischemia. Inadequate clot formation, on the other hand, can also precipitate organ injury either directly from hemorrhage into tissue or indirectly as a consequence of hemorrhagic shock. Coagulation therefore needs to be closely regulated to ensure that neither extreme is attained. This balance is achieved by regulating procoagulant, anticoagulant, and prolysins and antilysins.

The propensity to form intravascular clot has been summarized into Virchow's triad of endothelial injury, hypercoagulability and blood stasis. Flow of blood discourages coagulation by diluting and washing away any activated coagulation factors. Intact endothelium also discourages clot formation by preventing blood from coming into contact with the subendothelium and produces heparin, a cofactor for antithrombin III (AT-III). Endothelial cells also produce nitric oxide and prostacyclin to inhibit platelet activation and to discourage stasis by vasodilation. Endothelial cells express a membrane protein, thrombomodulin, which binds and changes the nature of thrombin from a procoagulant to an anticoagulant protease. After binding with thrombomodulin, thrombin loses its affinity for fibrinogen but activates protein C. The activated protein C forms a complex with protein S to inhibit factors VIIIa and Va. The importance of proteins S and C as anticoagulants is exemplified by factor V Leiden abnormality. In this condition, production of genetically altered factor V resistant to inhibition by protein C leads to the most common prothrombotic condition in Caucasian.

Coagulation is regulated by the positive and negative feedback mechansim. The process of positive feedback is repeated in many stages of coagulation. For example, kallikrein cleaves factor XII to accelerate contact activation and cleaves HMWK to liberate the nonapeptide bradykinin. The activated HMWK allows more prekallikrein (and factor XI) to interact with the activating surface [27]. An example of negative feedback is found in the conversion of factor XIIa to factor XIIf by kallikrein to turn off surface-bound coagulation. Factor XIa also cleaves the light chain of HMWK to limit its cofactor activity [43].

Plasma proteolytic inhibitors also participate in controlling the extent and speed of coagulation and fibrinolysis. Cl inhibitor is the major inhibitor of the intrinsic system, which inhibits factor XIIa and kallikrein [44]. α_1-antitrypsin inhibits factor XIa [45] and neutrophil elastase, and deficiency of α_1-antitrypsin results in emphysema due to the unopposed effects of elastase in the lung.

AT-III is the major inhibitor of factors IXa, Xa and thrombin by forming inactive AT-III-serine protease complexes. The inhibition is potentiated by heparin by its binding to a lysine group in AT-III [46]. It is known that approximately 40–50% reduction in AT-III may lead to thrombotic conditions. α_2-macroglobulin is a secondary inhibitor for many plasma coagulants and fibrinolytic enzymes, including kallikrein, thrombin and plasmin. α_2-macroglobulin-enzyme complexes possess some enzymatic activity and may be utilized for inhibition of certain enzymes protected from other inhibitors.

Abnormal hemostasis

Disorders of hemostasis may be encountered in the perioperative period, and they may arise from an abnormality in any of the phases of coagulation.

Spontaneous bleeding in the absence of trauma, however, is unusual and indicative of major defect in the hemostatic apparatus. Medical bleeding is a term that refers to excessive spontaneous or traumatic hemorrhage in the presence of some aberration of hemostasis. Bleeding is usually controlled once the underlying hemostatic defect is corrected. While postoperative bleeding may be exacerbated by preexisting hemostatic defects, its primary cause is usually surgical.

Congenital hemostatic disorders
von Willebrand disease

von Willebrand disease (vWD) is the most common congenital hemostatic disorder with a prevalence of 1% and is an autosomal dominant inherited disorder resulting from a quantitative or qualitative defects in vWF [47]. Since vWF mediates platelet adhesion to the subendothelial matrix, platelet dysfunction is the common finding. Additionally, vWF is a carrier for factor VIII and prevents its rapid enzymatic degradation. Patients with vWD therefore have a variable factor VIII deficiency that contributes to bleeding diathesis [48,49]. Laboratory tests reveal a prolonged bleeding time and activated partial thromboplastin time (aPTT). Diagnosis is made by ristocetin-induced platelet agglutination and by quantitation of vWF antigen. Bleeding in patients with a mild form of disease can be controlled with desmopressin (DDAVP), which stimulates the release of endogenous vWF from endothelial cells. The drug is ineffective in subtypes of the disease producing either normal quantities of functionally abnormal vWF or no vWF at all. Treatment of the latter forms requires administration of factor VIII/vWF concentrates in the form of either cryoprecipitate (CRYO) or commercially available alternatives that have been heat-treated to destroy human immunodeficiency virus (HIV).

Hemophilia A and B

Hemophilia A is an X-linked recessive disorder resulting in deficiency of coagulation factor VIII. It occurs in 1 in 10 000 live male births. Phenotypic expression varies with the degree of factor activity. Children with severe disease (factor VIII <1%) present with cephalhematoma at birth or neonatal bleeding after circumcision. Children with the moderate form of the disease (factor VIII 1–5%) often present with bleeding episodes into soft tissues and joints following mild trauma. Patients with mild disease (factor VIII > 5%) may be seen in adolescence with hemarthrosis and arthropathies involving weight-bearing joints or with serious bleeding following major trauma or surgery [50,51]. aPTT is usually prolonged, and specific factor assays are required to distinguish it from hemophilia B. Hemophilia B occurs less frequently (1 in 100 000 live births) and is due to factor IX deficiency. Treatment of acute bleeding episodes hinges on restoration of plasma factor levels. Rarer conditions that might be encountered are found elsewhere [52].

Acquired hemostatic disorders

Acquired disorders are more frequently encountered than their hereditary counterparts.

Vitamin K deficiency

Vitamin K is a fat-soluble vitamin that acts as a cofactor for γ-carboxylation of certain glutamic acid residues in prothrombin and factors VII, IX and X. Vitamin K deficiency can arise from inadequate dietary intake or defective intestinal absorption [53]. Prolonged administration of broad-spectrum antibiotics may cause vitamin K deficiency, as vitamin K–producing gut flora are destroyed. Early in its course, vitamin K deficiency presents with a prolonged prothrombin time (PT) and a normal aPTT owing to deficiency of factor VII with the shortest half-life [54]. When other vitamin K–dependent factors become depleted, aPTT is also prolonged. Parenteral vitamin K ameliorates the condition within 12–24 h. For a more rapid correction, fresh frozen plasma (FFP) is required.

Liver disease

The etiology of coagulation disorders in patients with chronic liver disease is multifactorial, and it affects all phases of coagulation [55,56]. Thrombocytopenia may result from reduced production and splenic sequestration and destruction of platelets. Synthesis of coagulation factors is also impaired by chronic liver disease, since the liver produces all coagulation factors except VIII and vWF. Liver disease may also impair the absorption and storage of vitamin K, resulting in vitamin K deficiency. The diseased reticuloendothelial component of the liver impairs the clearance of activated coagulation factors resulting in the hypercoagulable state and possibly consumptive coagulopathy. In addition, impaired clearance of tissue plasminogen activator, together with excessive activation of coagulation, triggers fibrinolysis.

Massive transfusion

Massive transfusion (greater than 10 units of packed red blood cells (RBCs) in 24 h) to correct accidental or iatrogenic hemorrhage can precipitate coagulopathy and exacerbate bleeding. This has been referred to as the 'bloody vicious cycle' [57]. The cause of coagulopathy following massive transfusion is multifactorial. Dilutional coagulopathy is the primary cause of coagulopathy in patients with acute bleeding, since a large quantity of coagulation factors and platelets can be lost. In uncomplicated major bleeding, dilutional coagulopathy is self-limiting once platelets and coagulation factors are replenished. The dilutional coagulopathy, however, can be compounded by complications of massive transfusion and impaired tissue perfusion. Metabolic acidosis is a common occurrence from acids in the transfused blood and tissue lactic acidosis, and impairs coagulation by inhibiting the enzymatic reactions involved in the coagulation cascade. Massive transfusion together with inadequate hepatic perfusion may lead to ionic hypocalcemia or citrate intoxication to impair coagulation [58]. Hypothermia can be another factor that may interfere with coagulation. Hypovolemia and inadequate tissue perfusion are the primary causes of hypothermia seen during massive transfusion [59], and exposure to cold environment and the use of cold resuscitating solutions are contributory factors. Hypothermia produces a number of detrimental effects on coagulation. It increases splenic and hepatic platelet sequestration [60], alters platelet morphology [61] and inhibits platelet function [62]. The coagulation cascade, an enzymatic process, is inhibited [63,64]. Decreasing the body temperature to 35°C, 33°C and 31°C prolongs PT, which is equivalent to that achieved by reducing factor IX activity to 39%, 16% and 2.5% of normal value, respectively [65]. It should be noted, however, that impaired coagulation in hypothermia may be protective, because normal coagulation in slow circulation at the capillary level may precipitate thrombosis. The role of hypothermia-induced vasoconstriction on clinical bleeding is unknown.

Drugs
Many patients are placed on inhibitors of coagulation to treat or prevent thrombotic events such as stroke, coronary thrombosis and deep venous thrombosis. These drugs affect hemostasis in a predictable way, and their detailed description is beyond the scope of this chapter.

Disseminated intravascular coagulation
Disseminated intravascular coagulation (DIC) has been extensively reviewed in the past [66,67]. Briefly, DIC is characterized by an excessive, uncontrolled activation of coagulation triggered by various stimuli, followed by secondary fibrinolysis. Bleeding is a consequence of depletion of coagulation factors and platelets, and fibrinolysis. Laboratory diagnosis is made by prolonged PT and aPTT, hypofibrinogenemia, thrombocytopenia, and the presence of a large quantity of fibrin(ogen) degradation products and D-dimer. DIC is managed by the treatment of underlying pathology and replacement therapy. Administration of FFP replaces coagulation inhibitors (i.e. AT-III) in addition to coagulation factors, and platelet infusion restores platelet function. The use of coagulation inhibitors (i.e. heparin) is still controversial.

Heparin-induced thrombocytopenia
Heparin-induced thrombocytopenia (HIT) is an IgG-mediated hypersensitivity reaction to heparin [68,69]. It is characterized by a decrease in platelet count and a propensity for intravascular venous or arterial coagulation. Heparin binds to platelets via PF4 and elicits IgG antibody production. These antibodies activate platelets by binding to platelet FCγIIa receptors by their Fc tails. HIT antibodies also facilitate thrombin generation by mediating tissue factor expression by endothelial cells and macrophages. While this condition is primarily prothrombotic, concurrent bleeding may occur in the face of severe thrombocytopenia.

Cardiopulmonary bypass

Cardiopulmonary bypass (CPB) is associated with a qualitative and quantitative platelet dysfunction characterized by an increase in bleeding time and a decrease in platelet aggregation and granular contents [70]. This defect is caused by the excessive activation of platelets by CPB and removal of aggregated platelets by the reticuloendothelial system [71]. The degree of platelet dysfunction is related to the duration of CPB, and bleeding time and platelet function return to normal after about 1 h of uncomplicated CPB.

Circulating anticoagulants

Circulating anticoagulants are immunoglobulins formed against any enzymes of the coagulation cascade, and the most common ones are antibodies against factor VIII. The lupus anticoagulant is an antibody against phospholipids, which was initially described in patients with systemic lupus erythematosus. Whilst excessive bleeding has been described in patients with lupus anticoagulant [72], the condition is primarily a prothrombotic one.

Evaluation of hemostasis

History and physical examination

History and physical examination are helpful in identifying patients with underlying coagulation disorders and assessing the risk of bleeding in the intra- and postoperative period. An inquiry should be made into bleeding tendencies following minor or major trauma, dental procedure or various types of surgery. A family history of bleeding may indicate an inherited coagulation disorder. Medication history is useful in identifying drugs or nutritional supplements that can affect coagulation. Coexisting medical conditions that may affect coagulation (e.g. congestive heart failure, renal dysfunction and cirrhosis) should be investigated. Certain malignancies may also be associated with bleeding dyscrasia. For example, 15% of patients with acute myelocytic leukemia develop DIC.

A physical examination might reveal evidence of underlying medical conditions. The presence of petechia and ecchymosis may suggest primary hemostatic defect. Stigmata of chronic liver disease (ascitis, hepatosplenomegally and jaundice) should alert the clinician of the possibility of hemostatic dysfunction.

Coagulation tests

Laboratory tests are conducted to confirm preliminary suspicions and to identify the site of the coagulation disorder, either at the coagulation proteins or at platelets.

Prothrombin time

In this test, tissue thromboplastin containing tissue factor and phospholipid is added to the citrated blood specimen, and the specimen is then recalcified. PT is the time to form the initial clot and is the expression of the extrinsic pathway. Since various sources of thromboplastin are used, a great variation is observed in its results. The International Normalized Ratio (INR) was introduced in an effort to overcome this shortcoming. It standardizes the measurement both with respect to values for normal patients and standard human thromboplastin sensitivity established by the World Health Organization. INRs obtained at different laboratories with different sources of thromboplastin are therefore comparable. PT monitors activities of factors V, VII, X, prothrombin and thrombin and is prolonged in defects of the extrinsic and common pathways. It is abnormal in vitamin K deficiency and is considered to be the most sensitive hepatic synthetic function test. It is also used to monitor the anticoagulant effects of coumadin.

Activated partial thromboplastin time

aPTT evaluates the intrinsic and common pathways. Phospholipid, calcium and a contact activator (e.g. kaolin or silica) are added to the citrated specimen, and clotting is activated via the intrinsic pathway. This is a reliable test with less than 10% variability and used to monitor heparin activity. Abnormal prolongation may be seen in the presence of circulating antibodies or when insufficient quantity of blood is mixed into the anticoagulant.

Thrombin time and reptilase time

Thrombin is added to the citrated specimen, and the time to clot formation is noted. Thrombin time (TT) is prolonged in hypofibrinogenemia, dysfibrinogenemia and in the presence of thrombin inhibitors such as heparin and FDPs. Reptilase time (RT) is a modification of TT. Reptilase, like thrombin, cleaves fibrinogen. Unlike thrombin, the cleavage fragments formed can spontaneously polymerize even in the presence of FDPs. Additionally, reptilase is not inhibited by AT-III and is unaffected by heparin. An abnormal TT in the presence of a normal RT suggests the presence of a thrombin inhibitor.

Bleeding time and platelet count

For bleeding time, a blood pressure cuff is applied to the upper arm and inflated to 40 mmHg in order to achieve a standardized venous pressure. One or two incisions are made on the forearm (9 mm long and 1 mm deep). A filter paper is used to blot the incision every 30 s until bleeding ceases. The bleeding time is a sensitive indicator of platelet dysfunction as long as platelet count is greater than $100\,000/mm^3$. Therefore, simultaneous determination of platelet count is important in interpretation of bleeding time. Bleeding time is prolonged in patients on aspirin and with vWD and Glazmann's thrombasthenia. It has a number of drawbacks. It is prolonged in the absence of platelet dysfunction in patients with anemia, severe hypofibrinogenemia and vascular defects. It is labor-intensive, and results may vary depending on location, technical expertise, and age and sex of patient.

Specialized platelet function tests

Platelet aggregometry measures platelet aggregation induced by ADP, thrombin and collagen. Flow cytometry utilizes monoclonal antibodies to determine platelet surface receptor density. A detailed discussion of these tests is beyond the scope of this chapter.

Platelet function analyzer

The platelet function analyzer (PFA) evaluates primary hemostasis by measuring the time required for whole blood to occlude an aperture in the membrane of the test cartridge, which is coated with platelet agonist. It requires only 500 μl of blood, and is conducted at 37°C. The test can be conducted at the patient's bedside and is simple, quick, reliable and reproducible [73].

Activated clotting time

Blood is added to a test tube containing an activator, such as kaolin or diatomaceous earth. The blood in the test tube is placed in a well where it is gently rotated to mix its contents and warmed to 37°C. The time to clot formation is the activated clotting time (ACT), and it monitors clot formation by the intrinsic pathway. Unlike aPTT, which is unreliable after a large dose of heparin, ACT is reliable even after a large dose of heparin given during CPB. ACT has the greatest utility in this setting and can be used as a bedside monitor for coagulation.

Preoperative screening tests

Determination of PT, aPTT, platelet count and bleeding time is commonly employed for screening surgical patients who may develop excessive bleeding. They are, however, very poor screening tools for the general population and do not per se predict the risk of bleeding. For example, Eisenberg *et al.* reviewed 750 patients who required general surgical or gynecological procedures [74]. Abnormal PT and/or aPTT results were obtained in 2.7% of 480 patients with no clinical history and signs of bleeding – an incidence similar to that occurring by chance (2.28%) – and none of the patients with prolonged PT developed bleeding complications. A similar observation was made by Velanovich in 520 patients undergoing elective surgical procedures, in which neither the PT nor the aPTT had independent or associated value in predicting surgical bleeding [75]. The lack of correlation between screening tests and the degree of bleeding in surgical patients is also found in bleeding time [76]. In a retrospective analysis on 1800 patients undergoing various surgical procedures, the bleeding time was prolonged in 110 (6%) patients. Of these, 66 ingested drugs that affect platelet function, 6 had uremia, 11 had blood count less than 100 000/L and 27 were with unknown etiology. 7 patients experienced postoperative bleeding: 3 patients experienced minor bleeding and 4 had bleeding unrelated with platelet dysfunction.

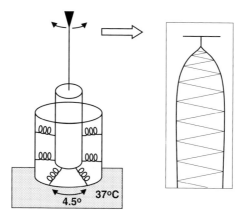

Figure 5.3 Schematic diagram of thromboelastography.

Thromboelastography

Thromboelastography (TEG) is a method of assessing whole blood coagulation, and technical aspects of the test have been extensively reviewed [77,78]. Briefly, a small quantity of blood (0.36 ml) is placed into a cuvette, and a central piston (pin) suspended by a torsion wire is lowered into the blood specimen (Figure 5.3). A rim of blood about 1 mm in its width is created between the cuvette and the piston. The cuvette rotates with a 4.5° angle in either direction at every 4.5 s, with a midcycle oscillatory pause of 1 s. Before clot formation, the pin is stationary. As clot begins to form, increasing elastic force of fibrin strands couples the pin and the cuvette, and oscillatory movement of the cuvette is transmitted to the pin. The torque experienced by the pin is plotted against time and displayed graphically on paper or digitally on a computer screen (Hemoscope). The reaction or gelation time (R) is the latency period between the initiation of the test (4 min from blood sampling time) and measurable fibrin formation (amplitude of 2 mm) (Figure 5.4). The clot formation time (K) begins from the initiation of clot formation to the

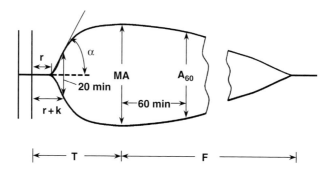

Figure 5.4 Typical thromboelastographic variables measured. (*Source*: Kang *et al.* [86] with permission.)

point where the clot reaches the viscoelastic property of 20 mm. R and K are prolonged in patients with coagulation factor deficiency thrombocytopemia and in the presence of anticoagulants (e.g. heparin). The alpha angle (α) measures the rate of clot formation and is affected by coagulation protein deficiencies and/or platelet dysfunction. Maximum amplitude (MA) is affected by platelet function and fibrinogen concentration. TEG parameters have been compared with conventional coagulation tests [79]. R and K times correlate with aPTT, and amplitude (A, mm) with the clot strength or shear elastic modulus, G [G (dynes cm^{-2}) = (5000A)/(100-A)]. A positive relation between maximum amplitude and platelets and fibrinogen has been demonstrated [80,81].

TEGs of various clinical conditions are shown in Figure 5.5 [82]. Deficiency of coagulation factors (e.g. hemophilia), hypocalcemia, hypothermia and heparin effect are seen as prolonged reaction time and slow clot formation rate. Thrombocytopenia is seen as small maximum amplitude, prolonged reaction time and slow clot formation rate, because platelet function is essential to the progression of the coagulation cascade. In patients with fibrinolysis, prolonged reaction time, slow clot formation rate and small maximum amplitude are accompanied by a gradual decrease in amplitude to zero, because the net amount of fibrin is reduced in the presence of active digestion of fibrins. Excessive activation of coagulation is seen as very short reaction time and rapid clot formation rate. Once DIC develops, all TEG variables deteriorate and a straight line is formed.

TEG has certain advantages over standard methods of coagulation monitoring. It is portable and the test can be performed at the patient's bedside. Results can be obtained fairly quickly: the onset of clot formation within a few minutes and platelet function within 45 min. While conventional coagulation tests end their observation once fibrin begins to form, TEG assesses dynamic changes of

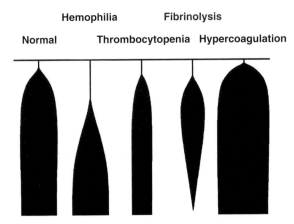

Figure 5.5 Thromboelastographic patterns of normal and disease states. (*Source*: Kang [82] with permission.)

the complete coagulation process, from coagulation to fibrinolysis. Further, if it is possible to make definitive differential diagnosis of coagulopathy by comparing multiple channels of TEG. For example, a comparison between TEG of untreated blood (0.36 ml) and that of blood treated with FFP (0.03 ml of FFP in 0.33 ml of whole blood) elucidates the presence of coagulation factor deficiency and beneficial effects of FFP administration. A similar comparison can be made by comparing TEGs of blood treated with other blood products (platelets and CRYO) and pharmacologic agents (epsilon-aminocaproic acid (EACA), protamine sulfate, aprotinin, DDAVP, etc.) [82–85].

Differential diagnosis of pathologic coagulation during liver transplantation is shown in Figure 5.6. Coagulation deteriorated rapidly on reperfusion of the grafted liver by prolonged clot formation rate, small amplitude and rapid decrease in amplitude. A blood specimen treated with EACA improved coagulation by a shortened reaction time, increased amplitude and disappearance of fibrinolysis, suggesting active fibrinolysis. The same blood specimen treated with protamine sulfate normalized the reaction time and increased amplitude with persistent fibrinolysis, indicating the heparin effect. This patient received EACA (250 mg) and protamine sulfate (25 mg) to normalize coagulation.

TEG has been proved valuable in intraoperative management of coagulation during liver transplantation, in which the etiology of bleeding is multifactorial and changes in coagulation are rapid and dramatic [86]. Its clinical effectiveness also has been shown in cardiac surgery and other major surgical procedures [87]. Most importantly, it is a valuable educational tool in understanding the global coagulation process.

Management of intraoperative coagulation

Clinical coagulation

Although major advances have been made in understanding coagulation in the past three decades, clinicians are often puzzled by the complexity of

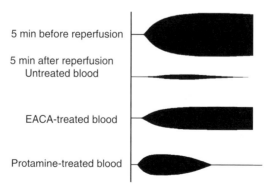

Figure 5.6 Differential diagnosis of fibrinolysis and heparin effect after reperfusion of the graft liver during orthotopic liver transplantation.

coagulation and lack of relationship between laboratory values and clinical presentation. This may stem from oversimplification of coagulation, analytic interpretation of coagulation instead of appreciation of global coagulation and, possibly, insufficient education of clinical coagulation. It is worthwhile to review coagulation in the perspective of clinicians.

Coagulation is a part of systemic inflammatory response. As described in the contact activation of coagulation, vascular injury leads to activation of Hageman factor, which activates kallikrein, bradykinin, fibrinolysis and the complement system. For example, tissue injury caused by various stimuli (laceration, thermal injury, ischemia, rejection, acidosis, etc.) activates in-flammation and coagulation to repair damaged tissue. Therefore, coagulation management should be directed to the treatment of underlying pathology.

Coagulation has five distinctive, equally important, interacting phases. However, major emphasis has been placed on the intrinsic and extrinsic system. The extent of vascular injury by the surgical team, local vasoconstric-tion and platelet aggregation may play a more important role in determining surgical blood loss, although its clinical significance has not been elucidated.

Hemostasis is a net balance between clot formation and fibrinolysis with positive and negative feedback, and is influenced by activities and inter-actions of procoagulants, anticogulants, lysins, antilysins, physiologic vari-ables, drugs and other physical chemical variables (Figure 5.7). Commonly used coagulation tests (PT, aPTT and platelet count) represent only a fraction of the coagulation balance and do not provide clinicians with necessary clinical information.

Another puzzling issue is that the surgical field appears to be 'wet' particu-larly at the end of a major surgical procedure, although coagulation profile at

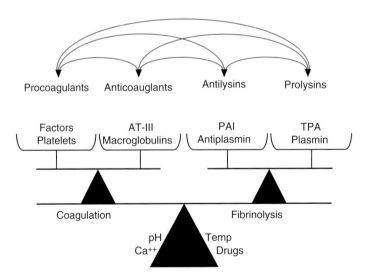

Figure 5.7 Hemostatic balance between clot formation and fibrinolysis.

this time may be relatively normal. It is speculated that this is a delayed bleeding phenomenon, possibly caused by the loss of incomplete clot formed in the presence of dilutional coagulopathy or by ongoing fibrinolysis after excessive activation of coagulation.

Coagulation management

Intraoperative hemorrhage can be life-threatening, and rapid and decisive intervention is essential. Surgical hemostasis is the most important part of coagulation management in most cases. The goal of medical management of coagulation is to maintain normal blood coagulability by frequent monitoring and specific therapy using blood components or pharmacologic agents, while avoiding thrombosis. The first step of coagulation management is maintaining optimal physiologic state (normovolemia, normothermia and normal electrolyte balance and acid–base state), since impaired tissue perfusion caused by the altered physiologic state triggers inflammatory response and coagulation. This is followed by replacement therapy and pharmacologic therapy.

Most clinicians agree that normal blood coagulability does not necessarily require normal quantity or activity of coagulation elements, and the reverse is also true. The hypothetical relationship between blood coagulability and coagulation profiles is shown in Figure 5.8 [88]. Normal blood coagulability is expected in patients with normal coagulation profiles and is well maintained until coagulation profiles or coagulation factors gradually decrease below the critical level. This is indirectly observed in hemophiliac patients in whom normal hemostasis is maintained unless factor VIII level reaches below 30%

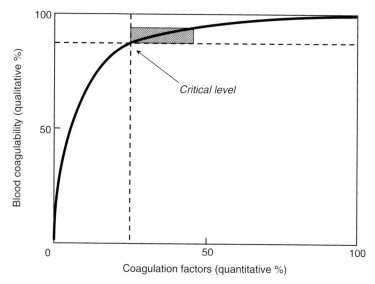

Figure 5.8 Hypothetical relationship between blood coagulability and coagulation profiles. (*Source*: Kang [88] with permission.)

of normal value, and platelet function is relatively normal until platelet count falls below 50 000/mm^3 [89,90]. Blood coagulability, however, is impaired rapidly and becomes a clinical concern once coagulation factor levels decrease below this critical level. If this relationship exists, normal blood coagulability can be achieved by maintaining coagulation profiles above the critical level (shaded area), while administering minimal quantity of blood products. This concept can be extended to patients undergoing surgical procedures with major bleeding (Figure 5.9). Intraoperatively, coagulability and coagulation profiles deteriorate by dilution and pathologic coagulation, and can be corrected by replacement therapy based on quantity of coagulation elements (open circles) or blood coagulability (solid circles). It is likely that patients with quantitative test–based replacement therapy receive more blood products while maintaining similar blood coagulability compared with their counterpart.

Monitoring of coagulation is an integral part of coagulation management, and serial determinations of PT, aPTT and platelet count are commonly employed. The conventional recommendation is to administer FFP to a patient with a prolonged PT. FFP contains approximately 400 mg of fibrinogen and 1 unit of clotting factors per 1 ml of solution. The labile factors (V and VIII) are easily destroyed in thawed FFP unless it is refrigerated. Common indications for use of FFP are: (1) reversal of the effects of coumadin in

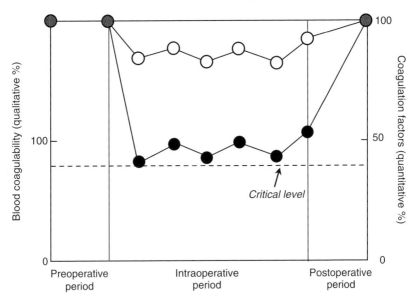

Figure 5.9 Blood coagulability and coagulation profiles during liver transplantation. Solid circles represent a hypothetical patient without coagulation monitoring and therapy, and open circles represent a patient with monitoring of coagulability and treatment. (*Source*: Kang [88] with permission.)

patients with active bleeding or anticipated surgical procedures; (2) documented or suspected factor deficiency; and (3) supplementation of depleted factors following massive transfusion or in patients with liver disease. The usual dose of 15–20 ml/kg is expected to raise coagulation factor levels by 2–3%. CRYO is rich in fibrinogen, factor VIII and vWF. It is indicated in vWD, hemophilia A, and the fibrinolytic state in which fibrinogen and factors V and VIII are selectively destroyed by plasmin.

Clinical effectiveness of FFP, however, is limited by the poor correlation between the laboratory values and clinical observation or blood loss as demonstrated in Figure 5.10 and 5.11 [91]. In patients undergoing liver transplantation, PT did not have significant relationship with the FFP use, and aPTT did not predict the perioperative RBC requirement. This poor correlation may be explained by a comparison of TEGs before and after heparin administration (Figure 5.12). Normal TEG pattern is observed before heparin administration. Bleeding, however, is expected to occur until clot is formed at the injured vessel, and the area under curve A represents blood loss. Heparin administration typically prolongs the reaction time and shifts the TEG to the right. The area under the curve or bleeding becomes larger and includes (B). Therefore, bleeding is greater with heparin administration, but the increase in the area under curve B may not be large enough to cause clinically significant bleeding.

The role of platelets is essential in hemostasis: platelets form the initial hemostatic plug, and coagulation process occurs on the surface of platelets. Although the number of platelets required for adequate hemostasis is controversial, current recommendation suggests that platelet count of greater than 50 000/ml be maintained during minor surgical procedures and greater than 100 000/ml during major surgical procedures and neurosurgery [92].

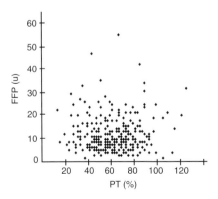

Figure 5.10 The relation between FFP requirement and prothrombin time during liver transplantation. (*Source*: Gerlach *et al.* [91] with permission.)

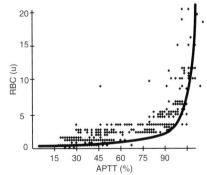

Figure 5.11 The relation between RBC requirement and aPTT during liver transplantation. (*Source*: Gerlach *et al.* [91] with permission.)

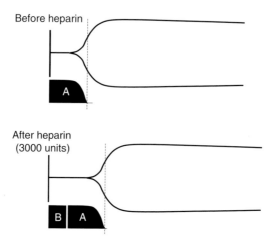

Before heparin

A

After heparin
(3000 units)

B A

Figure 5.12 The clinical significance of moderately prolonged clot formation.

Hemostatic drug therapy

Any therapeutic intervention that promotes hemostasis and reduces the need for transfusion of blood products is of obvious benefit. Drugs of different classes have entered the armamentarium of clinicians. The benefit of augmenting hemostasis, however, has to be weighed against the potential for thrombotic sequelae that may arise.

Antifibrinolytics

Lysine analogs

The lysine analogs, EACA and tranexamic acid (TXA), accelerate activation of plasminogen by inducing conformational change in the molecule, but inhibit fibrinolysis by blocking the lysine-binding site of plasmin. Antifibrinolytics have been shown to reduce blood loss and transfusion requirements in cardiac surgery [93,94], liver transplantation [95], prostate surgery [96] and in joint replacement surgery [97,98]. For cardiac surgery, either drug is given intravenously following the induction of anesthesia as a bolus followed by an infusion. The dose for EACA is 150 mg/kg bolus followed by 15 mg/kg/h, and for TXA it is 10 mg/kg followed by 1 mg/kg/h. It is noteworthy that a recent study showed that a small, single dose of EACA (< 500 mg) is effective in treating fibrinolysis during liver transplantation [99]. Since fibrinolysis is a natural protective mechanism against thrombosis, indiscriminate use of anti-fibrinolytics may lead to thrombosis.

Aprotinin

Aprotinin is a polypeptide serine protease inhibitor that reversibly binds to, and inactivates, a number of serine proteases including trypsin, chymotrypsin, plasmin, kallikrein, Hageman factor and most coagulation factors. As a result, it is expected to inhibit both coagulation and fibrinolysis [100]. It also prevents platelet activation during CPB and has been shown to preserve platelet GPIb receptors. Aprotinin is used in cardiac surgery to reduce blood loss and transfusion requirements, possibly by inhibiting excessive activation of coagulation and fibrinolysis. It is indicated when excessive blood loss is anticipated (e.g. redo cardiac surgery or patients on antiplatelet agents) or when blood transfusion is refused. Aprotinin is commonly given as 2 million KIU (kallikrein inactivation units) bolus followed by an infusion of 0.5 KIU/h. Aprotinin has been shown to reduce blood loss and transfusion requirements during liver transplantation [101]. However, recent literature questions the clinical effectiveness of aprotinin, and its use has been reduced in many centers. Although the incidence of thromboembolic complication was not different from patients who received placebo, fatal pulmonary embolism following administration of the drug has been reported [102]. Other possible side-effects are anaphylaxis and renal injury.

Desmopressin
DDAVP (1-deamino 8-d-arginine vasopressin) is a synthetic analog of the naturally occurring posterior pituitary hormone, vasopressin (antidiuretic hormone, ADH). It stimulates endothelial cells to release both factor VIII and subtypes of vWF, and their level can increase up to fourfold, peaking 30–60 min after an intravenous (IV) dose [103]. DDAVP improves hemostasis in patients with hemophilia A and vWD [104,105], and improves bleeding time in patients with uremia [106], congenital platelet defects [107], end-stage liver disease [108,109], and possibly those undergoing caridac surgery [110]. The dose of DDAVP is 0.3 µg/kg intravenously or subcutaneously; or 300 µg (150 µg in children) intranasally. It may be repeated 12–24 h after the initial dose. Tachyphylaxis may develop after the fourth dose.

Recombinant factor VIIa (rVIIa)
As described previously, factor VIIa-TF complex activates factor X to a small amount of Xa, and subsequently small amounts of thrombin are generated. This small quantity of thrombin activates factors V, VIII and IX and platelets to set the stage for platelet surface–mediated burst of thrombin generation. Factor VIIa has low affinity for platelet surfaces and does not attach to these surfaces in physiologic concentrations. However, in high concentrations, it does bind to the surface of activated platelets and directly activates factor X, resulting in platelet surface thrombin generation without factors VIIIa and IXa. Therefore, a high dose rFVIIa restores platelet surface thrombin generation and promotes clot formation in hemophlia A and B. In the USA, rFVIIa is approved for use in a subset of hemophilia patients in whom the presence of inhibitors substantially reduces the efficacy of conventional therapy with factor concentrates. Studies are ongoing to evaluate its utility in surgical patients.

References

1 Vasiiev JM, Gelfand IM. Mechanism of non-adhesiveness of endothelial and epithelial surfaces. *Nature* 1978; **274**: 710–11.
2 Mustard JF, Kinlough-Rathbone RL, Packham MA. The vessel wall in thrombosis. In: Colman RW, Hirsh J, Marder V. Salzman EW, eds. *Thrombosis and Hemostasis: Basic Principles and Clinical Practice*. Philadelphia: JB Lippincott, 1982, 703–15.
3 Mason RG, Mohammad SF, Chuang HY, Richardson PD. The adhesion of platelets to subendothelium, collagen and artificial surfaces. *Semin Thromb Hemost* 1976; **3**: 98–116.
4 Maclntyre DE, Pearson JD, Gordon JL. Localization and stimulation of prostacyclin production in vascular cells. *Nature* 1978; **271**: 549–51.
5 Marder VJ. Molecular bad actors and thrombosis. *N Engl J Med* 1984; **310**: 588–9.
6 Stead NW, Kinney 1, Lewis JG, Campbell EE, Shifman MA, Rosenberg RD, Pizzo SV. Venous thrombosis in a family with defective release of vascular plasminogen activator and elevated plasma factor VIII/von Willebrand's factor. *Am J Med* 1983; **74**: 33–9.
7 Kitchens CS. The anatomical basis of purpura. *Prog Hemost Thromb* 1980; **5**: 211–44.
8 Kaushansky K. Thrombopoietin: the primary regulator of platelet production. *Blood* 1995; **86**: 419–31.
9 Shattil SI, Bennett IS. Platelets and their membranes in hemostasis: physiology and pathophysiology. *Ann Intern Med* 1981; **94**: 108–18.
10 Marcus AJ, Weksler BB, Jaffe EA. Enzymatic conversion of prostaglandin endoperoxide H_2 and arachidonic acid to prostacyclin by cultured human endothehial cells. *J Biol Chem* 1978; **253**: 7138–41.
11 Shattil SJ, Hoxie JA, Cunningham MJ, Vrass LF. Changes in the platelet membrane glycoprotein IIb-IIIa complex during platelet activation. *J Biol Chem* 1985; **78**: 340–8.
12 Holmsen H, Weiss HJ. Secretable storage pools in platelets. *Ann Rev Med* 1979; **30**: 119–34.
13 White JG. Current concepts of platelet structure. *Am J Clin Pathol* 1979; **71**: 363–78.
14 Lyons RM, Stanford N, Majerus PW. Thrombin-induced protein phosphorylation in human platelets. *J Clin Invest* 1975; **56**: 924–36.
15 Pickett WC, Jesse RL, Cohen P. Initiation of phospholipase A_2 activity in human platelets by the calcium ionophore A23187. *Biochim Biophys Acta* 1977; **486**: 209–13.
16 Hamberg M, Svensson I, Samuelsson B. Prostaglandin endoperoxides: a new concept concerning the mode of action and release of prostaglandins. *Proc Nat Acad Sci* 1974; **71**: 3824–8.
17 Hamberg M, Svensson J, Samuelsson B. Thromboxanes: a new group of biologically active compounds derived from prostaglandin endoperoxides. *Proc Nat Acad Sci* 1975; **72**: 2994–8.
18 Gerrard JM, White JG. Prostaglandins and thromboxanes: "middlemen" modulating platelet function in hemostasis and thrombosis. *Prog Hemost Thromb* 1978; **4**: 87–125.
19 Phillips DR. An evaluation of membrane glycoproteins in platelet adhesion and aggregation. *Prog Hemost Thromb* 1980; **5**: 81–109.
20 Nurden AT, Caen JP. The different glycoprotein abnormalities in thrombasthenic and Bernard–Soulier platelets. *Semin Hematol* 1979; **16**: 234–50.
21 Packham MA, Mustard JF. Platelet adhesion. *Prog Hemost Thromb* 1984; **7**: 211–88.

22 Haslam RJ, Davidson MM, Fox JE, Lynham JA. Cyclic nucleotides in platelet function. *Thromb Haemost* 1978; **40**: 232–40.

23 Kaser-Glanzmann R, Jakabova M, George JN, Luscher EF. Stimulation of calcium uptake in platelet membrane vesicles by adenosine 3',5'-cyclic monophosphate and protein kinase. *Biochim Biophys Acta* 1977; **466**: 429–40.

24 Bucher D, Nebelin E, Thomsen J, Steflo J. Identification of gamma-carboxyglutamic add residues in bovine factors IX and X, and in a new vitamin K-dependent protein. *FEBS Lett* 1976; **68**: 293–6.

25 Mandle RJ Jr, Kaplan AP. Hageman factor substrates – human plasma prekallikrein: mechanism of activation of Hageman factor and participation in Hageman factor–dependent 11-fibrinolysis. *J Biol Chem* 1977; **252**: 6097–7001.

26 Ratnoff OD, Colopy JE. A familial hemorrhagic trait associated with deficiency of clot-promoting fraction of plasma. *J Clin Invest* 1955; **34**: 602–13.

27 Mandle RJ Jr, Colman RW, Kaplan AP. Identification of prekallikrein and high molecular weight kininogen as a complex in human plasma. *Proc Nat Acad Sci USA* 1976; **73**: 4179–83.

28 Cooper HA, Griggs TR, Wagner RH. Factor VIII recombination after dissociation by CaCl₂. *Proc Nat Acad Sci USA* 1973; **70**: 2326–9.

29 Bjorklid E, Storm E, Prydz H. The protein component of human brain thromboplastin. *Biochem Biophys Res Commun* 1973; **55**: 969–76.

30 Radcliffe R, Nemerson Y. Activation and control of factor VII by activated factor X and thrombin: isolation and characterization of a single chain form of factor VII. *J Biol Chem* 1974; **250**: 388–95.

31 Miletich JP, Jackson CM, Majerus PW. Properties of the Factor X binding site on human platelets. *J Biol Chem* 1978; **253**: 6908–16.

32 Doolittle RF, Goldbaum DM, Doolittle LR. Designation of sequences involved in the "coiled-coil" interdomainal connector in fibrinogen: constructions of an atomic scale model. *J Mol Biol* 1978; **120**: 311–25.

33 Blomback B, Blomback M. The molecular structure of fibrinogen. *Ann NY Acad Sci* 1972; **202**: 77–97.

34 Ferry JD. The conversion of fibrinogen to fibrin: events and recollections from 1942 to 1982. *Ann NY Acad Sci* 1983; **27**: 1–10.

35 Hermans J, McDonagh J. Fibrin: structure and interactions. *Semin Thromb Hemost* 1982; **8**: 11–24.

36 Folk JE, Finlayson JS. The epsilon-(γ-glutamyl) lysine crosslink and the catalytic role of transglutaminase. *Adv Protein Chem* 1977; **31**: 1–133.

37 McKee PA, Mattock P. Hill RL. Subunit structure of human fibrinogen, soluble fibrin, and cross-linked insoluble fibrin. *Proc Nat Acad Sci USA* 1970; **66**: 738–44.

38 Kaplan KL, Broekman MJ, Chernoff A, Lesznik GR, Drillings M. Platelet alpha-granule proteins: studies on release and subcellular localization. *Blood* 1979; **53**: 604–18.

39 Nachmias V, Sullender J, Asch A. Shape and cytoplasmic filaments in control and lidocaine-treated human platelets. *Blood* 1977; **50**: 39–53.

40 Lijnen HR, Collen D. Interaction of plasminogen activators and inhibitors with plasminogen and fibrin. *Semin Thromb Hemost* 1982; **8**: 2–10.

41 Alkjaersig N, Fletcher AP, Sherry S. The mechanism of clot dissolution by plasmin. *J Clin Invest* 1959; **38**: 1086–95.

42 Sakata Y, Aoki N. Cross-linking of alpha₂-plasmin inhibitor to fibrin by fibrin-stabilizing factor. *J Clin Invest* 1980; **65**: 290–7.

43 Scott CF, Silver LD, Purdon DA, Colman RW. Cleavage of human high molecular weight kininogen by factor XI, *in vitro*: effect on structure and function. *J Biol Chem* 1985; **260**: 10856–63.

44 Schapira M, Scott CF, Colman RW. Protection of human plasma kallikrein from inactivation by Cl inhibitor and other protease inhibitors: the role of high molecular weight kininogen. *Biochemistry* 1981; **20**: 2738–43.

45 Scott CF, Schapira M, James HL, Cohen AB, Colman RW. Inactivation of factor XIa by plasma protease inhibitors: predominant role of α_1-protease inhibitor and protective effect of high molecular weight kininogen. *J Clin Invest* 1982; **69**: 844–52.

46 Rosenberg RD, Damus PS. The purification and mechanism of action of human antithrombin-heparin cofactor. *J Biol Chem* 1973; **248**: 6490–505.

47 Murray EW, Lillicrap D. von Willebrand disease: pathogenesis, classification and management. *Transfus Med Rev* 1996; **10**: 93–110.

48 Wagner DD. Cell biology of von Willebrand factor. *Ann Rev Cell Biol* 1990; **6**: 217–46.

49 Bloom AL. von Willebrand factor: clinical features of inherited and acquired disorders. *Mayo Clin Proc* 1991; **66**: 743–5l.

50 Brinkhous KM, Graham JH. Hemophilia and the hemophilioid states. *Blood* 1954; **9**: 254–7.

51 Levine PH. Clinical manifestations and therapy of hemophilias A and B. In: Colman RW, Hirsh J, Marder V, Salzman EW, eds. *Thrombosis and Hemostasis: Basic Principles and Clinical Practice*. Philadelphia: JB Lippincott, 1987, 97–111.

52 Triplett DA. Coagulation and bleeding disorders: review and update. *Clin Chem* 2000; **46**: 1260–9.

53 Olson RE. Vitamin K. In: Colman RW, Hirsh J, Marder V, Salzman EW, eds. *Thrombosis and Hemostasis: Basic Principles and Clinical Practice*. Philadelphia: JB Lippincott, 1987, 846–60.

54 Green G, Poller L, Thompson SM, Dymock W. Factor VII as a marker of hepato-cellular synthetic function. *J Clin Pathol* 1976; **29**: 971–5.

55 Violi F, Ferro D, Quintarelli C, Saliola M, Corrado C, BalsanoF. Clotting abnormalities in chronic liver disease. *Dig Dis* 1991; **10**: 162–72.

56 Mammen EF. Coagulation defects in liver disease. *Med Clin N Am* 1994; **78**: 545–54.

57 Cosgriff N, Moore EE, Sauaia A, Kenny-Moynihan M, Burch JM, Galloway B. Predicting life-threatening coagulopathy in the massively transfused trauma patient: hypothermia and acidoses revisited. *J Trauma* 1997; **42**: 857–61.

58 Marquez J, Martin D, Virji MA, Kang YG, Warty VS, Shaw B Jr, Sassano JJ, Waterman P, Winter PM, Pinsky MR. Cardiovascular depression secondary to ionic hypocalcemia during hepatic transplantation in humans. *Anesthesiology* 1986; **65**: 457–61.

59 Bergenstein JM, Slakey DP, Wallace JR, Gottlieb M. Traumatic hypotension is related to hypotension, not resuscitation. *Ann Emerg Med* 1996; **27**: 39–42.

60 Hessel II, EA, Schmer G, Dillard DH. Platelets kinetics during deep hypothermia. *J Surg Res* 1980; **28**: 23–34.

61 White T, Krivit W. An ultrastructural basis for the shape changes induced in platelets by chilling blood. *Blood* 1967; **30**: 635–75.

62 Valeri CR, Feingold H, Cassidy G *et al*. Hypothermia-induced reversible platelet dysfunction. *Ann Surg* 1987; **205**: 175.

63 Rohrer MJ, Natale AM. Effect of hypothermia on the coagulation cascade. *Crit Care Med* 1992; **20**: 1402–5.

64 Kurrek MM, Reed RL. Effect of hypothermia on enzymatic activity of thrombin and plasmin. *Surg Forum*; 221–3.

65 Johnston TD, Chen Y, Reed RL. *Surg Forum* 1989; **40**: 199–201.

66 Sick RL. Disseminated intravascular coagulation and related syndromes: a clinical review. *Sem Thromb Hemost* 1989; **14**: 299–338.

67 Marder VJ, Martin SE, Frances CW, Colman RW. Consumptive thrombohemor-rhagic disorders. In: Colman RW, Hirsh J, Marder V, Salzman EW, eds. *Thrombosis and Hemostasis: Basic Principles and Clinical Practice*. Philadelphia: JB Lippincott, 1987, 975–1015.

68 Warkentin TE. An overview of the heparin-induced thrombocytopenia syndrome. *Semin Thromb Hemost* 2004; **30**: 273–83.

69 Comunale ME, Van Cott EM. Heparin-induced thrombocytopenia. *Int Anesthesiol Clin* 2004; **42**: 27–43.

70 George JN, Shattil SJ. The clinical importance of acquired abnormalities of platelet function. *N Engl J Med* 1991; **324**: 27–39.

71 Weerasinghe A, Taylor KM. The platelet in cardiopulmonary bypass. *Ann Thorac Surg* 1998; **66**: 2145–52.

72 Manoharan A, Gottlieb P. Bleeding in patients with lupus anticoagulant. *Lancet* 1984; **2**: 171.

73 Mammen EF, Comp PC, Gosselin R, Greenberg C, Hoots WK, Kessler CM, Larkin EC, Liles D, Nugent DJ. PFA-100 system: a new method of assessment of platelet dysfunction. *Semin Thromb Hemost* 1998; **24**: 195–202.

74 Eisenberg JM, Clarke JR, Sussman SA. Prothrombin and partial thromboplastin times as preoperative screening tests. *Arch Surg* 1982; **117**: 48–51.

75 Velanovich V. The value of routine preoperative laboratory testing in predicting postoperative complications: a multivariate analysis. *Surgery* 1991; **109**: 236–43.

76 Barber A, Green D, Galuzzo T, Ts'ao CH. The bleeding time as a preoperative screening test. *Am J Med* 1985; **78**: 761–4.

77 Kang Y. Thromboelastography in liver transplantation. *Semin Thromb Hemost* 1995; **21**: 34–44.

78 Mallett SV, Cox DJA. Thromboelastography. *BJA* 1992; **69**: 307–13.

79 Zuckerman L, Cohen E, Vagher JP, Woodward E, Caprini JA. Comparison of thromboelastography with common coagulation test. *Thromb Haemost* 1981; **46**: 752–6.

80 Gottumukkala VN, Sharma SK, Philip J. Assessing platelet and fibrinogen contribution to clot strength using modified thromboelastography in pregnant women. *Anesth Analg* 1999; **89**: 1453–5.

81 Khurana S, Mattson JC, Westley S, O'Neill WW, Timmis GC, Safian RD. Monitoring platelet glycoprotein IIb/IIIa-fibrin interaction with tissue-factor activated thromboelastography. *J Lab Clin Med* 1997; **130**: 401–11.

82 Kang YG. Monitoring and treatment of coagulation. In: Winter PM, Kang YG, eds. *Hepatic Transplantation, Anesthetic and Perioperative Management*. Philadelphia: Praeger Publisher, 1986: 151–73.

83 Kang YG, Lewis JH, Navalgund A, Russell MW, Bontempo FA, Niren LS, Starzl TE. Epsilon-aminocaproic acid for treatment of fibrinolysis during liver transplantation. *Anesthesiology* 1987; **66**: 766–73.

84 Kang Y, Scott V, DeWolf A, Roskoph J, Aggarwal S. In vitro effects of DDAVP during liver transplantation. *Transpl Proc* 1993; **25**: 1821–2.

85 Kang Y, DeWolf A, Aggarwal S, Campbell E, Martin LK. In vitro study on the effects of aprotinin on coagulation during orthotopic liver transplantation. *Transpl Proc* 1991; **23**: 1934–5.

86 Kang YG, Martin DJ, Marquez J, Lewis JH, Bontempo FA, Shaw BW Jr, Starzl TE, Winter PM. Intraoperative changes in blood coagulation and thrombelastographic monitoring in liver transplantation. *Anesth Analg* 1985; **64**: 888–96.

87 Shore-Lesserson L, Manspeizer HE, DePerio M, Francis S, Vela-Cantos F, Ergin MA. Thromboelastography-guided transfusion algorithm reduces transfusions in complex cardiac surgery. *Anesth Analg* 1999; **88**: 312–19.

88 Kang Y. Transfusion based on clinical coagulation monitoring does reduce hemorrhage during liver transplantation. *Liver Transpl Surg* 1997; **3**: 655–9.

89 Post M, Telfer MC. Surgery in hemophilic patients. *J Bone Joint Surg Am* 1975; **57**: 1136–45.

90 Miller RD, Robbins TO, Tong MJ, Barton SL. Coagulation defects associated with massive blood transfusions. *Ann Surg* 1971; **174**: 794–801.

91 Gerlach H, Slama KJ, Bechstein WO, Lohmann R, Hintz G, Abraham K, Neuhaus P, Falke K. Retrospective statistical analysis of coagulation parameters after 250 liver transplantations. *Semin Thromb Hemost* 1993; **19**: 223–32.

92 Consensus conference: platelet transfusion therapy. *JAMA* 1987; **257**: 1777–80.

93 Vander Salm TJ, Kaur S, Lancey RA, Okike ON, Pezzella AT, Stahl RF, Leone L, Li JM, Valeri CR, Michelson AD. Reduction of bleeding after heart operations through the prophylactic use of epsilon-aminocaproic acid. *J Thorac Cardiovasc Surg* 1996; **112**: 1098–107.

94 Katasaros D, Petricevic M, Snow NJ, Woodhall DD, Van Bergen R. Tranexamic acid reduces postbypass blood use: a double-blind, prospective, randomized study in 210 patients. *Ann Thorac Surg* 1996; **61**: 1131–5.

95 Boylan JF, Klinck JR, Sandler AN, Arellano R, Greig PD, Nierenberg H, Roger SL, Glynn MF. Tranexamic acid reduces blood loss, transfusion requirements, and coagulation factor use in primary orthotopic liver transplantation. *Anesthesiology* 1996; **85**: 1043–8.

96 Stefanini M, English HA, Taylor AE. Safe and effective, prolonged administration of epsilon-aminocaproic acid in the bleeding urinary tract. *J Urol* 1990; **143**: 559–61.

97 Benoni G, Fredin H. Fibrinolytic inhibition with tranexamic acid reduces blood loss and blood transfusion after knee arthroplasty: a prospective randomized, double-blind study in 86 patients. *J Bone Joint Surg Br* 1996; **78**: 434–40.

98 Hiippala ST, Strid LJ, Wennerstrand MI, Arvela JV, Niemela HM, Mantyla SK, Kuisma RP, Ylinen JE. Tranexamic acid radically decreases blood loss and transfusion associated with total knee arthroplasty. *Anesth Analg* 1997; **84**: 839–44.

99 Kang Y. Clinical use of synthetic antifibrinolytic agents during liver transplantation. *Semin Thromb Hemost* 1993; **19**: 258–61.

100 Kang Y, De Wolf AM, Aggarwal S, Campbell E, Martin LK. In vitro study of the effects of aprotinin on coagulation during orthotopic liver transplantation. *Transpl Proc* 1991; **23**: 1934–5.

101 Porte RJ, Molenaar IQ, Begliomini B, Groenland TH, Januszkiewicz A, Lindgren L, Palareti G, Hermans J, Terpstra OT. Aprotinin and transfusion requirements in orthotopic liver transplantation: a multicentre randomized double-blind study. *Lancet* 2000; **355**: 1303–9.

102 Baubillier E, Cherqui D, Dominique C, Khalil M, Bonnet F, Fagniez PL, Duval-destin P. A fatal thrombotic complication during liver transplantation after apro-tinin administration. *Transplantation* 1994; **57**: 1664–6.

103 Lethagen S, Harris AS, Sjorin E, Nilsson IM. Intranasal and intravenous adminis-tration of desmopressin: effect on F VIII/vWF, pharmacokinetics and reproduci-bility. *Thromb Haemost* 1987; **58**: 1033–6.

104 Mannucci PM, Ruggeri ZM, Pareti FI, Capitanio A. 1-deamino-8-D-arginine vaso-pressin: a new pharmacological approach to the management of hemophilia and von Willebrand's diseases. *Lancet* 1977; **1**: 869–72.

105 Kobrinsky NL, Israels ED, Gerrard JM, Cheang MS, Watson CM, Bishop AJ, Schroeder ML. Shortening of bleeding time by 1-deamino-8-D-arginine vasopres-sin in various bleeding disorders. *Lancet* 1984; **1**: 1145–8.

106 Steiner RW, Coggins C, Carvalho AC. Bleeding time in uremia: a useful test to assess clinical bleeding. *Am J Hematol* 1979; **7**: 107–17.

107 Rao AK, Ghosh S, Sun L, Yang X, Disa J, Pickens P, Polansky M. Mechanism of platelet dysfunction and response to DDAVP in patients with congenital platelet function defects: a double-blind placebo-controlled trial. *Thromb Haemost* 1995; **74**: 1071–8.

108 Mannucci PM, Vicente V, Vianello L, Cattaneo M, Alberca I, Coccato MP, Faioni E, Mari D. Controlled trial of desmopressin in liver cirrhosis and other conditions associated with a prolonged bleeding time. *Blood* 1986; **67**: 1148–53.

109 Kang Y, Scott V, DeWolf A, Roskoph J, Aggarwal S. In vitro effects of DDAVP during liver transplantation. *Transplant Proc* 1993; **25**: 1821–2.

110 Salzman EW, Weinstein MJ, Weintraub RM, Ware JA, Thurer RL, Robertson L, Donovan A, Gaffney T, Bertele V, Troll J. Treatment with desmopressin acetate to reduce blood loss after cardiac surgery: a double-blind randomized trial. *N Engl J Med* 1986; **314**: 1402–6.

CHAPTER 6

The Physiology of Anemia and the Threshold for Blood Transfusion

Joseph D Tobias

Introduction

Oxygen is the key component necessary for all aerobic processes. During the evolutionary process with the progression from unicellular and multicellular organisms to more complex forms, the process of diffusion becomes an ineffective means of delivering oxygen to the tissues due to constraints of time and distance. Although simple diffusion still functions at the oxygen–blood interface in the lungs and the blood–tissue interface at the capillary level, a functioning cardiovascular system and a fluid capable of delivering oxygen to the tissues is needed. Since oxygen is poorly soluble in water, most organisms have evolved a compound capable of binding oxygen and thereby increasing its solubility in the fluid milieu. In mammalian species, this compound is hemoglobin (Hb).

In humans and other mammalian species, the production of red blood cells (RBCs) is regulated to match the natural loss of RBCs as they age and are removed from the system in addition to any abnormal losses that occur due to hemorrhage or hemolysis. The process of erythropoiesis is regulated by erythropoietin (EPO), a hormone produced by the peritubular cells of the renal cortex and the liver [1]. The primary stimulus for the production and release of EPO is tissue hypoxia and a decrease in oxygen delivery to the tissue beds related either to anemia or a decreased oxygen saturation [2]. EPO concentrations can increase up to 1000-fold in the presence of hypoxia and increase exponentially as the Hb concentration decreases. However, in chronic disease states or during critical illness, the EPO response may be blunted, thereby making it inadequate to maintain a normal Hb concentration.

Causes of anemia and the compensatory mechanisms

In a general sense, anemia can be defined as a specific Hb concentration or hematocrit (Hct) value. Values defining anemia include an Hb concentration of less than 13 g/dl or a Hct less than 39% in an adult male and an Hb concentration of less than 12 g/dl or a Hct less than 36% in an adult female [3]. Although these definitions are generally accepted, they should not be confused with values that necessitate the administration of blood otherwise known as 'transfusion triggers' (see below). Additionally, although Hb and Hct concentrations are helpful in determining the presence or absence of anemia and the need for blood component therapy, factors such as the patient's ability to increase oxygen delivery to the tissues by increasing cardiac output and the status of the peripheral vascular system will affect the ultimate 'transfusion trigger'. The absolute Hb or Hct value can also be affected by various pathologic processes that may mask the presence of anemia. An acutely exsanguinating patient may have a normal Hb and Hct if intravenous (IV) fluids have not been administered to replace the lost blood. Alternatively, the Hb concentration may be low in a patient with a normal red cell mass who has received excessive IV fluids, or the Hb concentration may be normal when the anemia is masked by the concomitant association of dehydration. Although the measurement of the red blood cell mass is technically feasible, it requires the use of radiolabelled RBCs in addition to being time-consuming and costly, thereby eliminating it from the clinical arena [4].

The etiologies of a decreased red cell mass or anemia can be separated into three broad categories: (1) increased losses; (2) decreased survival time – increased destruction; and (3) decreased production. In the perioperative period or the acutely ill patient, more than one of the factors may come into play. Various factors may account for acute blood loss in the perioperative period or in the intensive care unit (ICU) patient including traumatic injury, intraoperative and postoperative surgical losses, and hemorrhage unrelated to the surgical procedure. In the latter case, gastrointestinal (GI) hemorrhage represents the most common site of acute blood loss either from esophageal varices or stress ulceration. Although the incidence of GI bleeding in the perioperative period is generally low [5,6], specific patient populations are at risk including thermal injury, trauma, mechanically ventilated and transplant patients [7,8]. Other associated factors shown to potentially increase the incidence of GI blood loss in the ICU setting include elevated serum creatinine, absence of enteral nutrition and choice of pharmacologic agent for GI prophylaxis [9].

Another concern regarding acute blood loss is that it is not always visible. Even intraoperatively, blood may accumulate in the peritoneal or thoracic cavity and be hidden from vision, thereby making alterations in vital signs – a relatively late indicator of acute blood loss – the first noticeable change. Bleeding from nonsurgical sites are more likely to be hidden, thereby mandating that diagnostic tests be repeated at frequent intervals to identify acute blood loss. Various 'hidden' sites of bleeding are present including intrathoracic, intra-abdominal, in the GI tract and retroperitoneal. Perhaps the most common 'hidden' cause of blood loss in the ICU setting is repeated laboratory analysis. The latter can be particularly problematic in infants and young children since the amount of blood drawn from central and arterial lines (sample amount plus the 'waste' amount as the line is cleared) can be significant. Limiting laboratory analyses to essential testing, minimizing the amount of blood needed by the use of specialized laboratory equipment if available, and returning the 'waste' to the patient can help minimize this 'hidden' blood loss. These practices are frequently implemented in adult Jehovah's Witness patients to limit iatrogenic blood loss.

Anemia may also result from decreased production or accelerated destruction of RBCs. Hemolysis of RBCs can occur in a variety of conditions related to both immune and nonimmune factors. The presence of hemolysis as the cause of anemia can be diagnosed by signs of increased RBC turnover including hemoglobinuria, hyperbilirubinemia and decreased serum haptoglobin concentrations. These findings coexist with evidence of increased RBC production (increased reticulocyte count) provided that the patient's bone marrow is functioning adequately. As mentioned previously, especially in the perioprative period or the critical care setting, the patient's ability to respond to acute blood loss either from hemolysis or hemorrhage by augmenting erythropoiesis may be blunted, thereby imposing a production problem on top of acute blood loss or increased destruction. When RBCs are destroyed, the Hb molecule is converted to bilirubin, which is then conjugated via the hepatic glucuronyl transferase system to make it water-soluble and allow for biliary excretion. Prior to conjugation, the bilirubin is known as unconjugated or indirect while after conjugation, it is known as direct. In the presence of hemolysis without associated hepatic disease, the release of bilirubin overcomes the hepatic glucuronyl transferase system resulting in an increase in the free (unconjugated or indirect) bilirubin. This results in the clinical findings of scleral icterus and jaundice. With significant and rapid hemolysis, the concentration of the serum protein that binds free Hb, haptoglobin, decreases. Analysis of the serum haptoglobin concentration is readily available from most hospital laboratories. As the free Hb increases, the haptoglobin level decreases. When the Hb concentration exceeds the haptoglobin binding capacity, free Hb is filtered in the urine. Clinically this may appear as hematuria as the red color of Hb is indistinguishable from that of blood. Although urine can be checked for the presence of Hb, a more rapid method is to check the urine for blood, which will be positive while microscopic examination will fail to reveal any RBCs, thereby making the pigment either Hb or myoglobin. Excessive hemoglobinuria can cause renal failure as the Hb pigment crystallizes in the urine causing tubular obstruction. Treatment includes reversal of the inciting process and alkalinization of the urine to increase the amount of Hb that can exist in solution as well as maintaining urine output.

Various pathologic conditions, both intrinsic and extrinsic to the RBC, may result in increased destruction. Disease processes that are intrinsic to the RBC include acute infectious conditions (malaria), abnormalities of the

Hb molecule (hemoglobinopathies such as sickle cell disease or thalassemia), abnormalities of the RBC membrane (spherocytosis, paroxysmal nocturnal hemoglobinuria), enzymatic deficiencies (pyruvate kinase deficiency) and immune-mediated hemolytic disorders. The latter are diagnosed by the presence of antibodies directed against the RBCs either on the surface of the RBCs themselves (direct Coombs positive hemolytic anemia) or in the serum (indirect Coombs positive). Extrinsic causes of hemolysis include trauma to the RBCs from mechanical devices (intra-aortic balloon pump, extracorporeal circulation or mechanical heart valve), the rapid infusion of hypotonic fluids, and mechanical problems during the administration of blood products that can occur with the use of excessive pressure on the blood bag, administration of rapid rates through small-bore IV lines, or with the use of excessive suction for intraoperative blood salvage. Increased RBC destruction can also be seen in a number of pathologic conditions that result in passive congestion of the spleen. This process, known as hypersplenism, results in splenomegaly and trapping of platelets and RBCs with their accelerated destruction within the spleen.

The third potential mechanism responsible for anemia is decreased production. The hallmark of this condition is anemia with an absent or low reticulocyte count. Decreased production may be the result of an inadequate substrate (deficiency of iron, folate or vitamin B_{12}) for the production of RBCs, primary bone marrow failure related to an acute illness or marrow infiltration from a neoplastic process. Although commonly present in the ICU population, substrate deficiency may go unrecognized and therefore untreated as the anemia is attributed to other causes [10]. Iron deficiency may be present in up to one-third of patients admitted to the ICU [10] while other investigators have demonstrated nutritional issues (iron, folate or vitamin B_{12} deficiency) responsible for anemia in more than 10% of the ICU population [11].

Physiologic response to anemia: the critical hemoglobin value

In the presence of anemia, compensatory mechanisms are called into play to maintain an adequate oxygen delivery to the tissues. These mechanisms can compensate for significant decreases in the Hb concentration; however, eventually a point is reached whereby the compensatory mechanisms become exhausted and the oxygen consumption of the tissues become dependent on oxygen delivery. This is known as the critical Hb.

In the normal state, oxygen transport to the tissues is dependent on both convection and diffusion. Convection is controlled by the oxygen content of the blood (CaO_2), cardiac output (CO) and the distribution of blood flow (within and between the tissue beds). The latter can be illustrated by the peripheral vasoconstriction with the resultant decrease of blood flow to the skin and muscles that occurs to maintain blood flow to the vital organs when there is a decrease in CO, blood volume or Hb concentration. Diffusion is the primary factor regulating the movement of oxygen from the alveoli to the Hb molecule in the pulmonary capillaries and the delivery of oxygen from the Hb molecule to the tissues at the capillary level. In the peripheral tissues, oxygen delivery is determined by the diffusion gradient (difference between the oxygen tension of the capillary blood and the tissue bed), oxygen conductance of the tissue and the oxyhemoglobin affinity (status of the oxyhemoglobin dissociation curve) [12,13]. As the other factors (diffusion gradients of oxygen from the alveoli to the Hb molecule in the pulmonary capillary system and from the Hb molecule to tissue bed) cannot be readily altered, the primary factor that increases the uptake of oxygen at the alveolar capillary level and augments the delivery of oxygen at the tissue level is a shift of the oxyhemoglobin dissociation curve.

Several factors can affect the position of the oxyhemoglobin dissociation curve including body temperature, acid–base status, 2,3-diphosphoglycerate (2,3 DPG) levels and the Hb molecule itself. The latter factor rarely comes into play except in situations where there is something other that normal adult Hb present. This can rarely be a hemoglobinopathy (generally a 1-amino acid substitution) whereby there is a permanent shift of the oxyhemoglobin dissociation curve. Such conditions are exceedingly rare and not amenable to therapy. More importantly, fetal Hb (with two α- and two γ-chains) results in altered binding of 2,3 DPG and thereby in an inherent shift to the left of the oxyhemoglobin dissociation curve. This leftward shift or increased affinity of the Hb molecule for oxygen results in improved oxygen uptake at the pulmonary capillary level. This factor improves the oxygen uptake *in utero* with the normal low PaO_2 of 30–40 mmHg. This leftward shift of the oxyhemoglobin dissociation curve due to fetal Hb is the major reason given for the recommendation that isovolemic hemodilution not be used until after 6–9 months of life, a time when fetal Hb has been replaced by adult Hb.

When considering the oxyhemoglobin dissociation curve, its position relative to the normal state can be expressed as the P_{50} value or the partial pressure of oxygen at which Hb is 50% saturated. In the normal state at a body temperature of 37°C with a pH of 7.4, the P_{50} is 26.6 mmHg. This value increases as the affinity of the Hb molecule for oxygen decreases (rightward shift) and decreases when the affinity of the Hb molecule for oxygen increases (leftward shift). Factors that result in a rightward shift of the curve serve to improve the unloading of oxygen at the tissue level. This mechanism does not become operative until the Hct reaches 20% [14]. The mechanism responsible for the shift is an increase in 2,3-DPG in erythrocytes.

Even with an effective compensatory mechanism, all organisms will have a critical Hb value below which oxygen consumption becomes flow-dependent, indicating that the oxygen delivery to the tissues is failing to meet the clinical need. Despite the universal presence of this critical Hb concentration, there is no specific Hb concentration that can be identified as the value below which this problem will occur. Several modifying factors may increase or decrease this critical Hb threshold. In various laboratory animals (dogs and baboons), Hb levels as low as 3–5 g/dl can be tolerated without adverse effects [15–17]. However, the importance of modifying features is illustrated by the fact that when dogs with experimentally induced critical coronary stenosis were subjected to isovolemic hemodilution, electrocadiographic (ECG) evidence of ischemia was noted and myocardial dysfunction occurred at a Hb concentration of 6–7 g/dl instead of 3–5 g/dl [18]. Tranfusion with RBCs corrected both the ECG changes and the myocardial dysfunction [19].

Several mechanisms, both convection and conduction (see above), are activated to maintain tissue oxygen delivery as the Hb concentration decreases. These include increased CO, increased oxygen extraction at the tissue level and a rightward shift of the oxyhemoglobin dissociation curve. In the awake state, increased CO is due primarily to an increase in both stroke volume and heart rate. In the anesthetized state, stroke volume changes without a significant change in heart rate [20]. This effect is postulated to result from the effects of the anesthetic agents on the autonomic and cardiovascular systems. An increase in heart rate during general anesthesia in response to anemia is more likely to be a sign of hypovolemia or inadequate anesthesia.

Factors responsible for the increased stroke volume include decreased systemic vascular resistance and increased venous return due to reduced whole-blood viscosity with improved microcirculatory flow [21,22]. The increased venous return is reflected by an elevation of left ventricular enddiastolic pressure [23]. The reduced viscosity of the blood also results in a reduction of the systemic vascular resistance, thereby reducing afterload and improving left ventricular ejection [24,25]. Myocardial contractility increases, most likely because of activation of cardiac sympathetic fibers [22]. If intravascular volume is maintained, the CO increase remains stable over a prolonged period of time without adverse hemodynamic consequences [26]. Although the sympathetic nervous system is activated, it may play only a minor role in the actual increase in CO. The increase in CO with hemodilution does not require an intact autonomic system, as laboratory studies in dogs have demonstrated that it occurs following either cardiac denervation or β-adrenergic blockage [21,27].

With a decrease in the Hb concentration, there will be a compensatory increase in the plasma component of the blood. This alteration in the relationship between the red cell mass and the plasma volume alters blood viscosity and hence microcirculatory flow. The ratio of shear stress (force required to move a fluid) to shear rate (rate at which a fluid flows) defines viscosity. Fluids with a higher viscosity require a higher shear stress (force) to move. Fluids are considered Newtonian if they maintain a constant viscosity regardless of the velocity of the flow. In such cases, a change in force causes a proportional change in flow rate. Blood is not Newtonian because changes in flow rate produce a change in viscosity and therefore not a linear increase in flow velocity. Viscosity also changes disproportionately to changes in Hct, in that change in Hct is followed by an exponential increase or decrease in blood viscosity.

As arterial oxygen content and delivery decline, the oxygen extraction ratio increases, thereby lowering the mixed venous oxygen saturation. In the resting state, peripheral oxygen extraction does not increase until the Hct decreases to less than 20–25% [27,28]. This relationship holds true provided that hypovolemia does not occur. Although a decrease in the mixed venous oxygen generally occurs at a Hct of 15–20%, more severe degrees of hemodilution may be tolerated in the presence of normal cardiovascular reserve. Van Woerkins *et al.* [22] demonstrated a constant mixed venous partial pressure of oxygen and oxygen saturation in dogs hemodiluted to a mean Hct of $9.3 \pm 0.3\%$ with an exchange of 50 ml/kg of blood. In this animal model, CO doubled resulting in increased flow to all organs except the liver and adrenals. The greatest increase in flow occurred to the heart and brain. The increased flow rates and CO maintained oxygen delivery down to a Hct of 9%. Similar stability with extreme degrees of hemodilution have been demonstrated in clinical investigations. In a cohort of eight pediatric patients with a mean age of 12 years, Fontana *et al.* demonstrated no adverse effects with hemodilution to a mean Hb of 3.0 g/dl [29]. Mixed venous oxygen saturation decreased from $90.8 \pm 5.4\%$ to $72.3 \pm 7.8\%$ while oxygen extraction increased from $17.3 \pm 6.2\%$ to $44.4 \pm 5.9\%$. No adverse effects were noted despite the extreme degree of hemodilution.

The compensatory mechanisms to maintain oxygen delivery during hemodilution may not be possible in patients with underlying cardiorespiratory dysfunction. The lowest tolerable Hb concentration at which a decrease in the mixed venous oxygen tension occurs will also be influenced by the use of anesthetic agents and neuromuscular blocking agents. Although these agents decrease peripheral oxygen consumption, they may also blunt the compensatory cardiovascular mechanisms [30,31].

Although it would be convenient to have a single, specific Hb value to use as a transfusion trigger in patients, several variables play into the decision to transfuse or not. Of significant importance are factors that alter the patient's ability to compensate for the low Hb by increasing CO or factors that place the patients at risk for coronary ischemia when these compensatory cardiovascular responses are activated. Spahn *et al.* [32] examined left ventricular function following left anterior descending (LAD) coronary artery occlusion (decrease by 95% of the vessel's cross-sectional area) and hemodilution in dogs. Only a marginal decrease in function occurred with hemodilution down to a Hct of $24.4 \pm 0.1\%$. They concluded that although myocardial function is preserved with moderate hemodilution, the critical level of isovolemic hemodilution in the presence of a critical stenosis of a coronary vessel is between a Hct of 15% and 25%. Other factors that might compromise coronary blood flow include factors that alter the myocardial oxygen delivery/demand ratio such as decreased mean arterial pressure and left ventricular hypertrophy. Therefore, the minimal safe Hct in patients with compromised cardiac function is defined as the Hct at which coronary blood flow can no longer increase sufficiently to meet myocardial demand, which may be a difficult or impossible parameter to measure in the clinical arena. While hemodilution appears safe in patients with normal myocardial function, problems may arise in the presence of compromised cardiovascular function or alterations in coronary anatomy, especially if combined with tachycardia, decreased perfusion pressure or decrease in the Hct to less than 20%.

Risk-benefit of blood transfusion

Although blood banking technology has improved dramatically over the past 20 years, there remains a significant potential for morbidity and even mortality with the use of blood and blood products. Much of the concern of the lay public regarding blood transfusion has focused on the potential for the transmission of infectious diseases, particularly the acquired immunodeficiency syndrome (AIDS). The current screening methods for donated blood and blood products have significantly decreased the risk of transmission of infectious agents. With the implementation of human immunodeficiency virus (HIV) testing of blood products in March 1985, the number of HIV infections related to blood products decreased to 5 per year compared to 714 reported in the year prior to testing [33]. Implementation of routine screening by use of the p24 antigen has further increased the identification of potentially infected blood products, thereby decreasing the risk of transmission of HIV to less than 1 per million units of blood products [34]. Similar success has been achieved with decreasing the risk of the transmission of hepatitis (A, B and C) from blood products. Risks of the transmission of these diseases is estimated at 1 in 220 000 units for hepatitis B, 1 in 1 million units for hepatitis A and 1 in 1 million units for hepatitis C.

Other complications related to blood product administration include both hemolytic and nonhemolytic transfusion reactions. Hemolytic complications may be immune- or nonimmune-mediated. The classic immune-mediated hemolytic transfusion reaction results from an incompatibility between the administered RBCs and the patient, mostly as the result of clerical errors. Its incidence is roughly 1 in 33 000 units with a fatality rate of 1 patient for every 500 000 units [35,36]. The signs and symptoms of a hemolytic transfusion reaction are related to activation of the patient's humoral system by the fragmented RBCs. They vary depending on the amount of incompatible blood that has been transfused. In a conscious and awake patient, the signs and symptoms include chest pain, dyspnea, nausea, vomiting, fever and chills. In anesthetized or unconscious patients, the only signs and symptoms may be hemoglobinuria, coagulopathy or cardiovascular disturbances. Treatment begins by immediately stopping the transfusion. Serious sequelae of a transfusion reaction include hemoglobinuria with renal failure and activation of the coagulation cascade with disseminated intravascular coagulation (DIC). Treatment includes maintenance of an alkaline diuresis with fluid administration, loop diuretics and mannitol. Cardiovascular instability is treated with fluid administration and direct-acting adrenergic agents as needed. Respiratory insufficiency related to acute respiratory distress syndrome may require endotracheal intubation and controlled ventilation. DIC and coagulation defects are treated as needed based on the platelet count, prothrombin time, partial thromboplastin time and fibrinogen level. Documentation of the occurrence of a transfusion reaction is made by obtaining serum for free Hb level and a direct Coombs test.

Nonimmune hemolytic reactions result from external forces that damage the RBCs prior to, or during, their administration. These problems can be prevented by appropriate handling and administration of blood products. RBC lysis can be caused by exposure to hypertonic or hypotonic IV fluids, thermal injury during blood transport or storage, and inappropriate methods (e.g. placing the blood in warm water) of warming the blood. The signs and symptoms of nonimmune hemolytic transfusion reactions are dependent on the quantity of hemolyzed blood that is administered and in many cases resemble those seen with hemolytic transfusion reactions. Treatment in severe cases is the same as for immune-mediated hemolytic transfusion reactions.

One of the more commonly encountered problems occurring during the administration of blood products is fever (greater than $1°C$ rise in core body temperature). The concern is that fever may be the first sign of an immune-mediated hemolytic transfusion reaction. When fever develops, the transfusion should be discontinued and the patient examined for other signs and symptoms of a hemolytic transfusion reaction. It is uncommon for fever to be the only sign of a transfusion reaction. Other possible causes of fever during transfusion include bacterial contamination of the blood product and a febrile nonhemolytic transfusion reaction (an FNHTR). An FNHTR occurs most commonly in patients who receive numerous transfusions and remains the most common cause of fever during a transfusion. The diagnosis is one of exclusion by eliminating the possibility of a hemolytic transfusion reaction and bacterial contamination of the transfused blood product. The incidence of an FNHTR is related to the patient's history of previous exposure to blood products and the specific component used (1% of packed RBCs vs. 20–30% of platelets). An FNHTR is an immune-mediated reaction related to the presence of antibodies in the recipient's plasma to white blood cell (WBC) antigens. The antibody–antigen reaction leads to the release of endogenous pyrogens from the WBCs. The incidence and symptoms of an FNHTR can be reduced by decreasing the WBC content of RBCs by using filters that remove leukocytes from the blood or by pretreating the patient with antihistamines and antipyretics. In many institutions, there has been a recent move toward the use of leukocyte-depletion filters for all packed RBCs to eliminate the occurrence of an FNHTRs. In many cases, this is performed in the blood bank since the use of these filters during transfusion can significantly slow the rate at which the blood is transfused.

Additional complications of transfusion, the incidence of which increase with the number of units administered, include hypothermia, metabolic alterations (hypocalcemia, acidosis, hyperkalemia), shift of the oxyhemoglobin dissociation curve and coagulation disturbances. With the administration of more than 10–15 ml/kg of any blood product over less than 1 h, use of a standard blood-warming device should be considered to avoid inadvertent hypothermia. After 2–3 weeks of storage, potassium concentrations of packed RBCs may reach levels of 20–30 meq/L. Although there is a limited amount of plasma contained in packed RBCs, its rapid administration (≥ 100 ml/min) can limit the time for potassium elimination and redistribution. The ECG should be monitored for signs of hyperkalemia during massive transfusions. In patients with renal dysfunction or preexisting hyperkalemia, RBCs can be washed prior to administration to remove the excess plasma and hence lower the potassium concentration. A second metabolic consequence of massive transfusion is hypocalcemia related to the binding of calcium by the citrate used as an anticoagulant. Following the transfusion of 15–25 ml/kg of packed RBCs, ionized calcium levels should be monitored and replacement therapy provided as needed. With a slower transfusion rate, the citrate is metabolized in the liver. Hepatic dysfunction may lead to a slower metabolism of citrate and thereby place the patient at greater risk of citrate toxicity. Signs and symptoms of hypocalcemia include a prolongation of the QT interval on the ECG, hypotension and impaired myocardial contractility. The latter effects may be magnified by associated acidosis and hypothermia. In addition to binding calcium, citrate also binds magnesium, leading to hypomagnesemia [37]. The latter may impair the normal regulatory responses to hypocalcemia including release of parathormone.

Packed RBCs also become more acidotic as time passes related to the citrate used as an anticoagulant and the normal metabolic processes of the RBCs and the production of lactate. With rapid administration, there may be inadequate time for the buffering of the acid load. Periodic measurement of arterial or venous blood gases and correction of the acidosis with sodium bicarbonate may be needed. The issues of hyperkalemia and acidosis have led some hospitals' blood banking committees to institute protocols suggesting the use of relatively fresh blood (less than 7–10 days) in neonates and infants who may be less able to tolerate and compensate the acid and potassium load.

Other patients may require the irradiation of blood products prior to their administration. The irradiation of blood products inactivates viable lymphocytes. Without such treatment, these lymphocytes can activate host defenses against the recipient leading to graft-versus-host disease. The latter may occur in patients with altered cellular immunity related to congenital defects (DiGeorge syndrome) or chemotherapeutic and immunosuppressive regimens. Irradiation of blood products should also be considered in premature and even term infants as cellular immune function may be immature. Irradiation of blood products requires appropriate equipment, which most blood banking facilities have and can be accomplished in a matter of minutes. No significant alteration in the integrity or composition of the blood product occurs other than an increase in the potassium concentration [38].

Recent clinical investigations have more thoroughly evaluated the potential role of blood product administration on the host's immune system. While the immunosuppressive effects of transfusion were once thought beneficial in the transplant recipient, given the decreased risk of rejection in previously transfused patients, it has now become apparent that the hidden danger of blood product administration may be its potential for causing immunosuppression and resulting in an increased incidence of nosocomial infections. Recent investigations into the potential adverse clinical impact of the immunomodulatory effects of blood products have demonstrated an increased incidence of nosocomial infections and cancer recurrence in transfused patients [39,40]. The increased incidence of infection in the postoperative arena has been demonstrated in patients undergoing orthopedic, abdominal and cardiac procedures [41–43]. These infections have been shown to increase morbidity and mortality as well as the length of ICU stay and hospital costs. Although the potential deleterious role of immunosuppression related to allogeneic blood products is not fully accepted by all experts in the field of transfusion medicine, these data appear to be striking enough that it should be given consideration when evaluating the risk/benefit ratio of transfusion therapy. Further credence to this phenomenon is provided by studies demonstrating that the leukocyte depletion of packed RBCs may be effective in eliminating these problems [44].

Summary

In higher organisms, diffusion is not capable of meeting the oxygen demands of the tissues because of the constraints of time and distance. Evolution has provided a mechanism whereby oxygen can be delivered to tissues by the means of a transfer system that includes an oxygen-binding component (Hb) and a pump – the cardiovascular system – to deliver this compound to the peripheral tissues. Although normal Hb levels range from 12 to 14 g/dl, like many other systems, a redundancy is built in to allow for protection when homeostasis is altered. Recent years have seen a move toward limitation of blood products. This interest was initially sparked by concerns of the transmission of infectious diseases from the administration of allogeneic blood products. Despite the increased safety of the blood pool with improved screening for the presence of infectious pathogens, a renewed interest in bloodless surgery has been created by data suggesting the potential immunosuppressive effects of allogeneic blood products with the potential for increased nosocomial infections and cancer recurrence.

As to what is the transfusion level or trigger Hb, each patient must be considered individually based on the association of comorbid features. In the absence of end-organ dysfunction or disease, clinical data suggest that patients may tolerate a Hb as low as 5–6 g/dl while higher values of 7–8 g/dl may be needed in patients with end-organ issues, especially cardiovascular disease and the risk of coronary ischemia.

References

1 Jelkmann W. Erythropoietin: structure, control of production, and function. *Physiol Rev* 1992; **72**: 449–89.
2 Ebert BL, Bunn HF. Regulation of the erythropoietin gene. *Blood* 1999; **94**: 1864–77.
3 Greenberg AG. Pathophysiology of anemia. *Am J Med* 1996; **101**: 7S–11S.
4 Vincent JL, Sakr Y, Creteur J. Anemia in the intensive care unit. *Can J Anaesth* 2003; **50**: S53–S59.
5 Pimentel M, Roberts DE, Bernstein CN *et al*. Clinically significant gastrointestinal bleeding in critically ill patients in an era of GI prophylaxis. *Am J Gastroenterol* 2000; **95**: 2801–6.
6 Devlin JW, Ben Menachem T, Ulep SK *et al*. Stress ulcer prophylaxis in medical ICU patients: annual utilization in relation to the incidence of endoscopically proven stress ulceration. *Ann Pharmacother* 1998; **32**: 869–74.
7 Czaja AJ, McAlhany JC, Pruitt BA Jr. Acute gastrointestinal disease after thermal injury: an endoscopic evaluation of incidence and natural history. *N Engl J Med* 1974; **291**: 925–9.
8 Schiessel R, Starlinger M, Wolf A *et al*. Failure of cimetidine to prevent gastroduodenal ulceration and bleeding after renal transplantation. *Surgery* 1981; **90**: 456–8.
9 Cook D, Heyland D, Griffith L *et al*. Risk factors for clinically important upper gastrointestinal bleeding in patients requiring mechanical ventilation. *Crit Care Med* 1999; **27**: 2812–17.
10 Streiff RR. Anemia and nutritional deficiency in the acutely ill hospitalized patients. *Med Clin North Am* 1993; **77**: 911–89.
11 Rodriguez RM, Corwin HL, Gettinger A *et al*. Nutritional deficiencies and blunted erythropoietin response as causes of the anemia of critical illness. *J Crit Care* 2001; **16**: 36–41.
12 Groebe K, Thews G. Basic mechanisms of diffusive and diffusion-related oxygen transport in biological systems: a review. *Adv Exp Med Biol* 1992; **317**: 21–33.
13 Trouwburst A, Van Woerkins ECSM, Tenbrinck R. Hemodilution and oxygen transport. *Adv Exp Med Biol* 1992; **317**: 431–40.
14 Sunder-Plassman L, Kessler M, Jesch F. Acute normovolemic hemodilution: changes in tissue oxygen supply and hemoglobin-oxygen affinity. *Bibl Haematol* 1975; **41**: 44–53.
15 Levine E, Rosen A, Sehgal L *et al*. Physiologic effects of acute anemia: implications for a reduced transfusion trigger. *Transfusion* 1990; **30**: 11–14.
16 Wilkerson DK, Rosen AL, Sehgal LR *et al*. Limits of cardiac compensation in anemia baboons. *Surgery* 1988; **103**: 665–70.
17 Geha AS. Coronary and cardiovascular dynamics and oxygen availability during acute normovolemic anemia. *Surgery* 1976; **80**: 47–53.

18 Geha AS, Baue AE. Graded coronary stenosis and coronary flow during acute normovolemic hemodilution. *World J Surg* 1978; **2**: 645–52.

19 Anderson HT, Kessinger JM, McFarland WJ Jr *et al.* The response of hypertrophied heart to acute anemia and coronary stenosis. *Surgery* 1978; **84**: 8–15.

20 Ickx BE, Rigolet M, Van der Linden P. Cardiovascular and metabolic response to acute normovolemic anemia: effects of anesthesia. *Anesthesiology* 2000; **93**: 1011–16.

21 Glick G, Plauth WH, Braunwald E. Role of the autonomic nervous system in the circulatory response to acutely induced anemia in unanesthetized dogs. *J Clin Invest* 1964; **43**: 2112–24.

22 Van Woerkins J, Trouborst A, Duncker DJ. Catecholamines and regional hemodynamics during isovolemic hemodilution alone and in combination with adenosine-induced controlled hypotension. *J Appl Phys* 1992; **72**: 760–9.

23 Guyton AC, Richardson TQ. Effect of hematocrit on venous return. *Circ Res* 1961; **9**: 157–65.

24 Crystal GJ, Rooney MW, Salem MR. Regional hemodynamics and oxygen supply during isovolemic hemodilution alone and in combination with adenosine-induced controlled hypotension. *Anesth Analg* 1988; **67**: 211–18.

25 Laks H, Pilon RN, Klovekorn WP *et al.* Acute normovolemic hemodilution: effects on hemodynamics, oxygen, transport, and lung water in anesthetized man. *Surg Forum* 1974; **180**: 103–9.

26 Bowens C, Spahn DR, Frasco PE *et al.* Hemodilution induces stable changes in global cardiovascular and regional myocardial function. *Anesth Analg* 1993; **76**: 1027–32.

27 Tarnow J, Eberlein HJ, Hess E *et al.* Hemodynamic interactions of hemodilution anaesthesia, propranolol pretreatment and hypovolemia – I: systemic circulation. *Basic Res Cardiol* 1979; **74**: 109–22.

28 Robertie PG, Gravlee GP. Safe limits of isovolemic hemodilution and recommendation for erythrocyte transfusion. *Int Anesthesiol Clin* 1990; **28**: 197–203.

29 Fontana JL, Welborn L, Mongan PD *et al.* Oxygen consumption and cardiovascular function in children during profound intraoperative normovolemic hemodilution. *Anesth Analg* 1995; **80**: 219–25.

30 Van der Linden P, De Hert S, Mathieu N *et al.* Tolerance to acute hemodilution: effect of anesthetic depth. *Anesthesiology* 2003; **99**: 97–104.

31 Gillies IDS. Anemia and anaesthesia. *Br J Anaesth* 1974; **46**: 589–602.

32 Spahn DR, Smith LR, McRae RL, Leone BJ. Effects of acute isovolemic hemodilution and anesthesia on regional function in left ventricular myocardium with compromised coronary blood flow. *Acta Anaesthesiol Scand* 1992; **36**: 628–36.

33 Selik RM, Ward JW, Buehler JW. Trends in transfusion-associated acquired immune deficiency syndrome in the United States. *Transfusion* 1993; **33**: 890–3.

34 Schreiber GB, Busch MP, Kleinman SH *et al.* The risk of transfusion-transmitted viral infections. *N Engl J Med* 1996; **334**: 1685–90.

35 Linden JV, Kaplan HS. Transfusion errors: cause and effects. *Trans Med Rev* 1994; **8**: 169–83.

36 Linden JV, Tourault MA, Schribner CL. Decrease in frequency of transfusion fatalities. *Transfusion* 1997; **37**: 243–4.

37 McLellan B, Reid R, Lane P. Massive blood transfusion causing hypomagnesemia. *Crit Care Med* 1984; **12**: 146–7.

38 Rivet C, Baxter A, Rock G. Potassium levels in irradiated blood. *Transfusion* 1989; **29**: 185–6.

39 Vamvakas EC. Transfusion-associated cancer recurrence and postoperative infection: meta-analysis of randomized, controlled clinical trials. *Transfusion* 1996; **36**: 175–86.

40 Amato AC, Pescatori M. Effect of perioperative blood transfusion on recurrence of colorectal cancer: meta-analysis stratified on risk factors. *Dis Colon Rectum* 1998; **41**: 570–85.

41 Innerhofer P, Walleczek C, Luz G *et al*. Transfusion of buffy coat-depleted blood components and risk of postoperative infection in orthopedic patients. *Transfusion* 1999; **39**: 625–32.

42 Houbiers JG, van de Velde CJ, Pahlplatz P *et al*. Transfusion of red cells is associated wit increased incidence of bacterial infection after colorectal surgery: a prospective study. *Transfusion* 1997; **37**: 126–34.

43 Ryan T, McCarthy JF, Rady MY *et al*. Early bloodstream infection after cardiopulmonary bypass: frequency rate, risk factors, and implications. *Crit Care Med* 1997; **25**: 2009–14.

44 Jensen LS, Kissmeyer Nielsen P, Wolff B *et al*. Randomized comparison of leucocyte-depleted versus buffy coat poor blood transfusion and complications after colorectal surgery. *Lancet* 1996; **348**: 841–5.

CHAPTER 7

Postoperative Management in Transfusion-Free Medicine and Surgery in the ICU

Jean-Louis Vincent

Introduction

Recent studies have shown that as many as 30% of intensive care unit (ICU) patients receive a transfusion at some point during their ICU stay [1,2], the rationale being that blood transfusion can help restore and maintain oxygen delivery. However, the decisions regarding when and how much to transfuse are largely subjective, with little objective evidence to support any particular global transfusion trigger. Traditionally many physicians have used cut-off values of a hemoglobin (Hb) concentration of < 10 g/dl or a hematocrit (Hct) of $< 30\%$ as transfusion triggers, although studies in patients who refuse blood transfusions have shown that most deaths related to anemia occur only when the Hb concentration falls below much lower levels [3]. With the concerns about possible negative effects of transfusion, particularly disease transmission and immunosuppression, many intensivists are reevaluating their reasons for transfusion and the traditional transfusion triggers have come under intense scrutiny. Indeed, with recent evidence suggesting that more restrictive transfusion protocols may be beneficial [1,4], and continuing concerns about blood use, availability, safety and quality, not to mention escalating costs and restrictions on who can donate blood, physicians and managers are paying increasing attention to the concept of transfusion-free medicine and surgery.

This chapter briefly discusses the impact of blood transfusion on oxygen transport, the concept of 'optimal' Hb with currently suggested transfusion thresholds, strategies to reduce iatrogenic blood loss and clinical strategies to reduce oxygen consumption.

Anemia in the ICU

Anemia is common in the ICU patient, and its etiology can be varied. Causes can be broadly divided as blood loss, reduced RBC production and increased

RBC destruction (hemolysis or sequestration), although in reality many ICU patients with anemia will have a mixture of these conditions. Hemorrhage is perhaps the most common cause of anemia occurring intra- and postoperatively in the ICU patient. However, while gastrointestinal hemorrhage or posttraumatic and postsurgical hemorrhage are usually clearly apparent, other less obvious forms of hemorrhage, for example intramuscular, retroperitoneal or intrapleural hemorrhage, may occur as complications of various ICU interventions including central venous catheterization and liver biopsy, and may be less easily detected.

Another important, and often neglected, cause of blood loss, which may contribute to transfusion requirements, especially in the ICU patient [5], is repeated blood sampling [5–8]. Early observational studies of phlebotomy in the USA reported an average blood sampling volume of 41.5 ml/day in medical-surgical ICUs [5]. A survey of ICUs in Great Britain found an average admitting day phlebotomy of 85.3 ml, followed by an average daily phlebotomy of 66.1 ml [9]. Corwin *et al.* [8] noted that in 142 transfused patients the average blood sampling volume was 61–70 ml/day, and that phlebotomy accounted for almost 30% of the total blood transfused. More recently, in the ABC study [1], the mean volume per blood draw was 10.3 ml, with an average total daily volume of 41.1 ml. A recent observational study of phlebotomy in German ICUs similarly found an initial median phlebotomy of 41.1 ml/day and reported that the total amount of diagnostic blood loss was the most significant independent predictor of later transfusion [10]. In the ABC study [1], there was a significant positive correlation between organ dysfunction and the number of blood draws and the total amount of blood drawn per day, possibly placing the sickest patients at increased risk for worse anemia and the attendant risks of transfusion [11].

Various strategies to limit such blood loss have been suggested [11] including the use of smaller (pediatric) sampling tubes [12,13], blood conservation devices [14], reduced volumes of discarded blood [15] and educational programs [16,17]. In a prospective controlled pilot clinical trial, introduction of a multifaceted blood conservation strategy with strategies combining small-volume phlebotomy tubes, point-of-care bedside microanalysis, closed no-waste sampling systems, elimination of standing daily repeat phlebotomies, iterative caregiver education, audit, feedback and academic detailing resulted in an 87.5% reduction of initial sample discard, 40.5% reduction in complete blood count phlebotomy volume, 26.4% reduction in chemistry phlebotomy volume and 31.2% reduction in coagulation phlebotomy volume, compared with the usual practice group. Patients treated with the restrictive diagnostic phlebotomy and blood conservation strategy were also significantly less likely to receive packed red blood cell (RBC) transfusions during their ICU stay [11]. Physicians need to be aware not only of the risks of iatrogenic blood loss and measures by which the volumes involved can be reduced but also of the possibility of being challenged to rationalize their request for a blood sample in the first place.

A recent study in nonbleeding ICU patients showed that Hb concentrations typically decline by at least 0.5 g/dl/day during the first 3 days of an ICU stay and continue to decline for patients with sepsis and higher severity of illness [18]. In patients who stayed longer than 3 days on the ICU, the fall in Hb was greater over the first 3 days than for subsequent days (0.66 ± 0.84 g/dl/day vs. 0.12 ± 0.29 g/dl/day, < 0.01), and after the third day was directly related to the severity of disease as assessed by the APACHE (acute physiology and chronic health evaluation) II and SOFA (Sequential Organ Failure Assessment) scores [18]. Interestingly, in nonseptic patients, the fall in Hb concentration levelled out after the third ICU day, while in septic patients, Hb concentrations continued to decrease (Figure 7.1). The reasons suggested by the authors for this difference between septic and nonseptic patients include increased blood taking and invasive procedures in these sicker patients, and decreased RBC survival and a blunted erythropoietin (EPO) response as a result of the active inflammatory response to infection [18].

Role of transfusion in resuscitation

The function of Hb is, in essence, to carry oxygen around the body and release it where it is (most) needed. The characteristics of Hb allow it to take on oxygen in the lungs and unload it at the tissue level. The oxygen-carrying capacity of Hb is represented by the familiar sinusoidal oxyhemoglobin dissociation curve. The amount of oxygen delivered to the tissues (DO_2) is the product of the cardiac output (CO) and the arterial oxygen content (CaO_2).

$$DO_2 = CO \times CaO_2$$

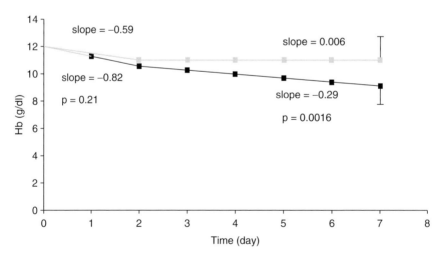

Figure 7.1 Changes in hemoglobin concentrations over time in septic (bottom line), and nonseptic (top line) patients. (*Source*: Reproduced from [18] with permission.)

Generally, the majority of oxygen is transported on Hb and the CaO_2 thus approximates to the Hb saturation. Increasing the concentration of Hb would be expected to increase DO_2 as has been demonstrated in several studies [19], and is the basic rationale behind blood transfusion [20]. However, while blood transfusion increases Hb concentration and DO_2, this does not necessarily mean that oxygen uptake (VO_2) and hence oxygen availability to the tissues is increased. Indeed, relatively few studies have evaluated the effect of blood transfusion on oxygenation parameters [21] and those that have, have shown no consistent effect on VO_2 [22,23]. The relationship 'increased hemoglobin = improved oxygenation' is thus not quite as simple as one might initially expect. First, the ability of Hb to download oxygen may vary in different disease processes, with, for example, microcirculatory factors such as RBC deformability and altered oxygen extraction capabilities influencing the transfer of oxygen from Hb in sepsis. Second, for transfused blood, the duration of storage prior to transfusion may limit the ability of Hb to deliver oxygen [24]. Third, by increasing viscosity, a rise in Hb may restrict micro-circulatory flow and limit the ability of Hb to reach the tissues [1].

However, severe anemia carries its own risks, including delayed wound healing and increased incidence of cardiac arrhythmias, and is associated with worse outcomes [25]. The problem is thus to determine at which point the risks of transfusion are outweighed by the risks of anemia – the so-called transfusion trigger. Until relatively recently, many physicians would have said their cut-off was an Hb concentration of around 10 g/dl, and below this level they were likely to transfuse. This common practice has, however, been challenged in recent years, largely by the results of a randomized controlled trial conducted between 1994 and 1997 in which a more restrictive transfusion protocol (transfusions given when the Hb concentration dropped below 7.0 g/dl and Hb concentrations maintained at 7.0–9.0 g/dl) was at least as, and possibly more, effective than a more conservative approach (transfusions given when the Hb concentration fell below 10.0 g/dl and Hb concentrations maintained at 10.0–12.0 g/dl) [4]. Although overall, 30-day mortality was similar in the two groups, the rates were significantly lower with the restrictive transfusion strategy among patients who were less acutely ill (APACHE II score of ≤ 20), and among younger patients (less than 55 years of age), except for patients with clinically significant cardiac disease. An observational study in Europe, the ABC study, conducted several years later in 1999, also noted that transfused ICU patients had higher mortality rates than patients who were not transfused [1], even when organ dysfunction scores were taken into account. In this study, a transfusion during the ICU stay increased the risk of death by a factor of 1.37 (95% confidence interval, 1.02–1.84).

However, another more recent observational study in Europe (the SOAP study), along the same lines as the ABC study, failed to demonstrate any increased mortality rates with transfusion [2]. These apparently conflicting results may, in fact, be related to the favorable effects of deleukocytation [26], which was only used regularly by 46% of ICUs in the ABC study, but is now instituted routinely in most European hospitals. A randomized controlled trial similar to that conducted by Hebert *et al.* [4] in the mid-1990s is currently ongoing to try to determine whether these early results still stand or whether widespread use of deleukocyted blood has reduced some of the adverse effects of transfusion on outcome.

Monitoring the adequacy of oxygenation

One of the challenges in assessing the need for transfusion is that, while all would agree that the prime goal of transfusion is to improve DO_2 and ensure that sufficient oxygen is delivered to cater for tissue requirements, we are hampered by the lack of a perfect, or even relatively good, means of measuring and monitoring tissue oxygenation, in particular regional oxygenation believed to be an important factor in the development of multiple organ failure. The need for transfusion will vary according to patients and depending on the underlying etiology of the shock, but as yet there is no precise means of determining when the desired goal, – restored and adequate tissue oxygenation – has been reached. Thus, while measurable global oxygenation parameters may be apparently normal, regional oxygenation may remain impaired. Importantly, attempts to increase CO and DO_2 to 'supranormal' levels with combinations of fluids, transfusions and vasoactive agents have been largely unsuccessful in mixed groups of critically ill patients [27,28], although many have a place in specific patients groups, stressing the need for full assessment and evaluation of each patient with treatment titrated to the individual.

Proposed markers to assess the adequacy of oxygenation include CO, mixed venous oxygen saturation (SvO_2) and blood lactate levels. Regional methods include gastric tonometry and more recent orthogonal polarization spectral (ops) imaging techniques, but these remain experimental at present.

Cardiac output

With a pulmonary artery catheter (PAC) in place, CO can be estimated by the thermodilution method. CO can now be monitored almost continuously using specially adapted PACs, equipped with a thermal filament positioned some 20 cm from the catheter tip. Although concerns have been raised about the safety of the PAC [29] and various less invasive methods are being promoted [30], these remain relatively untested and all have their limitations. In addition, many of the concerns related to PAC use can be abated if sufficient care is taken in placement and the data received are interpreted and applied correctly [31].

The CO can be said to represent total body blood flow, but offers no information on the blood flow reaching individual organs. In addition, CO varies significantly according to individual characteristics and oxygen requirements; for example, in sepsis a 'normal' or even high CO may be insufficient because of the increased oxygen requirements caused by the sepsis process. CO must therefore never be interpreted as an isolated parameter but in the light of various other factors including SvO_2.

SvO_2

SvO_2 is the oxygen saturation of the Hb in the mixed venous blood, and must be measured in the pulmonary artery. From the Fick equation, VO_2 is the product of the CO and the arteriovenous oxygen difference. If the amount of oxygen dissolved in the blood is ignored, the equation can be rearranged to:

$$SvO_2 = SaO_2 - [VO_2/(CO \times 13.9 \times Hb)]$$

where SaO_2 is the arterial oxygen saturation (13.9 is a constant value related to the amount of oxygen bound to 1 g Hb, multiplied by 10 to correspond with a VO_2 in ml/min). In the critically ill patient, a normal SvO_2 is considered to be about 70%. If the patient is not anemic or hypoxemic, the SvO_2 reflects the relationship between CO and VO_2. However, both anemia and hypoxemia are common in ICU patients, and SvO_2 must be seen as complementing rather than replacing CO data.

If a PAC is not in place, central venous oxygen saturation ($ScvO_2$) has been suggested as a surrogate marker of SvO_2. Indeed, Rivers *et al.* [32] showed improved survival in patients in whom resuscitation was targeted at $ScvO_2$ values.

O_2ER

An increase in tissue oxygen demands can be met by an increase in CO, in oxygen extraction or in both. In the normal, healthy individual increased oxygen demands are met by combined increases in both CO and oxygen extraction. In the critically ill patient, various processes such as sepsis can increase tissue oxygen demands, and if the CO is unable to respond adequately, tissue oxygen extraction will increase disproportionately to meet the patient's oxygen demands, with a resultant fall in the SvO_2. As DO_2 falls, oxygen extraction increases to maintain oxygen demand until this compensatory mechanism becomes insufficient and VO_2 starts to fall (VO_2/DO_2 dependency) with resulting inadequate tissue oxygenation.

The O_2ER is the ratio of VO_2 to DO_2 and is simple to calculate and independent of Hb concentration.

$$O_2ER = VO_2/DO_2 = (SaO_2 - SvO_2)/SaO_2$$

Plotting consecutive data points on a graph of cardiac index (CI) against O_2ER, and relating them to isopleths of VO_2 can be used to identify whether a patient has reached the point of VO_2/DO_2 dependency. The diagram can also be used to interpret CO values in various groups of patients and to evaluate a patient's response to treatment. In anemic patients, tolerance to anemia is due to increases in CI and O_2ER, which maintain VO_2. While a high CI in an anemic patient may appear adequate, the cardiac response may nevertheless be inadequate for the degree of anemia. The relationship be-tween CI and O_2ER can help interpret the CI in such situations [33]. In patients with anemia and normal cardiac function, a CI/O_2ER ratio < 10 suggests an inadequate CI, which is due either to hypovolemia or to altered myocardial function (Figure 7.2); if there is no evidence of altered cardiac function in these patients, it is likely that they are hypovolemic [33].

Patients with compromised cardiac function

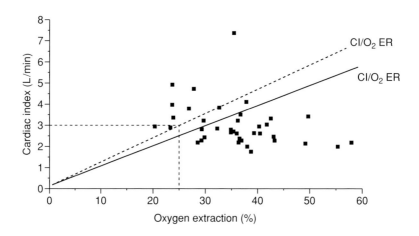

Patients with normal cardiac function

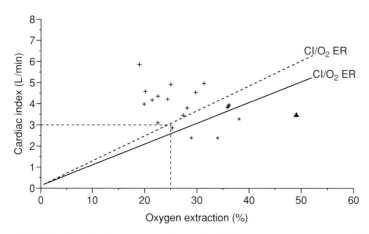

Figure 7.2 Relationship between cardiac index (CI) and oxygen extraction (O_2ER) in patients with compromised (upper panel) and normal (lower panel) cardiac function. * = three patients with concomitant hypovolemia; Δ = one patient with severe myocardial depression due to sepsis. (*Source*: Adapted from [33] with permission).

Blood lactate

As tissue oxygenation becomes inadequate and VO_2 becomes DO_2-dependent, anaerobic metabolism begins to play an increasingly important role and blood lactate levels rise [34]. While other causes of hyperlactatemia, including prolonged seizures, alcohol intoxication and extensive neoplastic disease, must be excluded, these are rare and a blood lactate level greater than 2 meq/L suggests inadequate tissue perfusion and oxygenation. Hyperlactatemia has been clearly associated with a poorer prognosis in various groups of critically ill patients [35], even in sepsis where other causes of hyperlactatemia may be present in addition to tissue hypoxia [36,37]. Importantly, serial blood lactate levels are of greater significance than any individual value.

Regional markers of tissue oxygenation

All of the above provide an indication of the global adequacy of tissue oxygenation, but no indication of local perfusion or oxygenation. In an attempt to provide more local data, gastric tonometry was developed, and calculation or measurement of gastric intramucosal pH (pHi) or PCO_2 has been extensively studied. However, while these measures have been shown to correlate with outcome [38–40], studies targeted at correcting these variables have shown no beneficial effects of such an approach on survival [41]. Other methods, including sublingual PCO_2 monitoring or OPS techniques, may prove to be of use, but are still experimental [42].

Reducing transfusion requirements

In certain patients, notably Jehovah's Witness (JW) patients, who refuse a blood transfusion, attempts must clearly be made to minimize blood loss, including iatrogenic loss. Techniques to limit intraoperative blood loss, including normovolemic hemodilution, controlled hypotensive anesthesia, meticulous hemostasis and red cell salvaging devices, have been dealt with in another chapter. The postoperative management of these patients may include other specific strategies to maximize DO_2 and minimize oxygen consumption, although there are few data, other than case reports and series, on the actual benefits of these strategies in anemic ICU patients.

Minimizing oxygen consumption

Deliberate mild hypothermia has been used to reduce oxygen consumption in JW patients, with a proposed target core temperature of 30–32°C [43]. While reducing oxygen consumption, blood viscosity is, however, increased, which may compromise DO_2, and hemodilution is thus often employed simultaneously. Neuromuscular blockade with sedation, intubation and mechanical ventilation can also reduce oxygen consumption. Neuromuscular blockade may be of particular use in the shivering patient as shivering can increase oxygen consumption considerably; however, the effects of neuromuscular blockade on oxygen consumption are not consistent in all patients [44]. In addition, prolonged paralysis or excessive sedation has its own risks, including an increased incidence of polyneuropathy.

Increasing cardiac output

As oxygen delivery is the product of CO and CaO_2, strategies to improve DO_2 can also include an increase in CO and dissolved oxygen. Intravascular volume and CO must be maintained at optimal to ensure adequate tissue perfusion and oxygenation. Dobutamine may be used to increase the force of contraction. Hyperbaric oxygen therapy can improve tissue DO_2 and has been used in severely anemic JW patients [45], although the potential benefit of such therapy must be weighed against the logistic problems and risks of this treatment modality that include oxygen toxicity and barotrauma. Hb-based oxygen carriers may have a place in the future management of such patients [46], and with recombinant technology are acceptable to most JW patients.

Erythropoietin

Under normal conditions, about 1% of circulating RBCs are renewed each day, but following acute blood loss, the rate of erythropoiesis can increase up to tenfold [47]. The principal regulator of erythropoiesis is the hormone EPO. Endogenous EPO stimulates the production and maturation of erythroid progenitor cells, and causes the premature release of a variety of cells, including reticulocytes, from the marrow. The most potent stimuli for EPO release are anemia and hypoxia. In the critically ill patient, the normal EPO response may be blunted [48,49], contributing to the anemia seen in these patients. These findings have led to the suggestion that EPO may be useful in the prevention of anemia in critically ill patients. In the only randomized controlled trial of EPO in adult ICU patients, 40 000 units of recombinant human EPO, given subcutaneously on day 3 of the ICU admission and weekly thereafter for a maximum of four doses, was associated with a reduced need for transfusion and an increase in Hb concentration [50]. The potentially beneficial effects of EPO on Hct may be particularly useful in JW patients [51]; however, this therapy is expensive and remains controversial, and further study is required to determine its effectiveness and optimal dosing in such patients.

Importantly, normal erythrocyte development also depends on adequate supplies of iron, folate and vitamin B12, and nutritional supplements of these products must be given routinely to such patients. Vitamin C may also help by improving iron absorption.

Conclusion

Anemia is common in the critically ill patient, particularly after surgery, and is associated with worse outcomes. However, strategies can be employed to limit the development of anemia including minimizing iatrogenic blood loss and oxygen consumption. Exogenous EPO and Hb-based oxygen carriers will be used increasingly in transfusion-free surgery, but further study is needed to determine their precise role.

REFERENCES

1 Vincent JL, Baron JF, Reinhart K *et al*. Anemia and blood transfusion in critically ill patients. *JAMA* 2002; **288**: 1499–507.
2 Vincent JL, Sakr Y, Le Gall J-R *et al*. Is red blood cell transfusion associated with worse outcome? Results of the SOAP study. *Chest* 2003; **124**: 125S (abstract).
3 Viele MK, Weiskopf RB. What can we learn about the need for transfusion from patients who refuse blood? The experience with Jehovah's Witnesses. *Transfusion* 1994; **34**: 396–401.
4 Hebert PC, Wells G, Blajchman MA *et al*. A multicenter, randomized, controlled clinical trial of transfusion requirements in critical care. *N Engl J Med* 1999; **340**: 409–17.
5 Smoller BR, Kruskall MS. Phlebotomy for diagnostic laboratory tests in adults: pattern of use and effect on transfusion requirements. *N Engl J Med* 1986; **314**: 1233–5.
6 Eyster E, Bernene J. Nosocomial anemia. *JAMA* 1973; **223**: 73–4.
7 Henry ML, Garner WL, Fabri PJ. Iatrogenic anemia. *Am J Surg* 1986; **151**: 362–3.
8 Corwin HL, Parsonnet KC, Gettinger A. RBC transfusion in the ICU: is there a reason? *Chest* 1995; **108**: 767–71.
9 Tarpey J, Lawler PG. Iatrogenic anaemia? A survey of venesection in patients in the intensive therapy unit. *Anaesthesia* 1990; **45**: 396–8.
10 von Ahsen N, Muller C, Serke S *et al*. Important role of nondiagnostic blood loss and blunted erythropoietic response in the anemia of medical intensive care patients. *Crit Care Med* 1999; **27**: 2630–9.
11 Fowler RA, Berenson M. Blood conservation in the intensive care unit. *Crit Care Med* 2003; **31**: S715–S720.
12 Foulke GE, Harlow DJ. Effective measures for reducing blood loss from diagnostic laboratory tests in intensive care unit patients. *Crit Care Med* 1989; **17**: 1143–5.
13 Smoller BR, Kruskall MS, Horowitz GL. Reducing adult phlebotomy blood loss with the use of pediatric-sized blood collection tubes. *Am J Clin Pathol* 1989; **91**: 701–3.
14 Silver MJ, Li YH, Gragg LA *et al*. Reduction of blood loss from diagnostic sampling in critically ill patients using a blood-conserving arterial line system. *Chest* 1993; **104**: 1711–15.
15 Rickard CM, Couchman BA, Schmidt SJ *et al*. A discard volume of twice the deadspace ensures clinically accurate arterial blood gases and electrolytes and prevents unnecessary blood loss. *Crit Care Med* 2003; **31**: 1654–8.
16 Rehm JP, Otto PS, West WW *et al*. Hospital-wide educational program decreases red blood cell transfusions. *J Surg Res* 1998; **75**: 183–6.
17 Merlani P, Garnerin P, Diby M *et al*. Quality improvement report: linking guideline to regular feedback to increase appropriate requests for clinical tests: blood gas analysis in intensive care. *Br Med J* 2001; **323**: 620–4.
18 Nguyen Ba V, Peres Bota D, Melot C *et al*. Time course of hemoglobin concentrations in non-bleeding ICU patients. *Crit Care Med* 2003; **31**: 406–10.

19 Gilbert EM, Haupt MT, Mandanas RY *et al*. The effect of fluid loading, blood transfusion and catecholamine infusion on oxygen delivery and consumption in patients with sepsis. *Am Rev Respir Dis* 1986; **134**: 873–8.

20 Steffes CP, Bender JS, Levison MA. Blood transfusion and oxygen consumption in surgical sepsis. *Crit Care Med* 1991; **19**: 512–17.

21 Hébert PC, Chin-Yee I. Should old red cells be transfused in critically ill patients? In: Vincent JL, ed. *2000 Yearbook of Intensive Care and Emergency Medicine*. Heidelberg: Springer, 2000: 494–506.

22 Spahn DR. The optimal and critical hemoglobin in health and acute illness. In: Sibbald WJ, Messmer K, Fink MP, eds. *Tissue Oxygenation in Acute Medicine*. Heidelberg: Springer, 1998: 263–75.

23 Lorente JA, Landin L, De Pablo R *et al*. Effects of blood transfusion on oxygen transport variables in severe sepsis. *Crit Care Med* 1993; **21**: 1312–18.

24 Marik PE, Sibbald WJ. Effect of stored-blood transfusion on oxygen delivery in patients with sepsis. *JAMA* 1993; **269**: 3024–9.

25 Carson JL, Duff A, Poses RM *et al*. Effect of anaemia and cardiovascular disease on surgical mortality and morbidity. *Lancet* 1996; **348**: 1055–60.

26 Hebert PC, Fergusson D, Blajchman MA *et al*. Clinical outcomes following institution of the Canadian universal leukoreduction program for red blood cell transfusions. *JAMA* 2003; **289**: 1941–9.

27 Hayes MA, Timmins AC, Yau EH *et al*. Elevation of systemic oxygen delivery in the treatment of critically ill patients. *N Engl J Med* 1994; **330**: 1717–22.

28 Gattinoni L, Brazzi L, Pelosi P *et al*. A trial of goal-oriented hemodynamic therapy in critically ill patients. *N Engl J Med* 1995; **333**: 1025–32.

29 Connors AF, Speroff T, Dawson NV *et al*. The effectiveness of right heart catheterization in the initial care of critically ill patients. *JAMA* 1996; **276**: 889–97.

30 Madan AK, UyBarreta VV, Aliabadi-Wahle S *et al*. Esophageal Doppler ultrasound monitor versus pulmonary artery catheter in the hemodynamic management of critically ill surgical patients. *J Trauma* 1999; **46**: 607–11.

31 Vincent JL, Dhainaut JF, Perret C *et al*. Is the pulmonary artery catheter misused? A European view. *Crit Care Med* 1998; **26**:1283–7.

32 Rivers E, Nguyen B, Havstad S *et al*. Early goal-directed therapy in the treatment of severe sepsis and septic shock. *N Engl J Med* 2001; **345**: 1368–77.

33 Yalavatti GS, De Backer D, Vincent JL. The assessment of cardiac index in anemic patients. *Chest* 2000; **118**: 782–7.

34 Vincent JL, Roman A, De Backer D *et al*. Oxygen uptake/supply dependency: effects of short-term dobutamine infusion. *Am Rev Respir Dis* 1990; **142**: 2–8.

35 Roumen RM, Redl H, Schlag G *et al*. Scoring systems and blood lactate concentrations in relation to the development of adult respiratory distress syndrome and multiple organ failure in severely traumatized patients. *J Trauma* 1993; **35**: 349–55.

36 Bakker J, Coffernils M, Leon M *et al*. Blood lactate levels are superior to oxygen-derived variables in predicting outcome in human septic shock. *Chest* 1991; **99**: 956–62.

37 Bakker J, Gris P, Coffernils M *et al*. Serial blood lactate levels can predict the development of multiple organ failure following septic shock. *Am J Surg* 1996; **171**: 221–6.

38 Doglio GR, Pusajo JF, Egurrola MA *et al*. Gastric mucosal pH as a prognostic index of mortality in critically ill patients. *Crit Care Med* 1991; **19**: 1037–40.

39 Friedman G, Berlot G, Kahn RJ *et al.* Combined measurements of blood lactate concentrations and gastric intramucosal pH in patients with severe sepsis. *Crit Care Med* 1995; **23**: 1184–93.

40 Levy B, Gawalkiewicz P, Vallet B *et al.* Gastric capnometry with air-automated tonometry predicts outcome in critically ill patients. *Crit Care Med* 2003; **31**: 474–80.

41 Gomersall CD, Joynt GM, Freebairn RC *et al.* Resuscitation of critically ill patients based on the results of gastric tonometry: a prospective, randomized, controlled trial. *Crit Care Med* 2000; **28**: 607–14.

42 Sakr Y, Dubois MJ, De Backer D *et al.* Persistent microcirculatory alterations are associated with organ failure and death in patients with septic shock. *Crit Care Med* 2004; **32**: 1825–31.

43 Mann MC, Votto J, Kambe J *et al.* Management of the severely anemic patient who refuses transfusion: lessons learned during the care of a Jehovah's Witness. *Ann Intern Med* 1992; **117**: 1042–8.

44 Russell WC, Greer R, Harper NJ. The effect of neuromuscular blockade on oxygen supply, consumption, and total chest compliance in patients with high oxygen requirements undergoing mechanical ventilation. *Anaesth Intens Care* 2002; **30**: 192–7.

45 McLoughlin PL, Cope TM, Harrison JC. Hyperbaric oxygen therapy in the management of severe acute anaemia in a Jehovah's Witness. *Anaesthesia* 1999; **54**: 891–5.

46 Creteur J, Vincent JL. Hemoglobin solutions. *Crit Care Med* 2003; **31**: S698–S707.

47 Schobersberger W, Hobisch-Hagen P, Fuchs D *et al.* Pathogenesis of anaemia in the critically ill patient. *Clin Intens Care* 1998; **9**: 111–17.

48 Krafte-Jacobs B, Levetown ML, Bray GL *et al.* Erythropoietin response to critical illness. *Crit Care Med* 1994; **22**: 821–6.

49 Rogiers P, Zhang H, Leeman M *et al.* Erythropoietin response is blunted in critically ill patients. *Intens Care Med* 1997; **23**: 159–62.

50 Corwin HL, Gettinger A, Pearl RG *et al.* Efficacy of recombinant human erythropoietin in critically ill patients: a randomized controlled trial. *JAMA* 2002; **288**: 2827–35.

51 Atabek U, Alvarez R, Pello MJ *et al.* Erythropoietin accelerates hematocrit recovery in post-surgical anemia. *Am Surg* 1995; **61**: 74–7.

CHAPTER 8

Anemia and Blood Conservation in the Critically Ill Patient

Aryeh Shander, Tanuja Rijhwani, Nimish Nemani, Carmine Gianatiempo

Anemia is a common finding in the intensive care unit (ICU) and blood transfusions are commonly used to treat it. A number of studies [1–6] to date have documented the prevalence of anemia in the critically ill patients and the high rate of blood transfusions administered in the ICUs. The prevalence of anemia as documented in some of these studies leads to red blood cell (RBC) transfusions in the range of 37–44% of patients during their ICU stay [2,7].

In a retrospective study by Corwin *et al.* [8], the authors report that a total of 23% of all patients admitted to the ICU had a length of stay greater than 1 week (19.6 ± 1.6 days). Of these patients, 85% received blood transfusions (9.5 ± 0.8 units per patient). These transfusions were not entirely due to acute blood loss. Patients were transfused at the rate of 2–3 units/week. Patients receiving blood transfusions were phlebotomized on average 61–70 ml/day. Almost one-third of all RBCs transfused were without a clear transfusion indication. Many blood transfusions appear to be administered because of an arbitrary 'transfusion trigger' rather than a physiologic need for blood.

Pathophysiology of intensive care unit – acquired anemia

Anemia in the ICU can be caused by a host of factors such as:
- frequent blood sampling for measurements of various laboratory parameters
- clinically apparent or occult blood loss from the gastrointestinal (GI) tract due to erosive upper GI mucosal disease or tissue trauma from suction of gastric contents
- blood loss due to trauma preceding admission to the ICU
- blood loss at the time of surgical procedures preceding or during the ICU stay

- inappropriately low circulating concentrations of erythropoietin (EPO) [9–14], the humoral regulator of RBC production
- diminished responsiveness of bone marrow precursor cells to EPO such as due to decreased availability of iron
- iron and other nutritional deficiencies

Rogiers *et al.* [12] obtained serial measurements of serum EPO levels by the ELISA method in 36 critically ill, nonhypoxemic patients who stayed more than 7 days in the ICU, including 22 patients with sepsis and 14 without. The control group was made up of 18 ambulatory patients with iron-deficiency anemia. A significant inverse correlation between serum EPO and hematocrit (Hct) levels was found in the control patients ($r = -0.81$, $p < 0.001$), but not in the critically ill patients ($r = -0.09$, NS), except in a subgroup of nonseptic patients without renal failure ($r = -0.61$, $p < 0.01$). The authors conclude that EPO levels can be inappropriately low in anemic critically ill patients, so that EPO deficiency may contribute to the development of anemia in these patients, not only in the presence of acute renal failure but also in the presence of sepsis.

von Ahsen *et al.* [14] studied 96 patients treated in a 24-bed medical ICU in a tertiary care university hospital for more than 3 days in an open prospective clinical study. Reticulocyte counts and EPO concentrations were inappropriately low for the degree of anemia, and plasma transferrin saturation was mostly $< 20\%$. The authors conclude that the erythropoietic response to anemia is blunted, probably as a consequence of an inappropriate increase in EPO production and possibly diminished iron availability.

Elliot *et al.* [11] in a prospective observational study performed on 25 critically ill patients examined the temporal relationships between serum EPO levels, hemoglobin (Hb) concentration and the inflammatory response in critically ill patients with and without acute renal failure (ARF). The control group included 82 nonhospitalized patients with normal renal function and varying Hb concentrations. EPO levels were markedly elevated in the initial phase of critical illness with ARF. In the chronic phase of critical illness, EPO levels were the same for patients with and without ARF, and could not be distinguished from noncritically ill patients with varying Hb concentrations. The authors add that exogenous EPO therapy is unlikely to be effective in the first few days of critical illness and that inappropriately low EPO levels persist for the duration of critical illness. Although endogenous EPO levels tend to be low in critically ill patients, these patients appear to retain responsiveness to the hormone. Prospective randomized trials [15–17] have demonstrated that administration of recombinant human erythropoietin (rHuEPO) can stimulate reticulocytosis and increase circulating Hb concentration in critically ill adults.

Disturbances in iron metabolism and availability are a major cause for anemia in critically ill patients and in patients with anemia of chronic disease [12]. In both groups of patients, laboratory studies typically reveal low serum iron concentration, low transferrin level, low transferrin saturation and elevated serum ferritin concentration (acute phase reactant); findings such as these are consistent with an acute phase response [9,15,18]. Despite evidence of adequate iron stores, circulating iron concentrations can be low, and less iron may be available to support erythropoiesis [19].

von Ahsen *et al.* [14] observed normal vitamin B12 levels but abnormally low folic acid concentrations in some anemic ICU patients, although RBC size was not increased. The significance of this low folic acid remains uncertain.

Rodriquez *et al.* [9] reported iron deficiency in 9% of ICU patients; 2% of the patients were deficient in vitamin B12, and another 2% suffered from folic acid deficiency.

Intensive care unit transfusion practice

Evidence suggests that there is considerable variability in RBC transfusion practices in critical care. The impact of anemia in the critically ill patients and the optimal therapy for anemia have not been clearly defined; hence, to date, no universal transfusion trigger exists.

Current guidelines for transfusion in the critically ill advise that, at an Hb of 7 g/dl, RBC transfusion is strongly indicated, whereas at Hb values above 10 g/dl, blood transfusion is seldom justified. For patients with Hb values in the 7–10 g/dl range, the transfusion trigger should be based on clinical indicators.

In a Canadian scenario, a national survey was conducted among critical care practitioners (n = 254) to characterize the contemporary RBC transfusion practice in the critically ill and to define clinical factors that influence these practices [20]. The participants were asked to fill out a questionnaire based on reviews of four separate clinical scenarios. Among the 76% respondents, internal medicine was the primary specialty for 56%; they were in practice for an average period of 8.4 ± 5.7 years and worked most often in combined medical-surgical ICUs (82%). There was a significant difference in baseline transfusion thresholds and transfusion practices among intensivists in Canada.

Hebert *et al.* performed a multicenter cohort study combined with a cross-sectional survey of physicians requesting RBC transfusions for patients in the cohort. The study population consisted of a cohort of 5298 consecutive patients admitted to six tertiary level ICUs. In addition, a survey was administered to 223 physicians requesting RBC transfusions in these units. Hb concentrations were collected, along with the number and reasons for RBC transfusions plus demographic, diagnostic, disease severity (APACHE (Acute Physiology and Chronic Health Evaluation) II score), ICU mortality and lengths of stay in the ICU. In the cohort study 25% of the critically ill patients received RBC transfusions. The overall number of transfusions per patient day in the ICU averaged 0.95 ± 1.39 and ranged from 0.82 ± 1.69 to 1.08 ± 1.27 between institutions ($P < 0.001$). Independent predictors of transfusion thresholds (pretransfusion Hb concentrations) included patient age, admission APACHE II score and the institution ($P < 0.0001$). A very significant institution effect ($P < 0.0001$) was detected that persisted even after multivariate adjustments for age, APACHE II score and within four diagnostic categories (cardiovascular disease, respiratory failure, major surgery and trauma) ($P < 0.0001$). The evaluation of transfusion practice using the bedside survey documented that 35% (202 of 576) of pretransfusion Hb concentrations were in the range of 9.5–10.5 g/dl and 80% of the orders were for 2 packed cell units. The most frequent reasons for administering RBCs were acute bleeding (35%) and the augmentation of oxygen delivery (25%). The authors conclude that institutional variability in transfusion practice exists and many intensivists continue to adhere to a 10.0 g/dl threshold, and opted to administer multiple units despite published guidelines to the contrary.

Evidence of clinical relevance of blood transfusions in critically ill patients

RBC transfusions are frequently advocated to increase oxygen delivery in critically ill patients. The immediate and long-term effectiveness of this mode of therapy in increasing oxygen delivery is questionable as stored RBCs have a depressed ability to unload oxygen peripherally as well as deform.

Marik and Sibbald [21] reported no improvement in systemic oxygen delivery for up to 6 h after transfusion in 23 critically ill patients with sepsis undergoing mechanical ventilation. In this prospective, controlled, interventional study, gastric intramucosal pH as measured by tonometry was used to assess changes in splanchnic oxygen availability. There was no increase in systemic oxygen uptake measured by indirect calorimetry in any of the patients studied for up to 6 h posttransfusion (including those patients with an elevated arterial lactate concentration). In those patients receiving blood that had been stored for more than 15 days, the gastric intramucosal pH consistently decreased following the RBC transfusion. The postulated mechanism as proposed by the authors is that the poorly deformable transfused RBCs cause microcirculatory occlusion in some organs, which may lead to tissue ischemia.

Efficacy of restrictive blood transfusion practice in critically ill patients

In a multicenter, prospective, randomized, pilot study, Hebert *et al.* evaluated the effects of a restrictive and a liberal RBC transfusion strategy on mortality and morbidity in critically ill patients. They studied [22] 69 normovolemic critically ill patients within 72 h of admission to one of five tertiary level ICUs with Hb values < 9.0 g/dl. After randomly allocating the patients to one of the two study groups, Hb values were maintained between 10.0 g/dl and 12.0 g/dl in the liberal transfusion group and between 7.0 g/dl and 9.0 g/dl in the restrictive group. In this small randomized trial, neither mortality nor the development of organ dysfunction was affected by the transfusion strategy, which suggests that a more restrictive approach to the transfusion of RBCs may be safe in critically ill patients. However, the study lacked power to detect small but clinically significant differences.

A subsequent large, prospective, multicenter trial, Transfusion Requirements in Critical Care (TRICC) [23], validated the results of this pilot study. Hebert *et al.* studied 838 critically ill patients to determine whether a restrictive strategy of RBC transfusion and a liberal strategy produced equivalent results in critically ill patients. The authors compared the rates of death from all causes at 30 days and the severity of organ dysfunction. Critically ill patients with euvolemia after initial treatment who had Hb concentrations of < 9.0 g/dl within 72 h after admission to the ICU were randomized for the study. The restrictive strategy of transfusion was defined as administering transfusions if the Hb concentration dropped below 7.0 g/dl and Hb concentrations were maintained at [at 7.0–9.0 g/dl. The liberal strategy was defined as administering transfusions when the Hb concentration fell below 10.0 g/dl and Hb concentrations were maintained at 10.0–12.0 g/dl. Overall, 30-day mortality was similar in the two groups (18.7% vs. 23.3%, $p = 0.11$). However, the rates were significantly lower with the restrictive transfusion strategy among patients who were less acutely ill – those with an Acute Physiology and Chronic Health Evaluation II score of 20 (8.7% in the restrictive strategy group and 16.1% in the liberal strategy group; $p = 0.03$) – and among patients who were less than 55 years of age (5.7% and 13% respectively; $p = 0.02$), but not among patients with clinically significant cardiac disease (20.5% and 22.9% respectively; $p = 0.69$). The mortality rate during hospitalization was significantly lower in the restrictive strategy group (22.3% vs. 28.1%, $p = 0.05$). The authors conclude that a restrictive strategy of RBC transfusion is at least as effective as, and possibly superior to, a liberal transfusion strategy in critically ill patients, with the possible exception of patients with acute myocardial infarction and unstable angina, although no definitive data was presented for that group of patients.

An additional *post hoc* cohort analysis of the TRICC trial was performed in 713 patients requiring mechanical ventilation. This *post hoc* analysis was performed in an attempt to address the controversy over whether the use of allogeneic blood transfusion for the treatment of anemia in these patients improves the weaning process [24]. The average duration of mechanical ventilation was 8.3 ± 8.1 days (95% confidence interval around difference, -0.79 to 1.68; $p = 0.48$), while duration of ventilator-free days was 17.5 ± 10.9 days and 16.1 ± 11.4 days (95% confidence interval around difference, -3.07 to 0.21; $p = 0.09$) in the restrictive strategy group versus the liberal strategy group, respectively. In the restrictive strategy group, 82% of the patients were considered successfully weaned and extubated for at least 24 h, compared to 78% for the liberal strategy group ($p = 0.19$). The relative risk of extubation success in the restrictive strategy group compared to the liberal strategy group, adjusted for the confounding effects of age, APACHE II score and comorbid illness, was 1.07 (95% confidence interval, 0.96–1.26; $p = 0.43$). The adjusted relative risk of extubation success associated with restrictive transfusion in the 219 patients who received mechanical ventilation for more than 7 days was 1.1 (95% confidence interval, 0.84–1.45; $p = 0.47$). In this study, there was no evidence that a liberal RBC transfusion strategy decreased the duration of mechanical ventilation in a heterogeneous population of critically ill patients.

Vincent *et al.* conducted a prospective observational study with two components: a blood sampling study and an anemia and blood transfusion study. The blood sampling study included 1136 patients from 145 western European ICUs, and the anemia and blood transfusion study included 3534 patients from 146 western European ICUs. Patients were followed up for 28 days or until hospital discharge, interinstitutional transfer or death. The main outcome measures included frequency of blood drawing and associated volume of blood drawn, collected over a 24-h period; Hb levels, transfusion rate, organ dysfunction (assessed using the SOFA (Sequential Organ Failure Assessment) score) and mortality, collected throughout a 2-week period. The mean (standard deviation, SD) volume per blood draw was 10.3 (6.6) ml, with an average total volume of 41.1 (39.7) ml during the 24-h period. There was a positive correlation between organ dysfunction and the number of blood draws ($r = 0.34$; $p < 0.001$) and total volume drawn ($r = 0.28$; $p < 0.001$). The mean Hb concentration at ICU admission was 11.3 (2.3) g/dl, with 29% (963/3295) having a concentration of < 10 g/dl. The transfusion rate during the ICU period was 37.0% (1307/3534). Older patients and those with a longer ICU length of stay were more commonly transfused. Both ICU and overall mortality rates were significantly higher in patients who had versus those who had not received a transfusion (ICU rates: 18.5% vs. 10.1% respectively; $\chi(2) = 50.1$; $p < 0.001$; overall rates: 29.0% vs. 14.9% respectively; $\chi(2) = 88.1$; $p < 0.001$). For similar degrees of organ dysfunction, patients who had a transfusion had a higher mortality rate. For matched patients in the propensity analysis, the 28-day mortality was 22.7% among patients with transfusions and 17.1% among those without ($p = 0.02$); the Kaplan–Meier log-rank test confirmed this difference. This study reveals the common occurrence of anemia and the large use of blood transfusion in critically ill patients. Additionally, this epidemiologic study provides evidence of an association between transfusions and diminished organ function as well as between transfusions and mortality.

Chohan *et al.* recently investigated RBC transfusion practice since the TRICC trial in a large Scottish teaching hospital ICU, and published their findings in *Vox Sanguinis*. The authors describe the current indications for transfusions, pretransfusion Hb concentrations, RBC use, distribution of daily Hb concentrations and the rate of onset of anemia in a large Scottish teaching ICU. They prospectively studied 176 patients who remained in the ICU during a 6-month period. The tertiary referral center where the study was performed had a case-mix of 50% surgical (including liver transplantation), 40% medical and 10% trauma patients. There were no postoperative cardiac surgery patients considered for the analysis. The outcomes evaluated were daily Hb concentrations, indications for transfusion (hemorrhage, nonhemorrhage, other such as hemolysis), Hb concentrations before and on the day after transfusion events, RBC usage (RBC units per ICU admission, RBC units per ICU day).

The authors found that the median RBC threshold in the absence of clinical hemorrhage was 7.8 g/dl. Of these 176 patients, 52% of patients staying in the ICU for longer than 24 h received an RBC transfusion. An Hb concentration of 9 g/dl was measured in 55% of patients; which occurred by day 1 and day 2 in 52% and 77% of these cases, respectively. Overall, the Hb concentration was 9 g/dl for 45% of all patient days. The total RBC use was 3.1 units per admission calculated as 0.47 units per patient day). Out of these more than 70% were administered for reasons other than hemorrhage; only 20% were prescribed for hemorrhage. The transfusion rates for the Chohan *et al.* study were higher than that observed in other studies.

The TRICC study recommended that all patients receive 1 RBC unit when the Hb concentration was < 7 g/dl. Chohan *et al.* practiced a transfusion trigger between 7–9 g/dl rather than 7 g/dl. Also 65% of transfusion events were in the absence of hemorrhage and were 2-unit transfusions. This strategy was reflected in the posttransfusion Hb concentrations, which were 9 g/dl in 50% of patients.

Chohan *et al.* and other practicing consultants had not agreed on a protocol for specific transfusion triggers covering all patients, but there was general consensus among the consultants based on the evidence from the TRICC study that supported the use of conservative transfusion triggers covering most patients. The patients in this study had greater illness severity and mortality as patients remaining for less than 24 h in the ICU were excluded. In addition, Hb concentration was not allowed to drop as low as 7 g/dl in most patients. Also, the authors did not use mortality as an outcome for the analysis.

The authors have raised important questions such as which clinical situations and subsets of patients warrant a transfusion trigger > 7 g/dl. Of utmost importance is to determine the transfusion threshold for patients with ischemic heart disease or in those weaned from a ventilator. Adequately powered randomized trials are needed to answer some of these questions.

Safety of restrictive blood transfusion practice in critically ill patients

Significant concern exists among intensivists regarding whether critically ill patients with cardiovascular disease can tolerate anemia in the face of limited cardiac reserve. A cohort of 357 critically ill patients with cardiovascular diseases from the TRICC who had an Hb concentration of < 9.0 g/dl within 72 h of admission to the ICU was analyzed [25]. Baseline characteristics in the restrictive (n = 160) and the liberal group (n = 197) were comparable, except for the use of cardiac and anesthetic drugs ($p < 0.02$). Average Hb concentrations (85 ± 6.2 vs. 103 ± 6.7 g/dl; $p < 0.01$) and RBC units transfused (2.4 ± 4.1 vs. 5.2 ± 5.0 units; $p < 0.01$) were significantly lower in the restrictive compared with the liberal group. Overall, all mortality rates were similar in both study groups, including 30-day (23% vs. 23%; $p = 1.00$), 60-day, hospital and ICU rates. Changes in multiple organ dysfunction from baseline scores were significantly less in the restrictive transfusion group overall (0.2 ± 4.2 vs. 1.3 ± 4.4; $p = 0.02$). In the 257 patients with severe ischemic heart disease, there were no statistically significant differences in all survival measures, but this is the only subgroup where the restrictive group had lower but nonsignificant absolute survival rates compared with the patients in the liberal group. The authors conclude that a restrictive RBC transfusion strategy generally appears to be safe in most critically ill patients with cardiovascular disease, with the possible exception of patients with acute myocardial infarcts and unstable angina.

Of particular concern is the significant increase in mortality noted in the liberal transfusion strategy group in the TRICC trial. The increased mortality rate in patients in the liberal group was not entirely accounted for by the higher incidence of pulmonary edema in this group. Other potential adverse effects related to allogeneic blood transfusion identified in critically ill patients, such as increased risk of nosocomial infection [26], inflammatory response [27], pulmonary and systemic vasoconstriction related to age of blood and nitric oxide binding [28,29], and immunosuppression [30], have not been accounted for in this study.

Concerns over the deleterious effects of anemia are being balanced by the increasing awareness of the untoward effects associated with the use of blood transfusion such as transmission of infectious (human immunodeficiency virus (HIV), hepatitis B virus (HBV), West Nile virus (WNV), SFV = Simian Foamy Virus, etc.) and noninfectious (transfusion reactions, administrative errors, transfusion-associated acute lung injury (TRALI), etc.) complications and immunomodulatory effects.

Strategies to prevent anemia in the intensive care unit

Prevention and arrest of bleeding

1 Close surveillance for blood loss:
   - Watch for signs and symptoms of bleeding
2 Rapid diagnosis and control of hemorrhage:
   - Therapeutic procedures should be anticipated and implemented as early as possible before loss of a patient's physiologic reserves
   - Surgical interventions should be simple, quick and well performed
3 Expeditious angiographic embolization:
   - Consider angiographic embolization as an adjuvant to a multimodality bleeding control strategy

- Early management of sepsis and septic shock (blood transfusion has not been shown to improve oxygen delivery in septic shock)
- Prompt management of disseminated intravascular coagulation (DIC)
4 Permissive moderate hypotension in the bleeding patient
5 Strict control of blood pressure after arrest of bleeding
6 Pharmacologic enhancement of hemostasis (systemic agents and topical hemostatic agents)
7 Autotransfusion/blood cell salvage:
- Intraoperative
- Postoperative
8 Hemostasis and anticoagulation management:
- Identification and management of coagulation disorders
- Individualized protamine/heparin management after cardiopulmonary bypass (CPB)
- Cautious thromboembolic prophylaxis
9 Prophylaxis of upper GI hemorrhage
10 Prophylaxis and management of infections

Minimization of iatrogenic blood loss

Average blood removal from a critically ill patient for testing can be more than 70 ml/day for days or even weeks, depending on the nature and severity of the illness [1]. Most patients have an indwelling catheter, which increases testing by as much as one-third [31].
1 Restricted diagnostic phlebotomy – several strategies can be employed to reduce blood testing while continuing optimal patient care:
- Use of pediatric sampling techniques, low-volume adult tubes and blood
- Conservation devices should be implemented in specific circumstances when repeated multiple sampling is required
- Point of care whole blood microsampling
- Noninvasive monitoring when possible
- Restrict use of indwelling lines; remove as early as possible
- In-line blood reservoirs; eliminate purge discard volume
2 Perform only essential tests
3 Coordinate and consolidate blood tests (multiple tests per sample)
4 Minimize volume of diagnostic blood sampling

Optimization of oxygen delivery
1 Assess tissue perfusion and tissue oxygenation
2 Judicious fluid replacement
3 Individualized volume and fluid management
4 Early optimization of tissue oxygenation and perfusion:
- Supplemental oxygen (increase FiO_2)
- Early optimization of cardiac output (CO)
- Hyperbaric oxygen (HBO therapy)

Minimization of oxygen consumption

- Consider adequate analgesia, sedation and muscle relaxants, mechanical ventilation where appropriate
- Consider moderate or mild hypothermia (32–33°C) when appropriate

Optimization of erythropoiesis

1 Early EPO therapy:

Critical illness is characterized by a blunted EPO production and response [9]. This blunted response appears to be a result of the inhibition of the EPO gene by inflammatory mediators [32,33].

In a prospective, randomized, double-blind, placebo-controlled, multicenter trial conducted by Corwin *et al.* between December 1998 and June 2001, the authors demonstrated the efficacy in critically ill patients on a weekly dosing schedule of rHuEPO to decrease the occurrence of RBC transfusion. A total of 1302 patients who had been in the ICU for 2 days and were expected to be in there for at least 2 more days and who met eligibility criteria were enrolled in the study; 650 patients were randomized to rHuEPO and 652 to placebo. Study drug (40 000 units of rHuEPO) or placebo was administered by subcutaneous (SC) injection on ICU day 3 and continued weekly for patients who remained in the hospital, for a total of 3 doses. The primary efficacy end point was transfusion independence, assessed by comparing the percentage of patients in each treatment group who received any RBC transfusion between study days 1 and 28. Patients receiving rHuEPO were less likely to undergo transfusion (60.4% placebo vs. 50.5% rHuEPO; $p < 0.001$; odds ratio 0.67; 95% confidence interval, 0.54–0.83). There was a 19% reduction in the total units of RBC transfused in the rHuEPO group (1963 units for placebo vs. 1590 units for rHuEPO) and reduction in RBC units transfused per day alive (ratio of transfusion rates 0.81; 95% confidence interval, 0.79–0.83; $p = 0.04$). Increase in Hb from baseline to study end was greater in the rHuEPO group (mean (SD), 1.32 2 g/dl vs. 0.94 (1.9) g/dl; $p < 001$). Mortality (14% for rHuEPO and 15% for placebo) and adverse clinical events were not significantly different. The authors concluded that in critically ill patients, weekly administration of 40 000 units of rHuEPO reduces allogeneic RBC transfusion and increases Hb.

2 Iron replacement:

Consider folic acid, vitamin B12 administration

3 Nutritional support

Tolerance of anemia

Many recent studies [23,34–37] have provided evidence against the 10/30 rule in critically ill patients as well as in the perioperative period. However, there is a gradual shift in the trend from transfusing to an arbitary Hb (10/30) to achieving a level of Hb necessary to meet the patient's tissue oxygen demands [38,39].

An assessment of human tolerance of severe acute anemia can be made from experiences in Jehovah's Witness patients. Thus, it is possible to demonstrate the feasibility of survival in the case of very low Hct [40–46].

Viele *et al.* [45] performed a MEDLINE search to review the medical and surgical reports involving Jehovah's Witnesses from 1970 through early 1993. The authors found 61 reports of untransfused Jehovah's Witnesses with Hb concentrations of = 8 g/dl or Hct values of 24%. These data have significant limitations but suggest that survival, without transfusion, is possible at low Hb concentrations, while mortality with an unknown incidence is encountered at Hb concentrations < 5 g/dl.

In an interventional study Weiskopf *et al.* [47] tested the hypothesis that acute isovolemic reduction of blood Hb concentration to 5.0 g/dl in healthy resting humans would produce inadequate cardiovascular compensation and result in tissue hypoxia secondary to inadequate oxygen transport in 11 preoperative patients and 21 nonsurgical volunteers with Hb as low as 5 g/dl. 'Critical' oxygen delivery (TO_2) was assessed by oxygen consumption (VO_2), plasma lactate concentration and ST changes on electrocardiogram. VO_2 increased slightly from a mean (SD) of 3.07 (0.44) ml of oxygen/kg/min to 3.42 (0.54) ml of oxygen/kg/min ($p < 001$) and plasma lactate concentration did not change (0.81 (0.11) mmol/L to 0.62 (0.19) mmol/L; $p = 0.09$). Acute isovolemic reduction of blood Hb concentration to 5.0 g/dl in conscious healthy resting humans does not produce evidence of inadequate systemic TO_2, as assessed by lack of change of VO_2 and plasma lactate concentration. Analysis of Holter readings suggests that at this Hb concentration in the resting healthy population, myocardial ischemia would occur infrequently.

Experiences from management of severely anemic Jehovah's Witness patients in the ICU

Jabbour *et al.* [48] report their experience in a two-stage hepatectomy done for a Jehovah's Witness patient who underwent live-donor liver transplant (LDLT) from his mother, also a Jehovah's Witness, without blood transfusion. The recipient had an unusually enlarged left lateral segment of the liver that was densely adherent to the spleen. Removing these adhesions in the presence of significant portal hypertension would have resulted in considerable blood loss. This was successfully avoided by leaving this portion of the liver attached to the spleen while proceeding with the hepatectomy. The right lobe of the liver from the donor was then implanted uneventfully. The remaining segment of the recipient liver was removed 2 weeks later without incident. Staging of procedures whenever feasible is a useful strategy that helps to better manage patients without the use of blood products.

Jabbour *et al.* [49] performed a retrospective chart review of 38 LDLTs: 8 in Jehovah's Witness patients (transfusion-free group) and 30 in non-Jehovah's Witness patients (transfusion-eligible group). All transfusion-free patients underwent preoperative blood augmentation with EPO, intraoperative cell salvage and acute normovolemic hemodilution. These techniques were used in only 7%, 80% and 10%, respectively, in transfusion-eligible patients. Perioperative clinical data and outcomes were reviewed. Preoperative liver disease severity was similar in both groups; however, transfusion-free patients had significantly higher Hct levels following EPO augmentation. Operative time, blood loss and postoperative Hcts were similar in both groups. No blood products were used in transfusion-free patients while 80% of transfusion-eligible patients received a median of 4.5 ± 3.5 units of packed RBC. ICU and total hospital stay were similar in both groups. The survival rate was 100% in transfusion-free patients and 90% in transfusion-eligible patients. These techniques may be widely applied to all patients for several surgical procedures.

Conclusion

Anemia still plagues the critically ill patient. Severity of illness in this group has led to increased transfusion rates across both continents. Persistence in variability of transfusion practice may add to the current risks of transfusion. Blood conservation begins with conserving the patient's own blood. Treating anemia with other available means and improving oxygen delivery with sufficient circulating volume should be entertained as first approach. Coupled with a restrictive transfusion practice, this strategy may have an overall beneficial outcome. Transfusion of blood products remains an option when time is not available and/or the clinical condition of the patient is too severe to implement the above treatments. Although relevant information is lacking on patients with active cardiac disease, available data suggest that these patients may be at higher risk of anemia, but it still remains to be seen if transfusion alters this risk one way or another.

References

1 Corwin H. RBC transfusion in the ICU. Is there a reason? *Chest* 1995; **108**: 767–71.
2 Vincent JL, Baron JF, Reinhart K, Gattinoni L, Thijs L, Webb A *et al*. Anemia and blood transfusion in critically ill patients. *JAMA* 2002; **288**: 1499–507.
3 Corwin HL, Gettinger A, Pearl RG, Fink MP, Levy MM, Abraham E *et al*. The CRIT study: anemia and blood transfusion in the critically ill – current clinical practice in the United States. *Crit Care Med* 2004; **32**: 39–52.
4 Shapiro MJ, Gettinger A, Corwin HL, Napolitano L, Levy M, Abraham E *et al*. Anemia and blood transfusion in trauma patients admitted to the intensive care unit. *J Trauma* 2003; **55**: 269–73; discussion 273–4.
5 Rao MP, Boralessa H, Morgan C, Soni N, Goldhill DR, Brett SJ *et al*. Blood component use in critically ill patients. *Anaesthesia* 2002; **57**: 530–4.
6 Nguyen BV, Bota DP, Melot C, Vincent JL. Time course of hemoglobin concentrations in nonbleeding intensive care unit patients. *Crit Care Med* 2003; **31**: 406–10.

7 Corwin HL. Anemia and blood transfusion in the critically ill patient: role of erythropoietin. *Crit Care* 2004; **8**(Suppl. 2): S42–S44.

8 Corwin HL, Parsonnet KC, Gettinger A. RBC transfusion in the ICU: is there a reason? *Chest* 1995; **108**: 767–71.

9 Rodriguez RM, Corwin HL, Gettinger A, Corwin MJ, Gubler D, Pearl RG. Nutritional deficiencies and blunted erythropoietin response as causes of the anemia of critical illness. *J Crit Care* 2001; **16**: 36–41.

10 Hobisch-Hagen P WF, Mayr A, Fries D, Jelkmann W, Fuchs D, Hasibeder W, Mutz N, Klingler A, Schobersberger W. Blunted erythropoietic response to anemia in multiply traumatized patients. *Crit Care Med* 2001; **29**: 743–7.

11 Elliot JM, Virankabutra T, Jones S, Tanudsintum S, Lipkin G, Todd S *et al*. Erythropoietin mimics the acute phase response in critical illness. *Crit Care* 2003; **7**: R35–R40.

12 Rogiers P, Zhang H, Leeman M, Nagler J, Neels H, Melot C *et al*. Erythropoietin response is blunted in critically ill patients. *Intens Care Med* 1997; **23**: 159–62.

13 Krafte-Jacobs B. Erythropoietin response to critical illness. *Crit Care Med* 1994; **22**: 821–6.

14 von Ahsen N, Muller C, Serke S, Frei U, Eckardt KU. Important role of nondiagnostic blood loss and blunted erythropoietic response in the anemia of medical intensive care patients. *Crit Care Med* 1999; **27**: 2630–9.

15 van Iperen C. Response of erythropoiesis and iron metabolism to recombinant human erythropoietin in intensive care unit patients. *Crit Care Med* 2001; **28**: 2773–8.

16 Corwin HL, Gettinger A, Rodriguez RM, Pearl RG, Gubler KD, Enny C *et al*. Efficacy of recombinant human erythropoietin in the critically ill patient: a randomized, double-blind, placebo-controlled trial. *Crit Care Med* 1999; **27**: 2346–50.

17 Corwin HL, Gettinger A, Pearl RG, Fink MP, Levy MM, Shapiro MJ *et al*. Efficacy of recombinant human erythropoietin in critically ill patients: a randomized controlled trial. *JAMA* 2002; **288**: 2827–35.

18 Baumann H, Gauldie J. The acute phase response. *Immunol Today* 1994; **15**: 74–80.

19 Weiss G, Wachter H, Fuchs D. Linkage of cell-mediated immunity to iron metabolism. *Immunol Today* 1995; **16**: 495–500.

20 Hebert PC, Wells G, Martin C, Tweeddale M, Marshall J, Blajchman M *et al*. A Canadian survey of transfusion practices in critically ill patients: transfusion requirements in critical care investigators and the Canadian Critical Care Trials Group. *Crit Care Med* 1998; **26**: 482–7.

21 Marik PE, Sibbald WJ. Effect of stored-blood transfusion on oxygen delivery in patients with sepsis. *JAMA* 1993; **269**: 3024–9.

22 Hebert PC, Wells G, Marshall J, Martin C, Tweeddale M, Pagliarello G *et al*. Transfusion requirements in critical care: a pilot study – Canadian Critical Care Trials Group. *JAMA* 1995; **273**: 1439–44.

23 Hebert PC, Wells G, Blajchman MA, Marshall J, Martin C, Pagliarello G *et al*. A multicenter, randomized, controlled clinical trial of transfusion requirements in critical care: transfusion requirements in critical care investigators – Canadian Critical Care Trials Group. *N Engl J Med* 1999; **340**: 409–17.

24 Hebert PC, Blajchman MA, Cook DJ, Yetisir E, Wells G, Marshall J *et al*. Do blood transfusions improve outcomes related to mechanical ventilation? *Chest* 2001; **119**: 1850–7.

25 Hebert PC, Yetisir E, Martin C, Blajchman MA, Wells G, Marshall J *et al*. Is a low transfusion threshold safe in critically ill patients with cardiovascular diseases? *Crit Care Med* 2001; **29**: 227–34.

26 Taylor R. Impact of allogeneic packed red blood cell transfusion on nosocomial infection rates in the critically ill patient. *Crit Care Med* 2002; **30**: 2249–54.

27 Johnson JL, Moore EE, Gonzalez RJ, Fedel N, Partrick DA, Silliman CC. Alteration of the postinjury hyperinflammatory response by means of resuscitation with a red cell substitute. *J Trauma* 2003; **54**: 133–9; discussion 139–40.

28 Fernandes CJ Jr, Akamine N, De Marco FV, De Souza JA, Lagudis S, Knobel E. Red blood cell transfusion does not increase oxygen consumption in critically ill septic patients. *Crit Care* 2001; **5**: 362–7.

29 Reiter CD, Wang X, Tanus-Santos JE, Hogg N, Cannon RO 3rd, Schechter AN *et al*. Cell-free hemoglobin limits nitric oxide bioavailability in sickle-cell disease. *Nat Med* 2002; **8**: 1383–9.

30 Goodnough LT, Brecher ME, Kanter MH, AuBuchon JP. Transfusion medicine: first of two parts – blood transfusion. *N Engl J Med* 1999; **340**: 438–47.

31 Low LL, Harrington GR, Stoltzfus DP. The effect of arterial lines on blood-drawing practices and costs in intensive care units. *Chest* 1995; **108**: 216–19.

32 Frede S, Fandrey J, Pagel H, Hellwig T, Jelkmann W. Erythropoietin gene expression is suppressed after lipopolysaccharide or interleukin-1 beta injections in rats. *Am J Physiol* 1997; **273**(3 Pt 2): R1067–R1071.

33 Jelkmann W. Proinflammatory cytokines lowering erythropoietin production. *J Interferon Cytokine Res* 1998; **18**: 555–9.

34 Carson JL, Duff A, Berlin JA, Lawrence VA, Poses RM, Huber EC *et al*. Perioperative blood transfusion and postoperative mortality. *JAMA* 1998; **279**: 199–205.

35 Waggoner JR 3rd, Wass CT, Polis TZ, Faust RJ, Schroeder DR, Offord KP *et al*. The effect of changing transfusion practice on rates of perioperative stroke and myocardial infarction in patients undergoing carotid endarterectomy: a retrospective analysis of 1114 Mayo Clinic patients – Mayo Perioperative Outcomes Group. *Mayo Clin Proc* 2001; **76**: 376–83.

36 Spiess BD, Ley C, Body SC, Siegel LC, Stover EP, Maddi R *et al*. Hematocrit value on intensive care unit entry influences the frequency of Q-wave myocardial infarction after coronary artery bypass grafting – The Institutions of the Multicenter Study of Perioperative Ischemia (McSPI) Research Group. *J Thorac Cardiovasc Surg* 1998; **116**: 460–7.

37 Carson JL, Willett LR. Is a hemoglobin of 10 g/dL required for surgery? *Med Clin North Am* 1993; **77**: 335–47.

38 Sehgal LR, Zebala LP, Takagi I, Curran RD, Votapka TV, Caprini JA. Evaluation of oxygen extraction ratio as a physiologic transfusion trigger in coronary artery bypass graft surgery patients. *Transfusion* 2001; **41**: 591–5.

39 Stehling L, Simon TL. The red blood cell transfusion trigger: physiology and clinical studies. *Arch Pathol Lab Med* 1994; **118**: 429–34.

40 Majeski J. Advances in general and vascular surgical care of Jehovah's Witnesses. *Int Surg* 2000; **85**: 257–65.

41 Grebenik CR, Sinclair ME, Westaby S. High-risk cardiac surgery in Jehovah's Witnesses. *J Cardiovasc Surg* (Torino) 1996; **37**: 511–15.

42 Kitchens CS. Are transfusions overrated? Surgical outcome of Jehovah's Witnesses. *Am J Med* 1993; **94**: 117–19.

43 Victorino G, Wisner DH. Jehovah's Witnesses: unique problems in a unique trauma population. *J Am Coll Surg* 1997; **184**: 458–68.

44 Ott DA, Cooley DA. Cardiovascular surgery in Jehovah's Witnesses: report of 542 operations without blood transfusion. *JAMA* 1977; **238**: 1256–8.

45 Viele MK, Weiskopf RB. What can we learn about the need for transfusion from patients who refuse blood? The experience with Jehovah's Witnesses. *Transfusion* 1994; **34**: 396–401.

46 Spence RK, Alexander JB, DelRossi AJ, Cernaianu AD, Cilley J Jr, Pello MJ *et al.* Transfusion guidelines for cardiovascular surgery: lessons learned from operations in Jehovah's Witnesses. *J Vasc Surg* 1992; **16**: 825–9; discussion 829–31.

47 Weiskopf RB, Viele MK, Feiner J, Kelley S, Lieberman J, Noorani M *et al.* Human cardiovascular and metabolic response to acute, severe isovolemic anemia. *JAMA* 1998; **279**: 217–21.

48 Jabbour N, Gagandeep S, Mateo R, Sher L, Henderson R, Selby R *et al.* Live donor liver transplantation: staging hepatectomy in a Jehovah's Witness recipient. *J Hepatobiliary Pancreat Surg* 2004; **11**: 211–14.

49 Jabbour N, Gagandeep S, Mateo R, Sher L, Strum E, Donovan J *et al.* Live donor liver transplantation without blood products: strategies developed for Jehovah's Witnesses offer broad application. *Ann Surg* 2004; **240**: 350–7.

CHAPTER 9

Feasibility of Transfusion-Free Medicine and Surgery in Clinical Practice

Nicolas Jabbour, Ryan Young, S Ram Kumar,
Rick Selby, Yuri Genyk

Introduction

This chapter will serve as an overall guide to understanding the availability, cost and usage of blood products in the surgical discipline. We will show how careful perioperative management of a patient can decrease or eliminate the need for blood transfusion during major surgery, including liver transplantation. This discussion will include techniques used during operative procedures, such as cell saver and acute normovolemic hemodilution (ANH), which play a role in minimizing the need for blood products. We also will address postoperative issues regarding careful use of blood testing and an understanding of the relationship between oxygen consumption and delivery. In addition, artificial blood products and their potential applications in the future will be considered. Finally, we will present a summary of our data from the University of Southern California's Transfusion-Free Surgery Program with a focus on liver transplantation. As patients with liver disease often develop significant coagulopathy, we expect that the successful practice of transfusion-free medicine applied in these cases can safely be extrapolated to other procedures as well to significantly limit homologous blood usage.

The cost-effectiveness of blood products: a surgical perspective

Traditional notions about blood transfusions, including arbitrary cutoff values of hemoglobin (Hb) and theories supporting multiple unit transfusions, should be challenged in light of a better understanding of blood products in surgical and medical practice. While the use of blood products can be life-saving, it comes at a price. Blood is a precious, fast-depleting commodity with a sizable price tag and significant adverse effects associated with it, like any other intervention in medicine.

The wide-ranging impact of transfusion-free surgery cannot be fully realized before considering the status of blood donation and transfusion in the USA. Reports from the National Blood Data Resource Center reveal that in 2001 approximately 14 million units of blood were used in the treatment of 5 million patients, most of whom were older than 65. As the population of the USA ages, these blood requirements will only continue to rise. If this trend is not met by supply – and that is not likely given the increasing exclusionary criteria placed on collected blood along with declining donation rates – shortages are predicted to occur by the year 2030. At the time of this publication, elective surgeries have been delayed and sometimes cancelled with relative frequency, even at major medical centers due to inadequate blood supply. This shortage of blood products has a deleterious effect on the public's well-being directly and indirectly, especially during unforeseen events such as trauma, acts of terrorism and war. Often, the survival of a trauma patient is related directly to the adequate availability of blood products.

The cost of the practice of blood transfusion includes more than just acquisition, banking, work-up and dispensation of blood. Additional indirect expenditures arise surrounding the administration of blood products, which encompass, for example, the work-up and treatment of side-effects of blood transfusion. Fever, the most common side-effect of homologous blood transfusion, occurs at a rate of 1–2% and, in many instances, requires extensive radiographic and microbiologic evaluations. Taking into account all of these factors, the burden blood transfusion bears to society can amount to several billion dollars a year. Surgery influences this value significantly since greater than half of all transfused blood is administered to surgical patients.

Financial concerns aside, transfusion-associated health risks are an important consideration as well. Screening has significantly reduced the rate of viral transmission but has not eliminated it (See Table 2.2) [1], and there has been little improvement in the risk of bacterial sepsis. The risk of clinically apparent sepsis following blood transfusion exceeds the risk of human immunodeficiency virus (HIV), hepatitis B virus (HBV) and hepatitis C virus (HCV) transmission [2]. Transmission of prion-associated diseases, such as Creutzfeldt–Jakob disease, and of parasitic infections, such as Leishmaniasis or Chagas' disease, has been documented in small but significant numbers. ABO incompatibility occurs at a rate of 1 in 33 000 and acute anaphylaxis at 1 in 20 000–50 000 [1]. Transfusion-related acute lung injury (TRALI) is another rare, poorly understood, but potentially fatal, complication of blood transfusion.

Additionally, the immunomodulatory effects of allogeneic blood can have adverse consequences. A number of studies have indicated that homologous blood transfusions may increase the risk of postoperative bacterial infection [1,3,4]. In a meta-analysis of prospective trials comparing transfused versus nontransfused patients, Hill *et al.* [5] showed that transfused patients, especially trauma victims, were 3.45 times more likely to develop a postoperative bacterial infection. In a prospective study of transfusion in intensive care units (ICUs), Shorr *et al.* [6] showed by multivariate analyses that packed red blood cell (RBC) transfusion independently increases the risk of ventilator-associated pneumonia. Several studies also have documented a strong association between blood transfusion and cancer recurrence, although a causal relation has not been established. In a meta-analysis, Vamvakas [7] reported a 3.6 times increase in risk of cancer recurrence with blood transfusion in head and neck cancers, 2.4 times in gastric cancers, and 1.6 times in prostate cancers. Similarly, while examining colorectal cancers, Amato *et al.* [8] reported a 1.68 times increase in odds of recurrence with blood transfusion, irrespective of all patient or disease-specific factors. The risk of recurrence was directly related to the number of units transfused, with transfusion of greater than 3 units resulting in double the risk associated with transfusion of 1 or 2 units. Following transfusion of at least 2 units of allogeneic blood, the serum of patients begins to show a significant increase in vascular endothelial growth factor and a concomitant drop in endostatin, thereby rendering it favorable for angiogenesis [9] – a potential mechanism that mediates cancer recurrence. This angiogenic potential of the serum has been documented *in vitro* by a significant increase in endothelial cell proliferation and whole-assay angiogenesis [9].

We, therefore, believe that blood product transfusions are similar to organ transplantation and must be treated with as much care, attention and consideration, and must be used only when absolutely indicated (Figure 9.1). The goal of utilizing blood products should be limited to improving tissue oxygenation and facilitating coagulation.

Preoperative optimization of the surgical patient

Preoperative optimization is not a novel surgical practice. A number of patient variables have been studied in association with surgical outcome. Much focus has been placed on the link between a patient's nutritional status and the morbidity and mortality from surgical procedures. Interestingly, the need for transfusion during surgery has also been linked to a patient's nutritional status. Stephenson *et al.* [10] categorized 99 patients with end-stage liver disease requiring liver transplantation into mild, moderate and severe malnutrition based on subjective global assessment of nutritional status. After correcting for several patient variables such as age, sex, platelet count, serum creatinine and Hb levels, those with severe malnutrition were found to require significantly more packed RBC transfusion than those in the mild and moderate categories.

Traditionally, less emphasis has been placed on a patient's hematological status prior to surgery. Patients who are anemic prior to surgery are clearly more likely to receive transfusions than those who are not. In fact, in a multivariate analysis conducted in the study described above, the only other factor predictive of intraoperative transfusion was preoperative Hb levels [10]. We believe in extensively evaluating the integrity of the

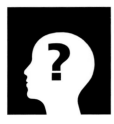 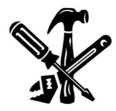 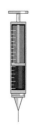

Decision-making
Indication
Timing of surgery
Two-stage procedure

Technical
Surgical Skills
Cell saver
ANH

Drug therapy
Erythropoietin
Factor VIIa
Aminocaproic acid
Aprotinin
Artificial blood?

Figure 9.1 Overall strategy to reduce the need for blood transfusion in surgical practice.

hematologic system prior to surgery, just as we would the cardiovascular or respiratory systems. The surgical community is not in the habit of enhancing hematologic values prior to surgery, a fact partially due to the perception of safety and universal availability of blood products. Anemia and coagulopathy should be addressed decisively preoperatively to improve the patient's Hb levels prior to surgery and to minimize operative blood loss. Clotting disorders as a result of vitamin K deficiency, for example, secondary to biliary obstruction, long-term parenteral nutrition, etc. should be alleviated via supplementation. When coagulopathy due to liver disease prevents response to this intervention, components of the clotting pathway may need to be replenished directly (as discussed in Chapter 5).

Anemia, with a wide array of causative factors such as chronic disease, bone marrow suppression, malnutrition, iron deficiency and hemolysis, can be a particular challenge to manage. One of the preferred approaches to managing preoperative anemia is directly enhancing the patient's red cell mass, which, in many ways, can be considered equivalent to autologous donation without the use of blood banking. We view the patient's bone marrow as an untapped well of blood products and reason that before asking of the general public, the patient can and should serve as a source of this precious product. By carefully and adequately stimulating the bone marrow, patients can produce an average of 1 unit of blood per week [11], resulting in more than 5 units of blood within 4–6 weeks.

To stimulate the bone marrow, it is important to understand the cause of anemia and also provide the bone marrow with the elements necessary for synthesis. Recombinant human erythropoietin (rHuEPO) has gained widespread popularity to enhance the possibility of autologous donation in a number of orthopedic surgical procedures [12,13] as well as for Jehovah's Witness patients [14,15,16]. Subcutaneous (SC) administration of rHuEPO (with a half-life of 19–22 h) has been preferred to the intravenous (IV) route (with half-life of 4–5 h) due to its increased ability to maintain effective stimulatory levels in the blood, cost-effectiveness and greater convenience of application [17]. In addition, a dosing interval of 72 h has been reported to result in greater reticulocyte responses than an interval of 24 h, with a maximum absolute dose of 900 IU/kg/week [18]. Bone marrow stimulation with rHuEPO can be employed in most patients even in the presence of malnutrition, liver disease or portal hypertension. However, in response to inflammation either from chronic or acute infections or neoplasm, the stimulatory effect of rHuEPO may be blunted. Kalantar-Zadeh *et al.* [19] examined erythropoietic responsiveness in a cohort of patients with anemia secondary to end-stage renal disease, a condition normally treated with rHuEPO. During a 13-week period, patients were given, on average, 217 U/kg of rHuEPO along with iron supplementation. Patients with higher Malnutrition Inflammation Scores (MIS) and increased inflammatory markers, such as IL-6, were found to have greater resistance to treatment. Ozguroglu *et al.* [20] studied the effect of endogenous EPO in 40 anemic cancer patients and in 20 otherwise healthy patients with iron deficiency anemia. They found a diminished response in the cancer patients at all observed Hb levels. In addition, because the anemic cancer patients were found to have higher measured levels of EPO than 34 cancer patients without anemia, the study attributed the findings to a blunted response to EPO. Anecdotally, we can document our own experience with this refractoriness to rHuEPO in a 76-year-old Jehovah's Witness male with renal cell carcinoma, malnutrition, mild anemia and a high fever that remained unresponsive to treatment. He was started on rHuEPO (300–1000 IU/kg/week) and iron (iron sulfate 325 mg PO TID for 12 days followed by iron dextran 100 mg IV QD for 12 days). After a full week of therapy, his iron profile remained abnormal, and no response was observed even after 4 weeks of therapy (Figure 9.2). We proceeded with surgery starting at a hematocrit (Hct) of 28%. The tumor was completely resected with minimal blood loss. He recovered well postoperatively, with the fever and tumor-induced inflammatory response subsiding immediately. Without any further rHuEPO therapy, his Hct steadily increased. Although the precise pathophysiology of this widely observed clinical effect has not been elucidated, it is believed that inflammatory cytokines, such as IL-1 and TNFα, directly inhibit erythropoiesis and induce iron sequestration by the reticuloendothelial system, promoting the synthesis of ferritin at the expense of RBC formation [21].

In addition to stimulation, supplemental minerals and vitamins are required for efficient erythropoiesis. Several studies have evaluated the effects of iron supplementation. EPO has been shown to hasten the depletion of iron stores by phelobotomy in iron-replete adults [22]. Physiologically normal amounts of mobilizable iron are frequently insufficient to meet the needs of the expanded

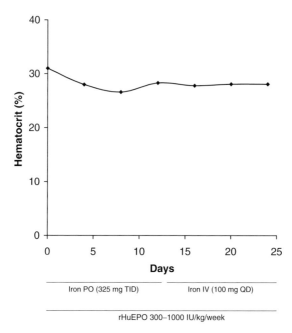

Figure 9.2 Cancer-related refractoriness of anemia to rHuEPO therapy.

pool of transferrin receptors on RBC precursors, resulting in relative iron deficiency and limiting rHuEPO-driven erythropoiesis [22]. Iron requirements (in mg) can be estimated by multiplying the factor of 150 by the amount of desired elevation in Hb (in g/dl). Pretreatment iron stores can be evaluated by measuring serum iron, total iron-binding capacity, transferrin saturation and ferritin levels. A functional iron deficiency occurs when transferrin saturation falls below 20%, serum ferritin declines to less than 100 μg/L or the proportion of hypochromic RBCs rises above 10%. Daily 200 mg doses of oral elemental iron, or 900 mg of iron sulfate, can be given during the first 4–6 weeks of treatment. The enteral route of supplementation, however, may not meet the requirements of a highly promoted erythropoiesis and may be poorly tolerated by patients. As a result, additional IV iron dextran or iron saccharate at a dose of 200 mg/week for 3–4 weeks may help meet the accelerated needs. Administration of parenteral iron, however, is associated with rare but potentially serious complications including life-threatening anaphylactoid reactions and possibly acute iron toxicity [23], a risk that may be even smaller with the use of the saccharate form. In our experience with three Jehovah's Witness patients with end-stage liver disease and major upper gastrointestinal (GI) variceal bleeding, we have elevated Hct levels from a low of 16% to 48% in the 3 months prior to surgery. Similarly, vitamin B12 and folate levels also must be monitored during rHuEPO therapy.

Attempts must be made preoperatively to minimize sources of blood loss. For example, in patients with massive esophageal varices or severe portal hypertension, minimizing preoperative blood loss may be just as important as the correction of anemia. A discriminatory use of a transjugular intrahepatic portosystemic shunt (TIPS) may be indicated in such select cases.

Intraoperative approach to transfusion-free surgery

There are some cardinal principles that need to be adhered to intraoperatively to minimize blood loss and preclude the need for transfusions. These include sound surgical judgment, accurate surgical technique, application of ANH and cell salvage techniques, management of anesthesia and optimization of the coagulation system.

Surgical judgment

Perioperative decision-making and judgment are as important as the surgical technique and are crucial to successful outcomes. Good decision-making involves flexibility and the acknowledgment that operative procedures should not proceed under unfavorable circumstances. Under conditions of foreseeable uncontrolled hemorrhage, for example, alternative methods and approaches must be pursued.

To illustrate this, we will use the case of a 35-year-old Jehovah's Witness male with end-stage liver disease (CPT score of 8 and stage 3 on the UNOS waiting list) secondary to primary sclerosing cholangitis [24]. Prior GI bleeding from esophageal and gastric varices had reduced his Hct to 16%. TIPS, rHuEPO, folic acid and iron supplementation raised his Hct to 49%. His platelet count was 49 000/cmm prior to a scheduled live-donor liver transplant (LDLT) using the right lobe of his mother. At the start of the procedure, 6 units of blood were removed as part of ANH, which was made feasible by the preoperative elevation in the patient's Hct. Intraoperatively, an unusually large left lateral segment of liver was encountered and found to be adherent to the spleen (Figure 9.3A, B, C). Attempts to ligate the upper polar branch of the splenic artery led to significant hemorrhage from perisplenic collaterals, likely due to severe portal hypertension. Consequently, we decided to approach the procedure in stages. A partial hepatectomy was performed and the donor lobe was implanted successfully with a total blood loss of 2900 cc, of which 850 cc was reinfused using the cell saver. Despite this blood loss, his Hct at the end of surgery was 45%, due to the judicious intraoperative use of ANH and cell-saver techniques. With recovery of the implanted liver, the patient's coagulopathy spontaneously corrected and platelet count recovered (Figure 9.3D). In 2 weeks, he was taken back for removal of the remaining left lateral segment of the liver and partial splenectomy. Notwithstanding a complicated course and a major surgical undertaking, the patient was discharged in 3 weeks

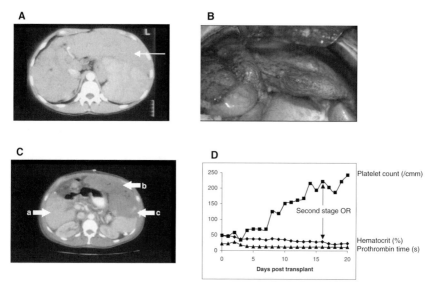

Figure 9.3 Staging hepatectomy during live-donor liver transplant (LDLT) in Jehovah's Witness recipient. This 35-year-old male was in end-stage liver failure due to primary sclerosing cholangitis. (A) A preoperative CT scan demonstrates a large left lateral segment of the liver (arrow), (B) which was confirmed at surgery. Due to severe hemorrhage from splenic collaterals during hepatectomy, the procedure was staged. A partial hepatectomy was performed leaving behind the left lateral segment adherent to the spleen and the donor lobe implanted. (C) Postoperative CT scan on day 15 showing (a) the transplanted right lobe of the liver, (b) the devascularized left lateral segment of the cirrhotic liver and (c) the ischemic upper pole of the spleen. Following recovery of the implanted liver and (D) improvement in his hematologic and coagulation parameters, he was taken back to the operating room for completion hepatectomy and partial splenectomy. He had an uncomplicated recovery. Portions of the figure republished with permission from [24].

with completely normal liver function, without the administration of any blood products during the course of his treatment. He is doing well 4 years later. The concept of a two-stage procedure is not a new one. However, in this particular scenario, the risk of uncontrolled bleeding had to be weighed against the septic complications due to the remaining segment of liver and the partially infarcted spleen, and the time interval required for the transplanted liver to recover before proceeding with the next surgery.

With the routine application of highly innovative technology to the practice of medicine, less focus is directed toward clinical management and thought processes involved in overall patient care. Clearly, there is no substitute for good surgical judgment, and astute clinical management continues to play a pivotal role in patient outcome.

Surgical technique

As long as a patient's Hb is sufficient to provide tissues with adequate oxygen, the only indication for blood transfusion is to replace operative blood loss. Transfusion is not a therapeutic goal in itself. Of all the indications for intraoperative blood product utilization, most are related directly to the amount of blood lost. Surgeons, therefore, are the only health care providers who can effectively decrease the use of blood products. To provide a safe, transfusion-free surgical practice, therefore, surgical techniques should be driven by a zero tolerance for blood loss. Precise technique and meticulous hemostasis must be the cornerstones of any surgical procedure. The patient's coagulation system should not be relied upon, and simple physical packing, even of minor bleeding, should not be considered sufficient. We recommend resorting to more dependable measures such as argon beam electrocautery and suture ligation.

We have been amply rewarded by the application of these principles to liver transplant recipients in end-stage liver disease with severe coagulopathy and portal hypertension. Of the 120 live-donor hepatectomies performed at our center over the last 4 years, only one patient required transfusion of 1 unit of packed RBCs due to hemorrhage from spontaneous slippage of a vascular clamp on the vena cava (Figure 9.4). In addition, over 80% of liver resections are performed at our center without the use of any blood products. As a result of broadening the use of these technical principles from Jehovah's Witness patients to all patients, our surgical center has, during the past few years, seen significant reductions in blood product usage in several other

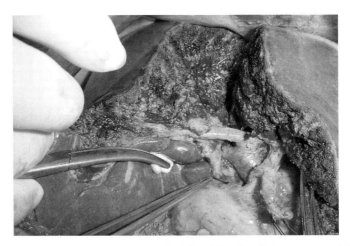

Figure 9.4 Operative picture showing right lobe of the liver being transected during live-donor liver transplantation (LDLT). Note that transection of the liver parenchyma is performed without vascular control. Hemostatsis is achieved with surgical clips. The average blood loss during partial hepatectomy at our center is under 400 cc.

procedures including pancreatic resection, complicated biliary surgery and orthopedic procedures. We believe that application of these principles across nature or type of procedure should be feasible and should result in diminished blood product utilization following any surgical procedure.

Intraoperative cell salvage

Intraoperative cell salvage (ICS) serves as an effective tool in blood conservation by allowing the retrieval and reuse of blood lost in the operative field. Several studies have documented the intact structure and function of RBCs recycled in this fashion. Electron microscopy has revealed only minor alterations in RBC morphology with ICS [25]. The RBCs maintain near normal survival [26] as well as 2,3 diphosphoglycerate concentration [27]. ICS is regarded as a reliable method of autotransfusion and is embraced even by Jehovah's Witness patients if administered via a contained system continuous with the patient at all times. ICS has been successfully employed to reduce the need for allogeneic blood in a wide variety of surgical procedures including gynecologic [28], cardiac [29], orthopedic [30] and liver transplant [31] surgery. A meta-analysis by Huet *et al.* [32] showed that with the use of ICS, exposure of orthopedic surgery patients to homologous blood products was reduced by 61%. McGill *et al.* [33], in a randomized controlled trial, documented that when undertaken with ICS, patients undergoing coronary artery bypass were 0.47 times less likely to require blood products.

However, the use of ICS brings with it a new set of important considerations prior to its integration into any program. Probably the most controversial issue surrounding ICS is cost. The cell-saver device, associated components and disposables, and the services of a perfusionist add up to a significant financial undertaking. Several studies have evaluated the ICS economic burden in comparison to blood transfusions [34,35]. Shuhaiber *et al.* [36] evaluated the impact of introducing ICS into a community hospital for use in abdominal aortic aneurysm repairs. The authors retrospectively looked at 93 elective and 25 emergent aortic aneurysm repairs: 33% of elective repairs and 84% of emergent repairs exclusively received allogeneic blood, while the rest received some combination of allogeneic and autologous blood. The use of ICS did not statistically significantly reduce the need for allogeneic blood or impact the length of hospital stay or postoperative Hb levels. However, the incorporation of ICS doubled the expenditure associated with blood product utilization.

In a study of orthotopic liver transplants, Kemper *et al.* [37] compared the cost of ICS based on the duration of the surgery with the absolute cost of transfusing equivalent amounts of allogeneic packed RBCs. On an average, autologous ICS cost $1048/patient, while an equivalent amount of allogeneic blood was calculated at $429/patient. Their case-by-case analysis revealed that in only three patients (4.8%) who received between 16.4 and 46.6 units of recycled cells did the use of ICS result in cost savings. In stark contrast, other studies that have looked at all surgical patients in a general hospital setting [38] or exclusively abdominal trauma victims [39] have reported significant financial savings with the use of ICS. A retrospective review [40] of patients who underwent elective abdominal aortic aneurysm repair examined the cost-effectiveness of a standby cell saver for all patients. Factoring in the expenses associated with acquisition, laboratory services, administration and overheads, the authors computed a cost of $169 for 1 unit of autologous blood that compared favorably with $155 for 1 unit of allogeneic blood. From this data, the authors concluded that operations involving at least 1000 ml blood loss with cell salvage of at least 750 ml would benefit from ICS.

Szpisjak *et al.* [41] examined the economic factors involved in the incorporation of an intraoperative autotransfusion service using four differing economic models. The fully outsourced model evaluated the cost when the entire service was outsourced; in the partially outsourced model, the equipment and disposables were provided by the hospital while the technician was contracted; the new employee model involved hiring a full-time technician exclusively for the ICS service; and in the cross-trained model, the equipment and disposables were provided by the hospital and the technician was an employee who was cross-trained in the operation of ICS. Their analysis assumed a maximum of one case per day using ICS and a fixed cost of ICS per use. The authors found that the fully outsourced model was the most economical for caseloads below 55 cases annually, beyond which the cross-trained model was predicted to generate the lowest cost (Figure 9.5). In

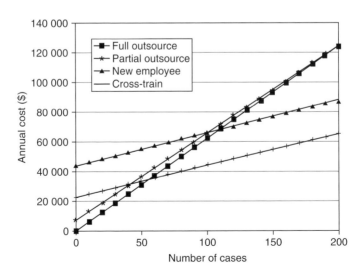

Figure 9.5 Annual cost of incorporation of intraoperative cell salvage (ICS) technology using four economic models. (*Source*: Reproduced with permission from [41].)

reality, the cost analysis of ICS is complex and depends on a variety of factors including the type of cell-salvage device, nature of surgical procedures, amount of blood loss and annual caseload. More importantly, studies of cost are an index of the direct financial burden. What cannot be included in these analyses is the price of allogeneic blood transfusion, far more important than the mere cost of it. For all the reasons we have discussed earlier, ICS will certainly ease the burden on the need for blood products and, we believe, may even lead to an eventual financial benefit.

Another important consideration with the use of ICS is that only RBCs are salvaged. The blood that is recycled is depleted of clotting factors and platelets. Large-volume ICS may, therefore, lead to a coagulopathy if clotting factors are not appropriately replenished. If heparin is used in the ICS circuit to prevent clotting, the returned blood cells must be washed carefully of any residual heparin. Some of the other complications associated with the use of ICS include air embolism, infection and disseminated intravascular coagulation (DIC) [28]. To minimize these risks, ICS is contraindicated in patients with intra-abdominal infections and in cases with potential for contamination with gastric or amniotic fluid. Certain local clotting agents, such as gelatin sponges, powders or collagen-hemostatic material, should also be avoided in conjunction with ICS (Table 9.1).

Caution also should be exercised with the use of ICS in patients with malignancy. Animal studies have suggested that tumor cells are capable of maintaining viability even after filtration and centrifugation in ICS [42], and there is hence at least a theoretical potential for systemic dissemination of malignant cells. In a study of 408 patients who underwent radical retropubic prostatectomy for cancer, Davis *et al.* [43] monitored prostate-specific antigen (PSA) levels postoperatively as a surrogate for cancer recurrence. They found no difference in recurrence rates between patients who received ICS, autologous blood or no transfusion at all. Furthermore, there is evidence that the application of specific techniques may even reduce the likelihood of malignant cell transmission.

Hansen *et al.* [44] investigated the effect of irradiating salvaged blood that contains neoplastic cells *in vitro*. Tumor cells obtained from a number of cell lines and solid tumors, such as breast, colon, pancreatic and prostate cancers, were added to washed RBCs. At a radiation dose of 50 Gy, they documented complete eradication of the proliferative capacity and DNA metabolism of all neoplastic cells, even when the mixtures contained 10^7-10^{10} tumor cells prior to irradiation. The erythrocytes remained unaffected, maintaining their 2,3 DPG and ATP levels, as well as their rheologic properties and structural integrity. Leukocyte-depletion filters (LDFs) also have been studied *in vitro* to limit reinfusion of cancer cells. Edelman *et al.* [45] ran suspensions containing 10^6 cells from renal cell, prostate and transitional cell carcinoma cell lines through a standard ICS, a standard blood filter and an LDF. The LDF, but not the other two, was effective at completely eliminating tumor cells from the suspension. Both irradiation and LDF come at an additional

Table 9.1 Common hemostatic agents and their use with intraoperative cell salvage (ICS).

Agent	Type	Source	Use with ICS	Precaution
AVITENE	Collagen (powder and web)	Med-Chem	No	Flush wound with large amount of saline after product activated before resuming ICS
COLLOSTAT	Collagen powder	Vitaphore	No	Flush wound with large amount of saline after product activated before resuming ICS
COLLOSTAT	Collagen matrix sponge	Vitaphore	Yes	Avoid direct aspiration into ICS suction
GELFOAM	Gelatin powder	Upjohn	No	Flush wound with large amount of saline after product activated before resuming ICS
GELFOAM	Gelatin sponge	Upjohn	No	Flush wound with large amount of saline after product activated before resuming ICS
HELISTAT	Absorbable collagen sponge	Colla-tec, Inc.	Yes	Avoid direct aspiration into ICS suction
HEMOPAD	Nonwoven collagen pad	Astra	No	Flush wound with large amount of saline after product activated before resuming ICS
INSTAT	Collagen sponge	J&J	No	Flush wound with large amount of saline after product activated before resuming ICS
SURGICEL	Collagen fabric	J&J	Yes	Avoid direct aspiration into ICS suction
THROMBOGEN	Bovine thrombin spray	J&J	Yes	Avoid direct aspiration into ICS suction
THROMBOSTAT	Bovine thrombin spray	Parke Davis	Yes	Avoid direct aspiration into ICS suction

expense, but they may be justifiable when the use of ICS may be lifesaving in, for example, a Jehovah's Witness patient, to avoid the alternative of potentially life-threatening anemia.

In sum, while the technology of ICS is rapidly evolving, significant controversy surrounds the utility of ICS, and several precautionary measures need to be undertaken for its successful use. We believe that a judicious expansion of the application of ICS will significantly assist in the maturation of a transfusion-free program.

Acute normovolemic hemodilution

A promising complement to ICS is ANH. It is normally considered if the potential for blood loss exceeds 20% of the patient's blood volume [46]. ANH involves collection of blood and its replacement with a colloid or crystalloid infusion just prior to incision, followed by reinfusion of the collected blood at the conclusion of the surgery. By inducing a moderate isovolemic anemia during surgery, the blood lost is diluted, and by withdrawing and later reinfusing whole blood, ANH spares not only the red cell mass but platelets and clotting factors as well. Experience with ANH has revealed that normovolemic anemia is well tolerated in most patients. We demonstrate in Figure 9.6 the physiologic changes with ANH in various cardiovascular parameters in one of our patients. As the Hct falls (usually to the low 20s), cardiac output (CO) rises while the central venous pressure (CVP) is maintained at its initial level throughout surgery. In addition to the increased CO,

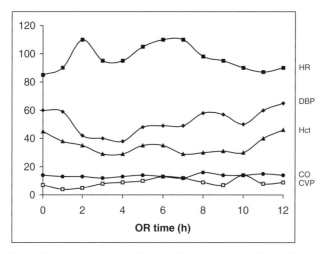

Figure 9.6 Physiologic changes in cardiovascular parameters observed in a patient following acute normovolemic hemodilution (ANH). HR, heart rate (beats/min); DBP, diastolic blood pressure (mmHg); Hct, hematocrit (%); CO, cardiac output (L/min); CVP, central venous pressure (mm water); OR, operating room.

the main compensatory responses seen include an increased oxygen extraction at the tissue along with a rightward shift of the oxyhemoglobin dissociation curve (see Chapter 6).

Under anesthesia, these responses can occur without significant elevations in heart rate. Several studies have corroborated these findings in cardiovascular parameters. Weiskopf *et al.* [47] studied 32 healthy volunteers in whom ANH was instituted to Hb levels of 5 g/dl. Oxygen consumption, plasma lactate concentration and electrocardiographic (ECG) changes were monitored. Even after 2.4 h of isovolemic anemia, there was no evidence of inadequate oxygenation, no change was observed in right or left side filling pressures, nor was a significant alteration seen in lactate levels. The ECG findings were mostly normal, except for ST elevations in two patients, which resolved without sequelae. A mild increase in oxygen consumption was detected, but the compensatory responses were mainly due to an increased heart rate (75%) and CO (25%). In a meta-analysis of the effect of normovolemic anemia following surgery in Jehovah's Witness patients [48], the risk of postoperative mortality was found to be significantly higher in patients with underlying cardiovascular disease. Consequently, ANH is not recommended in patients with myocardial disease or in infants and neonates.

ANH offers a few advantages over preoperative autologous donation (PAD). There are added benefits of greater convenience and reduced expense. Blood collection as part of ANH is performed only once, on the day of surgery in the operating room, whereas PAD can involve multiple clinic visits depending on the quantity of blood desired. This additional administrative cost when coupled with the extra expenditure associated with discarded or unused blood units [49] diminishes the appeal of PAD. Nor does PAD guarantee against clerical errors or mishandling leading to a host of other complications. Furthermore, the quality of blood used in PAD often can be compromised in manners that are unlikely to occur within ANH. For example, stored blood can develop abnormal 2,3 DPG levels and other biochemical alterations that can reduce the oxygen-carrying capacity. Finally, ANH has the potential of gaining acceptance among Jehovah's Witnesses because collected blood can be kept within an extracorporeal circuit that is in continuity with the patient.

Anesthesia management

Vital to the management and maintenance of a patient's hematologic system is clear communication with the anesthesiologist. The role of anesthesiologists in blood management is critical, especially given their involvement in ICS and ANH. The explicit goals of anesthesia during transfusion-free surgery should include the maintenance of normovolemic status and the potential need for hyperoxic ventilation and controlled hypotensive anesthesia. For example, a low CVP may markedly reduce blood loss during parenchymal transection for liver resection. In a similar fashion, blood loss during spinal surgery can be curtailed significantly by relative hypotensive anesthesia. Avoidance of hypothermia can help avoid temperature-related coagulopathy.

Coagulation management

Meticulous surgical technique aside, an understanding and an optimization of the coagulation system during surgery are essential to minimize blood loss. This approach must go beyond the standard coagulation tests, such as prothrombin time (PT), partial prothrombin time (PTT) and platelet count, which reflect the quantity of clotting factors but convey little in regard to the quality of clot formation. While these basic measurements suffice in most patients, in select instances, more sophisticated monitoring may be required. For example, fibrinolysis can be a major cause of coagulopathy unresponsive to conventional treatment in patients with end-stage liver disease. However, the diagnosis of fibrinolysis cannot be made by the usual coagulation tests, mandating the need for a thomboelastogram (Figure 9.7) (see Chapter 5).

Until recently, the correction of coagulopathy implied the infusion of blood products such as fresh frozen plasma (FFP), cryoprecipitate (CRYO) and platelets. Recently, significant inroads have been made into the understanding of, and ability to manipulate, several other factors that play a major role in enhancing coagulation. As mentioned above, in end-stage liver failure patients with reticent coagulopathy, the use of epsilon-aminocaproic acid (EACA) to limit fibrinolysis may be of significant benefit. In a randomized, prospective study, the use of both EACA and tranexamic acid (TXA) significantly reduced blood loss, transfusion requirements and sternal closure times in children undergoing corrective surgery for cyanotic heart disease [50]. A recent multicenter, randomized study examined the effectiveness of aprotinin in orthotopic liver transplantation [51]. Porte *et al.* divided 137 patients with similar clinical characteristics, preoperative laboratory parameters and surgical variables into three groups based on preoperative administration of high-dose aprotinin, regular-dose aprotinin and placebo. High-dose aprotinin, which served to inhibit kallekrein, and regular-dose aprotinin, at a plasmin-inhibiting level, were administered at a loading dose of 2×10^6 KIU (kallekrein-inhibiting units), followed by an infusion of 1×10^6 KIU/h and 0.5×10^6 KIU/h respectively, until 2 h after graft reperfusion. Aprotinin administration resulted in significant reduction in blood loss by 60% in the high-dose group and 44% in the regular-dose group ($p = 0.03$), with a concomitant fall in the need for homologous and autologous blood ($p = 0.02$) and blood products ($p = 0.01$). All of these benefits were observed in the absence of any prothrombotic complication.

Recombinant activated factor VII (rFVIIa) was initially introduced as an alternative therapy for hemophiliacs with inhibitors for human factors. Extracted from transfected hamster kidney cells, rFVIIa is characterized by an amino acid sequence and biological activity that are identical to activated human factor VII. rFVIIa binds to exposed tissue factor at sites of injury only, thereby promoting the formation of a localized clot, without increasing the

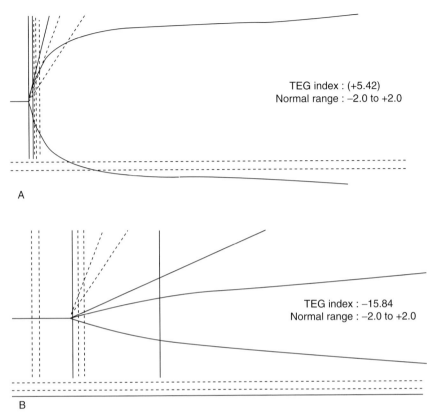

Figure 9.7 Thromboelastogram (TEG) evaluates quality of blood clot formation. The tracing in A shows generation of a good quality clot as evidenced by the rapid and widely separated lines with a positive TEG index. To the contrary, the tracing in B shows a slow rising and narrow tracing with a negative TEG index, indicating clinically significant fibrinolysis. Of note, both patients had comparable results on the standard coagulation tests.

risk of systemic thrombosis. Its initial role in the management of hemophilia has been expanded upon in recent years (an off-label use outside of the Food and Drug Administration (FDA)-approved indication) to include liver disease, drug-induced coagulopathy, platelet disorders such as Glanzmann thrombasthenia, pregnancy-related clotting disorders and DIC [52]. More recently, rFVIIa has shown significant promise for the control of bleeding in several surgical procedures such as liver transplantation, trauma [53], vascular surgery [54] and prostatectomy [55]. Egan *et al.* [56] retrospectively reviewed the records of six children who underwent cardiac surgery, which was complicated by persistent bleeding unresponsive to conventional therapy consisting of aprotinin, FFP and CRYO. Two IV doses of rFVIIa given 2 h apart significantly curtailed the bleeding. The authors, hence, support the use of rFVIIa as a safe tool for hemostasis that may serve to limit the need for repeat thoracotomy in this population.

Given that most clotting factors are synthesized by the liver, and that FVIIa, with a half-life of less than 2 h, is depleted most rapidly in liver failure, rFVIIa is thought to hold significant promise in liver transplantation [57,58]. In an open-label, pilot study on six patients undergoing liver transplantation, the use of a single 80 fg/kg dose of rFVIIa resulted in a significant reduction in blood loss and the requirement of both packed RBCs and FFP compared to matched controls [57]. We have reviewed our experience with the use of rFVIIa in ten Jehovah's Witness patients undergoing liver transplantation between 2001 and 2003 [59]. Eight of the patients had decompensated cirrhosis, secondary to hepatitis C, one had alpha-1 antitrypsin deficiency, and one had cryptogenic cirrhosis, with a CPT score of 11 and MELD scores spread between 14 and 38. Six patients underwent cadaveric liver transplants, while the remainder received live-donor liver lobes. The administration of rFVIIa intravenously at induction of anesthesia, in conjunction with ANH and ICS, was helpful in these patients with severe coagulopathy who refuse blood products. Two patients died, who both had dialysis-dependent renal failure as well, and it is highly likely that the negative outcome may have been related to uremic platelet dysfunction or von-Willebrand factor (vWF) deficiency, in addition to coagulopathy from liver failure.

One of the major concerns surrounding the use of such potent clotting factors is the propensity to develop a prothrombotic state, especially in patients who have undergone vascular interventions. We have encountered only one portal vein thrombosis 1 month following an LDLT in a Jehovah's Witness patient in whom rFVIIa was used intraoperatively. In this particular instance, the donor had two separate portal veins requiring back-table reconstruction with the patient's jugular and facial vein branches. The short half-life of FVIIa, and the need for four separate venous anastomosis to reconstruct the portal vein in this patient, made a contributing role for rFVIIa very unlikely. Nonetheless, the potential for prothrombotic complications must be borne in mind when potent clotting factors are used to treat reticent coagulopathy.

Postoperative care

Appropriate postoperative management of the hematologic system begins with prevention and early recognition of blood loss. Any sudden drop in Hct or ongoing blood loss from drains should warrant consideration of active bleeding and be dealt with promptly. Further work-up, including laboratory testing, should not delay institution of appropriate interventions. Phlebotomy represents a major and underappreciated source of blood loss, especially in the ICU setting. Restricting investigations to the absolute essential, avoidance of blood draw from large-bore or high-flow lines, and minimizing the quantity of blood drawn by using pediatric collection tubes can significantly limit iatrogenic postoperative anemia. MacIsaac et al. [60] investigated the effects of a blood-conserving device on anemia in a randomized trial of 160 patients. After matching for age, sex and severity of illness, the use of the venous arterial management protection plus (VAMP Plus) system reduced the amount of blood used for lab testing by 53% when compared with routine blood draws from standard arterial lines.

There is an increasing body of evidence that moderate degrees of anemia are well tolerated by a majority of patients in the postoperative recovery phase. Hebert et al. [61] conducted a randomized trial examining the relationship between transfusion strategies and patient outcomes. Among 838 patients with Hb levels less than 9 g/dl within 72 h of admission to an ICU, approximately half were managed using a liberal strategy of transfusing blood for Hb values below 10 g/dl, while the rest were assigned to a more restrictive strategy of transfusion for levels below 7 g/dl. The overall in-hospital mortality was significantly lower in the restrictive group, as was 30-day mortality among patients under 55 years of age or those less acutely ill. The overall 30-day mortality was similar between both groups. Patients with cardiac disease, however, represent a unique population for whom additional consideration is warranted. In an investigation of the effect of anemia on surgical morbidity and mortality in patients with cardiovascular disease, the cases of 1958 Jehovah's Witnesses who declined transfusions were reviewed by Carson et al. [48]. They found that mortality increased from 1.3% in patients with Hb levels exceeding 12 g/dl to 33.3% in those with Hb levels less than 6 g/dl.

The adverse effects of blood transfusion are particularly more pronounced in the postoperative period. In a prospective, multicenter study of 4892 ICU patients, Corwin et al. [62] reported that 44% received at least 1 unit of packed RBCs. Only 19% of the 213 participating hospitals followed established guidelines governing transfusion, and low Hb value (at a mean of 8.6 g/dl) was cited 90% of the times as the reason for the transfusion. Blood transfusion was associated with a significantly increased incidence of acute respiratory distress syndrome, pneumonia and infection. In addition, after correcting for baseline Hb levels and severity of illness, transfusion had a strong correlation with prolonged hospitalization and increased mortality.

Studies that have evaluated the role of rHuEPO in the postoperative period have produced mixed results [63], largely related to the heterogeneity of the patients studied and the high degree of variability among drug administration protocols. Animal studies have documented improved erythropoiesis with the use of rHuEPO post laparotomy [64]. In two large, randomized, prospective studies, Corwin et al. [65,66] showed that the use of rHuEPO resulted in significantly higher Hb levels and reduced blood transfusion requirements. No improvement was observed, though, in the duration of hospitalization or mortality. Gabriel et al. [67] observed that in patients with multiple organ

A Normal postoperative course

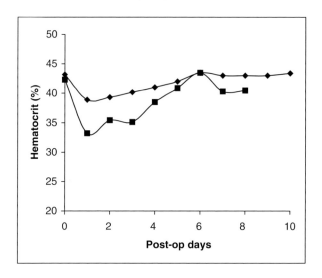

B Complicated postoperative course

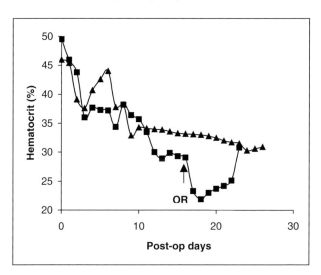

Figure 9.8 Response to rHuEPO in the postoperative period. (A) The two patients who had an uncomplicated course had a predicted improvement in hematocrit (Hct) levels. (B) Patient 1 (▲) developed intra-abdominal sepsis and his Hct did not respond to rHuEPO until control of the sepsis; patient 2 (■) had an unrecognized splenic infarct and its appropriate management at surgery rapidly restored the erythropoietic capability of rHuEPO.

dysfunction, despite increased cytokine levels, rHuEPO resulted in increased reticulocyte counts, though it did not translate into a reduction in transfusion requirement. Still *et al.* [68] also observed no change in transfusion requirements despite rHuEPO administration. In our experience, the preoperative effectiveness of rHuEPO is retained during the postoperative period. Not surprisingly, postoperative complications can diminish the responsiveness to rHuEPO. Figure 9.8 shows the postoperative Hct levels in four liver transplant recipients on rHuEPO. Patients in (A) had an uncomplicated course, with a predicted improvement in Hct levels. Postoperative infectious complications in patients in (B) resulted in a transient unresponsiveness to rHuEPO. Appropriate management of the complications rapidly restored the erythropoietic capability of rHuEPO.

Additional goals that complement reducing blood loss and improving Hb levels in the postoperative period include augmenting oxygen delivery and reducing oxygen consumption. Oxygen delivery can be improved by increasing the inhaled oxygen content (via supplemental oxygen, mechanical ventilation or hyperbaric oxygen), maintaining adequate intravascular volume and optimizing cardiac performance. Appropriate cardiac and respiratory support, control of fevers and shivering, and bed rest with sedation or complete paralysis in selected instances can help minimize oxygen consumption. To illustrate this, we review the case of a 65-year-old Jehovah's Witness male admitted to our center for a cadaveric liver transplant. Preoperatively, he was markedly coagulopathic and anemic due to severe liver disease and hepatorenal syndrome, for which he underwent intraoperative dialysis. Postoperatively, his Hct fell to 13% and remained refractory to rHuEPO, iron and folic acid supplementation. As a result of his anemia, he developed cardiac arrhythmia refractory to medical therapy. Unable to improve his oxygen delivery further, we directed our attention towards decreasing oxygen consumption. Ventilatory support (which accounted for over 30% of the oxygen consumption in this patient) through a tracheostomy was implemented. His arrhythmia resolved spontaneously. He continued to improve, and once his Hct reached 20%, ventilatory support was successfully weaned and he was discharged 3 months after the transplant with normal liver and kidney function.

In another 67-year-old Jehovah's Witness female, the stump of the right hepatic artery ruptured postoperatively following right hepatic resection. Bleeding was controlled surgically, and her postoperative Hct was 12%. She was left intubated and paralyzed in order to decrease her oxygen consumption, while allowing the bone marrow to recover. Her Hct gradually improved with supportive measures (Figure 9.9) and she was extubated and discharged within 3 weeks without any further complications.

While we do not advocate these measures as an alternative to homologous blood transfusion, these examples show how manipulating oxygen delivery and consumption may be lifesaving if timely blood transfusion is not possible such as in Jehovah's Witness patients or when compatible blood may not be readily available.

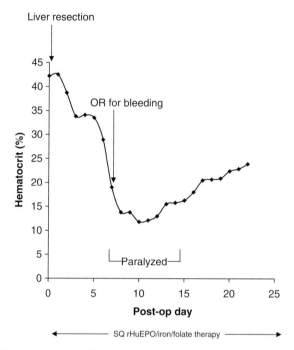

Figure 9.9 Balancing oxygen delivery and consumption. Spontaneous recovery of hematocirt (Hct) in a 67-year-old Jehovah's Witness female following paralysis and ventilatory support after a right hepatectomy was complicated by bleeding, refractory anemia and hypoxic complications.

Feasibility and results of transfusion-free surgery: University of Southern California experience

While few reports of bloodless liver transplantation exist in the literature, we have performed 27 such procedures between 1999 and 2004 (3 pediatric patients and 24 adults) [69,70]. We have reviewed the adult experience [71] comparing 16 live-donor and 8 cadaveric transplantations (Table 9.2). All patients received preoperative blood augmentation with rHuEPO, intraoperative ANH and ICS. All 16 patients survived in the live-donor group, while 6 of 8 survived in the cadaveric group (75% survival) – the two deaths being related to intraoperative graft failure in one and severe coagulopathy and anemia postoperatively in the other. Figure 9.10 illustrates the trend in postoperative Hb levels in two patients. The patient in A had an uneventful postoperative course associated with a quick recovery of his Hb level. He was discharged home within 1 week and is well at 4-year follow-up. The patient in B had a complicated postoperative period requiring multiple

Table 9.2 University of Southern California experience with liver transplantation in 24 Jehovah's Witness adults.

Parameter	Live donor (n = 16)	Cadaveric donor (n = 8)
Preoperative variables		
Age (years)	44.5 (17–62)	53 (47–66)
No. with prior GI bleed	8 (50%)	2 (29%)
No. with prior abdominal surgery	6 (38%)	1 (14%)
TIPSS	5 (31%)	2 (29%)
Ascites	11 (69%)	5 (71%)
Encephalopathy	8 (50%)	5 (71%)
Bilirubin (mg/dl)	4.9 (0.9–22.5)	11.4 (1.3–33.1)
Albumin (gm/dl)	3.1 (2.1–4.2)	2.4 (1.9–3.6)
Hematologic profile		
Pre-op hematocrit (%)	42.8 (34.9–49.5)	35.8 (26.9–45.3)
End of surgery hematocrit (%)	37.8 (23.5–48.5)	24.4 (17.4–34.8)
Discharge hematocrit (%)	32.7 (21.1–43.4)	26 (20.9–33.9)
Pre-op PT (s)	14.3 (11.4–19.7)	20.0 (14.3–24.9)
Highest post-op PT (s)	22.3 (13.3–30.5)	18.4 (15.3–23.6)
Pre-op platelets (/cmm)	96.1 (48–182)	49.8 (21–119)
Lowest post-op platelets (/cmm)	46.8 (14–101)	25 (10–34)

abdominal explorations for persistent intra-abdominal infection. During this course, his Hct fell to a low of 12%. With aggressive and appropriate intervention, his abdominal sepsis was controlled resulting in rapid improvement in Hb levels and complete recovery without sequelae. He continues to do well 3 years later. This case serves to illustrate patient response to appropriate therapy even in the face of severe anemia, and reiterates that surgery or any other necessary intervention should not be withheld solely because of profound anemia.

We also have reviewed our experience with 38 LDLTs between 1998 and 2001, 8 in Jehovah's Witness patients (the transfusion-free TF group) and the remainder in the transfusion-eligible (TE) group [69]. Patients in the TF group were approached utilizing the transfusion-free principles reviewed in this chapter, including preoperative rHuEPO administration, ANH, ICS and rFVIIa supplementation, all of which were used sparingly in the TE group. All donor hepatectomies were completed without any intraoperative complication or the use of blood products. Preoperative liver disease severity was similar in both groups, as was the hospital course, including operative times and hospital stays (Table 9.3). TF patients began with significantly higher Hct levels following EPO augmentation and had similar levels postoperatively. In the TE group, 80% of patients received a median of 4.5 ± 3.5

A

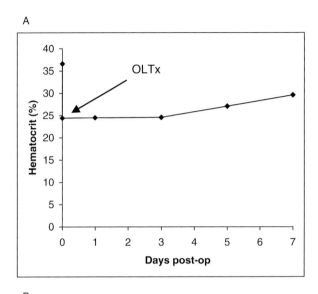

B

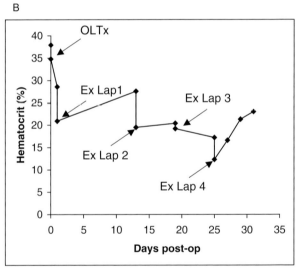

Figure 9.10 Trend in postoperative hematocrit (Hct) levels in two patients following orthotopic liver transplantation (OLTx). The patient in (A) had an uneventful recovery with a prompt improvement in Hct. The patient in (B) had a complicated postoperative course requiring multiple abdominal explorations (Ex Lap) for persistent intra-abdominal sepsis. With aggressive interventions to control the septic process, his Hct rapidly improved.

units of packed RBCs. Survival was 100% in the TF group and 90% in the TE group. We believe that a comprehensive understanding of every aspect of transfusion-free surgery, including preoperative optimization, intraopera-

Table 9.3 Comparison of pre-, intra- and postoperative outcomes following live-donor liver transplants (LDLTs) in 8 transfusion-free (TF) and 30 transfusion-eligible (TE) patients at the University of Southern California.

Parameter	Transfusion-free (TF) group (n = 8)	Transfusion-eligible (TE) group (n = 30)
Preoperative variables		
Hematocrit (%)	43.8 (34.5–49.5)	35.3 (24.2–48.1)
Platelets (/cmm)	102 (41–172)	113 (26–594)
Prothrombin time (s)	14.0 (11.3–21.2)	16.1 (10.2–64.8)
Albumin (gm/dl)	3.1 (2.1–3.9)	3.0 (2.0–4.2)
Total bilirubin (mg/dl)	7.5 (1.2–22.5)	4.4 (0.3–32.4)
CPT score	8 (5–13)	8.4 (5–12)
Intraoperative variables		
Beginning hematocrit (%)	43.8 (34.5–49.5)	35.6 (28.0–48.1)
Ending hematocrit (%)	37.5 (29.4–46.4)	35.3 (23.4–47.5)
Units transfused	0	4.5 (0–14)
Postoperative variables		
ICU stay (days)	5.0 (2–9)	5.8 (2–18)
Hospital stay (days)	17.5 (8–27)	19.5 (8–71)
Need for reoperation	2 (25%)	9 (30%)
Survival (%)	100	90

tive judgment and efficient blood conservation, and postoperative management has significantly contributed to this success. The advent of LDLT has further expanded the possibilities of performing transplants prior to the onset of end-stage liver disease and therefore increased the feasibility of achieving favorable outcomes.

   The techniques used in adult liver transplantation have also been applied to two pediatric Jehovah's Witness patients to avoid blood transfusion [70], although Jehovah's Witness children may be transfused (see Chapter 1). These two children were 6 months and 3 years of age and had end-stage liver disease secondary to biliary atresia. The first patient had undergone a Kasai procedure following which he developed rapidly deteriorating liver failure and GI bleeding. The second patient had previously received a live-donor liver at another institution that was lost to chronic rejection. Preoperative rHuEPO use improved their Hct levels significantly to 37.1% and 31.5%. Intraoperative coagulopathy was managed by the use of aprotinin, desmopressin and rFVIIa. Despite the small size and low total blood volume of these patients, ANH and cell saver were used without complication. The Hct level was maintained at 29% at the end of surgery. Both patients recovered uneventfully, had an uncomplicated postoperative course and are well at 2 1/2-year follow-up. The use of blood-sparing techniques may be uniquely

Table 9.4 Perioperative hematologic profiles of 107 consecutive patients who underwent transfusion-free major surgical procedures at the University of Southern California (values are expressed as mean with range in parentheses).

Parameter	All cases	(-)ANH/(-)CS	ANH only	CS only	(+)ANH/(+)CS
Number of patients (%)	107 (100%)	33 (31%)	18 (17%)	27 (25%)	29 (27%)
Hematocrit (%)					
Preoperative	40.6 (22.1–54.3)	38.3 (25.2–50.6)	40.0 (32.7–47.8)	41.3 (22.1–54.3)	42.8 (32.1–49.5)
Postoperative	34.6 (18.7–46.4)	32.6 (20.1–42.1)	35.6 (28.5–43.0)	34.2 (18.7–42.8)	36.2 (24.7–46.4)
Change	−6.0	−5.7	−4.4	−7.1	−6.6
Platelet count (cells/cmm)					
Preoperative	253 (41–940)	315 (112–940)	261 (96–417)	244 (117–662)	186 (41–342)
Postoperative	204 (34–479)	243 (100–479)	207 (63–293)	205 (88–462)	160 (34–410)
Change	−49	−72	−55	−39	−26
Estimated blood loss (ml)	502 (100–2900)	414 (100–2400)	393 (100–1000)	490 (100–2000)	683 (100–2900)
Operating time (h)	4.7 (1.5–15.0)	3.4 (1.5–7.0)	4.9 (2.0–10.5)	3.7 (1.5–10.0)	6.8 (2.0–15.0)
Units of blood removed for ANH	N/A	N/A	2.2 (1.0–4.0)	N/A	2.5 (1.0–7.0)
Volume of CS (ml)	N/A	N/A	N/A	97.2 (0–375)	159.5 (0–850)

Note: ANH, Acute normovolemic hemodilution.
CS, Cell saver.

relevant in the pediatric population since many blood-borne infections do not become apparent until many decades after transfusion.

We hope the concepts refined in part by our experience in liver transplantation can be applied more broadly to surgery in general, as is the case in our own center. By August 2001, we had performed 107 major procedures (procedures with a predicted blood loss of more than 500 cc) at our institution after the commencement of the transfusion-free program in January 1997 – 58 (54%) were men and 49 (46%) women, with a mean age of 52.5 years. The use of ANH and ICS was decided on a case-by-case basis by the operating surgeon (Table 9.4). The mean Hct level at admission was 41% and at discharge, 35%. There was a 6.5% intraoperative complication rate, 33% overall morbidity, and no mortality, consistent with reported numbers in all patients undergoing these procedures. The mean ICU stay of 3 days and hospital stay of 9 days were also no different from the general population. Our experience has established that even in procedures that have historically been associated with the risk of significant blood loss, transfusion-free surgery is uniformly achievable.

Trends in transfusion-free surgery

Ongoing intense investigation into the understanding and application of oxygen-carrying blood substitutes is bound to further reduce our dependence on allogeneic blood products. Blood substitutes that can serve the function of tissue oxygenation may have significant utility, while at the same time eliminate the risk of transmission of infections, allow longer shelf lives, and lead to a predictable supply and availability with universal compatibility. The use of blood substitutes may also allow for greater intraoperative normovolemic hemodilution. Blood substitutes are being evaluated for use in trauma, during sickle cell crises and in the perfusion of ischemic tissues. Two oxygen carriers in particular are the focus of laboratory research – Hb-based oxygen carriers and perfluorocarbons.

Hb-based compounds have a high oxygen affinity and *in vivo* half-lives of 3–12 h. Initial trials showed some promise with the use of stroma-free Hb. However, the lack of 2,3 DPG regulation caused an inadequate release of oxygen. Further, stroma-free Hb has renal toxicity and an affinity for nitric oxide, which has the potential to result in hypertension. Current studies focus on modifying or genetically engineering Hb to overcome these problems. Surface-modified Hb was designed to increase vascular retention by conjugating Hb with larger molecules such as dextran or polyethylene glycol. Cross-linking or polymerization of the Hb reduces subunit dissociation and toxicity. In preliminary studies, recombinant Hb serves the function of oxygen delivery well, with significantly fewer side-effects and decreased nitric oxide affinity. In addition, a liposome-encapsulated form of Hb also has been developed, which closely emulates native RBCs.

Perfluorocarbons are hydrocarbons whose hydrogen atoms have been re-placed with fluorine. They have a high potential for oxygen solubility and can transport carbon dioxide as well. However, they have a short half-life of 2–4 h, a high viscosity and a flu-like syndrome associated with their admin-istration. Also, perfluorocarbons have low oxygen capacities, with oxygen pressures as high as 500 mmHg required to achieve an oxygen content of 15 ml/dl, which is still considerably lower than the content of whole blood. Perfluorocarbons are excreted by the reticuloendothelial system and the lungs.

In addition to these oxygen-carrying blood substitutes, synthetic coagula-tion factors also play an important role in the future of blood product utiliza-tion. The clinical success observed with rFVIIa has triggered a multitude of studies evaluating recombinant proteins that shift the procoagulant/ anticoagulant balance toward a more procoagulant state at the site of blood loss. Newer agents in laboratory trials have the potential to decrease blood loss even in the absence of an obvious underlying hemostatic defect or in the setting of coagulopathies resulting from dilution and consumption as in trauma and surgery [72]. The availability of these transfusion-sparing hemostatic agents will further facilitate the practice of transfusion-free medicine.

Conclusion

Transfusion-free medicine and surgery is an attainable goal. Its realization begins with the comprehension of the significant downsides to the use of allogeneic blood and blood products. As our experience with a high-risk patient population undergoing major surgery has documented, a more focused application of some relatively easily enforced clinical interventions can go a long way in achieving the goal of transfusion-free medicine. The pace of ongoing research relating to clotting factors and blood substitutes will almost certainly make this goal well within the clinician's reach in the not so far future.

References

1 Carson JL, Altman DG, Duff A, Noveck H, Weinstein MP, Sonnenberg FA *et al*. Risk of bacterial infection associated with allogeneic blood transfusion among patients undergoing hip fracture repair. *Transfusion* 1999; **39**: 694–700.

2 Wagner SJ. Transfusion-transmitted bacterial infection: risks, sources and inter-ventions. *Vox Sang* 2004; **86**: 157–63.

3 Duffy G, Neal KR. Differences in post-operative infection rates between patients receiving autologous and allogeneic blood transfusion: a meta-analysis

of published randomized and nonrandomized studies. *Transfus Med Rev* 1996; **6**: 325–8.

4 Vamvakas EC. Possible mechanisms of allogeneic blood transfusion-associated postoperative infection. *Transfus Med Rev* 2002; **16**: 144–60.

5 Hill GE, Frawley WH, Griffith KE, Forestner JE, Minei JP. Allogeneic blood transfusion increases the risk of postoperative bacterial infection: a meta-analysis. *J Trauma* 2003; **54**: 908–14.

6 Shorr AF, Duh MS, Kelly KM, Kollef MH, CRIT Study Group. Red blood cell transfusion and ventilator-associated pneumonia: a potential link? *Crit Care Med* 2004; **32**: 666–74.

7 Vamvakas EC. Perioperative blood transfusion and cancer recurrence: meta-analysis for explanation. *Transfusion* 1995; **35**: 760–8.

8 Amato AC, Pescatori M. Effect of perioperative blood transfusions on recurrence of colorectal cancer: meta-analysis stratified on risk factors. *Dis Colon Rectum* 1998; **41**: 570–85.

9 Patel HB, Nasir FA, Nash GF, Scully MF, Kakkar AK. Enhanced angiogenesis following allogeneic blood transfusion. *Clin Lab Haematol* 2004; **26**: 129–35.

10 Stephenson GR, Moretti EW, El-Moalem H, Clavien PA, Tuttle-Newhall JE. Malnutrition in liver transplant patients: preoperative subjective global assessment is predictive of outcome after liver transplantation. *Transplantation* 2001; **72**: 666–70.

11 Goodnough LT, Monk TG, Andriole GL. Erythropoietin therapy. *N Engl J Med* 1997; **336**: 933–8.

12 Sans T, Bofil C, Joven J, Cliville X, Simo JM, Llobet X *et al*. Effectiveness of very low doses of subcutaneous recombinant human erythropoietin in facilitating autologous blood donation before orthopedic surgery. *Transfusion* 1996; **36**: 822–6.

13 Price TH, Goodnough LT, Vogler WR, Sacher RA, Hellman RM, Johnston MF *et al*. Improving the efficacy of preoperative autologous blood donation in patients with low hematocrit: a randomized, double-blind, controlled trial of recombinant human erythropoietin. *Am J Med* 1996; **101**: 22S–27S.

14 Sarac TP, Clifford C, Waters J, Clair DG, Ouriel K. Preoperative erythropoietin and blood conservation management for thoracoabdominal aneurysm repair in a Jehovah's Witness. *J Vasc Surg* 2003; **37**: 453–5.

15 Nelson CL, Stewart JG. Primary and revision total hip replacement in patients who are Jehovah's Witnesses. *Clin Ortho* 1999; **369**: 251–61.

16 Bennett DR, Shulman IA. Practical issues when confronting the patient who refuses blood transfusion therapy. *Am J Clin Pathol* 1997; **107**: S23–S27.

17 Ng T, Marx G, Littlewood T, Macdougall I. Recombinant erythropoietin in clinical practice. *Postgrad Med J* 2003; **79**: 367–76.

18 Cazzola M, Mercuriali F, Brugnara C. Use of recombinant human erythropoietin outside the setting of uremia. *Blood* 1997; **89**: 4248–67.

19 Kalantar-Zadeh K, McAllister CJ, Lehn RS, Lee GH, Nissenson AR, Kopple JD. Effect of malnutrition-inflammation complex syndrome on EPO hyporesponsiveness in maintenance hemodialysis patients. *Am J Kid Dis* 2003; **42**: 761–73.

20 Ozguroglu M, Arun B, Demir G, Demirelli F, Mandel NM, Buyukunal E *et al*. Serum erythropoietin level in anemic cancer patients. *Med Oncol* 2000; **17**: 29–34.

21 Weiss G. Pathogenesis and treatment of anaemia of chronic disease. *Blood Rev* 2002; **16**: 87–96.

22 Brugnara C, Chambers LA, Malynn E, Goldberg MA, Kruskall MS. Red blood cell regeneration induced by subcutaneous recombinant erythropoietin: iron-deficient erythropoiesis in iron-replete subjects. *Blood* 1993; **81**: 956–64.

23 Goodnough LT, Skikne B, Brugnara C. Erythropoietin, iron, and erythropoiesis. *Blood* 2000; **96**: 823–33.

24 Jabbour N, Gagandeep S, Mateo R, Sher L, Henderson R, Selby R *et al.* Live donor liver transplantation: staging hepatectomy in a Jehovah's Witness recipient. *J Hepatobiliary Pancreat Surg* 2004; **11**: 211–14.

25 Paravicini D, Wasylewski AH, Rassat J, Thys J. Red blood cell survival and morphology during and after intraoperative autotransfusion. *Acta Anaesthesiol Belg* 1984; **35**: 43–9.

26 Ray JM, Flynn JC, Bierman AH. Erythrocyte survival following intraoperative autotransfusion in spinal surgery: an in vivo comparative study and 5-year update. *Spine* 1986; **11**: 879–82.

27 Williamson KR, Taswell HF. Intraoperative blood salvage: a review. *Transfusion* 1991; **31**: 662–75.

28 Yamada T, Yamashita Y, Terai Y, Ueki M. Intraoperative blood salvage in abdominal uterine myomectomy. *Int J Gynaecol Obstet* 1997; **56**: 141–5.

29 Rosengart TK, Helm RE, DeBois WJ, Garcia N, Krieger KH, Isom OW. Open heart operations without transfusion using a multimodality blood conservation strategy in 50 Jehovah's Witness patients: implications for a "bloodless" surgical technique. *J Am Coll Surg* 1997; **184**: 618–29.

30 Huo MH, Paly WL, Keggi KJ. Effect of preoperative autologous blood donation and intraoperative and postoperative blood recovery on homologous blood transfusion requirement in cementless total hip replacement operation. *J Am Coll Surg* 1995; **180**: 561–7.

31 Williamson KR, Taswell HF, Rettke SR, Krom RA. Intraoperative autologous transfusion: its role in orthotopic liver transplantation. *Mayo Clin Proc* 1989; **64**: 340–5.

32 Huet C, Salmi LR, Fergusson D, Koopman-van Gemert AW, Rubens F, Laupacis A. A meta-analysis of the effectiveness of cell salvage to minimize perioperative allogeneic blood transfusion in cardiac and orthopedic surgery – International Study of Perioperative Transfusion (ISPOT) Investigators. *Anesth Analg* 1999; **89**: 861–9.

33 McGill N, O'Shaughnessy D, Pickering R, Herbertson M, Gill R. Mechanical methods of reducing blood transfusion in cardiac surgery: randomised controlled trial. *BMJ* 2002; **324**: 1299–306.

34 Guerra JJ, Cuckler JM. Cost effectiveness of intraoperative autotransfusion in total hip arthroplasty surgery. *Clin Orthop* 1995; **315**: 212–22.

35 Simpson MB, Georgopoulos G, Eilert RE. Intraoperative blood salvage in children and young adults undergoing spinal surgery with predeposited autologous blood: efficacy and cost effectiveness. *J Pediatr Ortho* 1993; **13**: 777–80.

36 Shuhaiber JH, Whitehead SM. The impact of introducing an autologous intraoperative transfusion device to a community hospital. *Ann Vasc Surg* 2003; **17**: 424–9.

37 Kemper RR, Menitove JE, Hanto DW. Cost analysis of intraoperative blood salvage during orthotopic liver transplantation. *Liver Transpl Surg* 1997; **3**: 513–17.

38 Keeling MM, Gray LA Jr, Brink MA, Hillerich VK, Bland KI. Intraoperative auto-transfusion: experience in 725 consecutive cases. *Ann Surg* 1983; **197**: 536–41.

39 Smith LA, Barker DE, Burns RP. Autotransfusion utilization in abdominal trauma. *Am Surg* 1997; **63**: 47–9.

40 Goodnough LT, Monk TG, Sicard G, Satterfield SA, Allen B, Anderson CB, Thompson RW, Flye W, Martin K. Intraoperative salvage in patients undergoing elective abdominal aortic aneurysm repair: an analysis of cost and benefit. *J Vasc Surg* 1996; **24**: 213–18.

41 Szpisjak DF, Potter PS, Capehart BP. Economic analysis of an intraoperative cell salvage service. *Anesth Analg* 2004; **98**: 201–5.

42 Homann B, Zenner HP, Schauber J, Ackermann R. Tumor cells carried through autotransfusion: are these cells still malignant? *Acta Anaesthesiol Belg* 1984; **35**: 51–9.

43 Davis M, Sofer M, Gomez-Marin O, Bruck D, Soloway MS. The use of cell salvage during radical retropubic prostatectomy: does it influence cancer recurrence? *BJU Int* 2003; **91**: 474–6.

44 Hansen E, Knuechel R, Altmeppen J, Taeger K. Blood irradiation for intraoperative autotransfusion in cancer surgery: demonstration of efficient elimination of contaminating tumor cells. *Transfusion* 1999; **39**: 608–15.

45 Edelman MJ, Potter P, Mahaffey KG, Frink R, Leidich RB. The potential for reintroduction of tumor cells during intraoperative blood salvage: reduction of risk with use of the RC-400 leukocyte depletion filter. *Urology* 1996; **47**: 179–81.

46 Napier JA, Bruce M, Chapman J, Duguid JK, Kelsey PR, Knowles SM *et al.* Guidelines for autologous transfusion – II: perioperative haemodilution and cell salvage. British Committee for Standards in Haematology Blood Transfusion Task Force, Autologous Transfusion Working Party. *Br J Anaesth* 1997; **78**: 768–71.

47 Weiskopf RB, Viele MK, Feiner J, Kelley S, Lieberman J, Noorani M *et al.* Human cardiovascular and metabolic response to acute, severe isovolemic anemia. *JAMA* 1998; **279**: 217–21.

48 Carson JL, Duff A, Poses RM, Berlin JA, Spence RK, Trout R *et al.* Effect of anemia and cardiovascular disease on surgical morbidity and mortality. *Lancet* 1996; **348**: 1055–60.

49 Etchason J, Petz L, Keeler E, Calhoun L, Kleinman S, Snider C *et al.* The cost effectiveness of preoperative autologous blood donations. *N Engl J Med* 1995; **332**: 719–24.

50 Chauhan S, Das SN, Bisoi A, Kale S, Kiran U. Comparison of epsilon-aminocaproic acid and tranexamic acid in pediatric cardiac surgery. *J Cardiothorac Vasc Anesth* 2004; **18**: 141–3.

51 Porte RJ, Molenaar IQ, Begliomini B, Groenland TH, Januszkiewicz A, Lindgren L *et al.* Aprotinin and transfusion requirements in orthotopic liver transplantation: a multicenter randomised double-blind study. *Lancet* 2000; **355**: 1303–9.

52 Midathada MV, Mehta P, Waner M, Fink LM. Recombinant factor VIIa in the treatment of bleeding. *Am J Clin Pathol* 2004; **121**: 124–37.

53 Kenet G, Walden R, Eldad A, Martinowitz U. Treatment of traumatic bleeding with recombinant factor VIIa. *Lancet* 1999; **354**: 1879.

54 Stratmann G, Russell IA, Merrick SH. Use of recombinant factor VIIa as a rescue treatment for intractable bleeding following repeat aortic arch repair. *Ann Thorac Surg* 2003; **76**: 2094–7.

55 Friederich PW, Henny CP, Messelink EJ, Geerdink MG, Keller T, Kurth KH *et al.* Effect of recombinant activated factor VII on perioperative blood loss in patients undergoing retropubic prostatectomy: a double-blind placebo-controlled randomised trial. *Lancet* 2003; **361**: 201–5.

56 Egan JR, Lammi A, Schell DN, Gillis J, Nunn GR. Recombinant activated factor VII in paediatric cardiac surgery. *Intens Care Med* 2004; **30**: 682–5.

57 Hendriks HG, Meijer K, de Wolf JT, Klompmaker IJ, Porte RJ, de Kam PJ *et al.* Reduced transfusion requirements by recombinant factor VIIa in orthotopic liver transplantation: a pilot study. *Transplantation* 2001; **71**: 402–5.

58 Nonthasoot B, Nivatvongs S. Multiple doses of recombinant factor VIIa in orthotopic liver transplantation: a case report. *Transpl Proc* 2003; **35**: 427–8.

59 Jabbour N, Gagandeep S, Cheng PA *et al.* Recombinant human coagulation factor VIIa in Jehovah's witness patients undergoing liver transplantation. *Am Surgeon* 2005; **71**: 175–9.

60 MacIsaac CM, Presneill JJ, Boyce CA, Byron KL, Cade JF. The influence of a blood-conserving device on anaemia in intensive care patients. *Anaesth Intens Care* 2003; **31**: 653–7.

61 Hebert PC, Wells G, Blajchman MA, Marshall J, Martin C, Pagliarello G *et al.* A multicenter, randomized, controlled clinical trial of transfusion requirements in critical care: transfusion requirements in critical care investigators – Canadian Critical Care Trials Group. *N Engl J Med* 1999; **340**: 409–17.

62 Corwin HL, Gettinger A, Pearl RG, Fink MP, Levy MM, Abraham E *et al.* The CRIT study: anemia and blood transfusion in the critically ill: current clinical practice in the United States. *Crit Care Med* 2004; **32**. 39–52.

63 Pajoumand M, Erstad BL, Camamo JM. Use of epoietin alfa in critically ill patients. *Ann Pharmacother* 2004; **38**: 641–8.

64 Levine EA, Rosen AL, Sehgal LR, Gould SA, Egrie JC, Sehgal HL *et al.* Treatment of acute postoperative anemia with recombinant human erythropoietin. *J Trauma* 1989; **29**: 1134–8.

65 Corwin HL, Gettinger A, Pearl RG, Fink MP, Levy MM, Shapiro MJ *et al.*, EPO Critical Care Trials Group. Efficacy of recombinant human erythropoietin in critically ill patients: a randomized controlled trial. *JAMA* 2002; **288**: 2827–35.

66 Corwin HL, Gettinger A, Rodriguez RM, Pearl RG, Gubler KD, Enny C *et al.* Efficacy of recombinant human erythropoietin in the critically ill patient: a randomized, double-blind, placebo-controlled trial. *Crit Care Med* 1999; **27**: 2346–50.

67 Gabriel A, Kozek S, Chiari A, Fitzgerald R, Grabner C, Geissler K *et al.* High-dose recombinant human erythropoietin stimulates reticulocyte production in patients with multiple organ dysfunction syndrome. *J Trauma* 1998; **44**: 361–7.

68 Still JM Jr, Belcher K, Law EJ, Thompson W, Jordan M, Lewis M *et al.* A double-blinded prospective evaluation of recombinant human erythropoietin in acutely burned patients. *J Trauma* 1995; **38**: 233–6.

69 Jabbour N, Gagandeep S, Mateo R, Sher L, Strum E, Donovan J *et al.* Live donor liver transplantation without blood products: strategies developed for Jehovah's Witnesses offer broad application. *Ann Surg* 2004; **240**: 350–7.

70 Jabbour N, Gagandeep S, Thomas D, Stapfer M, Mateo R, Sher L, Selby R, Genyk Y. Transfusion-free techniques in pediatric live-donor liver transplantation. *J Pediatr Gastroenterol Nutr* 2005; **40**(4): 521–3.

71 Jabbour N, Gagandeep S, Mateo R. *et al.* (in press) Transfusion-free surgery: single institution experience of 27 consecutive liver transplants in Jehovah's witnesses. *J Am Coll Surg*.

72 Chiu J, Ketchum LH, Reid TJ. Transfusion-sparing hemostatic agents. *Curr Opin Hematol* 2002; **9**: 544–50.

CHAPTER 10

The Changing Transfusion Practice of Neonatal and Pediatric Surgery

Pamela J Kling, Nicolas Jabbour, S Ram Kumar

Abstract

The use of erythrocyte transfusions to treat anemia in neonatal and pediatric surgery patients has changed dramatically over the last decade. The drug recombinant human erythropoietin (rHuEPO) has been shown to decrease transfusion numbers in many disease states in adults and children. rHuEPO has also been used perioperatively in children. We discuss perioperative anemia, strategies that can be successfully employed to limit need for transfusion therapy and their application to specific situations in pediatric surgery.

Introduction

About two-thirds of all erythrocyte transfusions have traditionally been administered in the perioperative period [1]. In 1988, an NIH Consensus Development Panel reported that data do not support utilization of a single perioperative transfusion criterion of hemoglobin (Hb) less than 10.0 g/dl and recommended ongoing study of transfusion criteria [1]. A practice parameter developed by the Task Force of the College of American Pathologists agreed with this conclusion by stating that 'in the perioperative period, a decision to transfuse at single arbitrary hemoglobin value is particularly inappropriate' [2]. Although few prospective studies have investigated perioperative transfusion criteria, a recent review suggests that an Hb transfusion threshold of 8.0 g/dl should be used in surgical patients without risk factors for tissue ischemia, and 10.0 g/dl could be justified in those at risk for ischemia [3]. In current surgical practice, very few randomized clinical trials examining transfusion triggers are found [4]. In pediatric surgery patients, even less information about transfusion criteria is known. Against this background, we will provide here an overview of the special considerations relevant to transfusion in the pediatric population, some strategies that can effectively curtail the need for transfusion and the application of these strategies in children who are surgical patients.

Transfusion considerations specific to the pediatric population

A large body of the current understanding of transfusion requirements and outcomes in children has been extrapolated from the adult literature. While common ground does exist between these two populations of patients, children present with some unique problems related to anemia. Children, for example, have smaller circulating blood volumes compared to phlebotomy losses (Table 10.1).

Transfusion in infants is associated with some unique effects that may be quite different from those in adults, such as its possible role on retinopathy of prematurity [5]. A large number of transfusion-related microbial infectious complications are discovered, or many manifest, many years after the incident transfusion, which poses a more serious hazard in infants and children with their long expected life span. Lastly, several interventions, including the use of artificial oxygen carriers, or 'blood substitutes', have not been adequately studied in pediatric patients. For all these reasons, a comprehensive knowledge of the problem of anemia and steps that can effectively restrict transfusion requirements in the pediatric population is in order.

Strategies to limit need for transfusion

The use of recombinant human erythropoietin

Anemia can be caused in the pediatric population by a variety of reasons, the most common of which is prematurity. A combination of the need to support rapid growth in the neonatal period and the shorter half-life of neonatal red blood cells (RBCs) in comparison to adult cells places an enormous demand on the neonatal marrow. However, plasma erythropoietin (EPO) levels are lower in the premature neonate compared to older children with comparable degrees of anemia, and the rise in EPO levels correlates poorly with falling Hb levels [6]. Hence, the use of rHuEPO for anemia of prematurity has a sound physiologic basis. Several studies have documented a reduction in [7,8], or in instances complete avoidance of [9], packed cell transfusion in low–birth weight infants in whom rHuEPO is started in the early postnatal life. Significant work has also examined optimization of response to rHuEPO by altering timing of therapy and iron supplementation [10,11].

Table 10.1 Limitations of treating anemia in neonates compared to adults.

	Neonates	Adults
Circulating blood volume	40–320 ml	>3500 ml
Hematocrit on admission	36–46%	36–46%
Phlebotomy loss first 24 h in ICU	3–10 ml	12–28 ml
First 24 h phlebotomy in ICU as % blood volume	0.9–25%	<0.8%
Weekly phlebotomy in ICU as % blood volume	6–50%	<2.5%

Table 10.2 Evidence for efficacy of rHuEPO in decreasing erythrocyte transfusions in pediatric patients.

Indication	U/kg/week	Randomized/ controlled trials	Retrospective/ descriptive reports
Anemia of prematurity	300–1500	++	±
Renal failure	50–150	++	±
Oncologic disease	450–1200	±	±
Autologous marrow transplant	900–1400	±	±
Allogenic marrow transplant	1050–1400	±	±
Cardiac surgery (pre & post)	300–1200	+	±
Pre-op autologous transfusion	200–900	*	±
Pre-op to raise Hct	200–300	*	+
Post-op	450–900	*	*
Burn patients	50–350	*	±
PICU patients	900–1500	*	±

Note: (++), multiple randomized/controlled trials supporting efficacy at decreasing transfusions; (+), one randomized/controlled trial supporting efficacy; (±), under randomized/ controlled trials indicates equal number supporting and refuting efficacy; (±), under retrospective/descriptive studies indicates data supporting rHuEPO efficacy; (*) indicates no study found in that category.
Source: [12–26].

Based on the foregoing evidence, extension of the application of rHuEPO to the perioperative population to limit transfusion has met with some success, although studies commonly lack appropriate randomization and control. Table 10.2 summarizes the evidence for efficacy of rHuEPO in pediatric patients, showing which indications are supported by randomized, controlled trials and which are supported by retrospective or descriptive reports. Recent descriptive reports suggest that rHuEPO may facilitate autologous donation of blood in children undergoing craniosynostosis and orthopedic repairs [19,20]. rHuEPO may be effective for autologous donation in children as small as 6–10 kg weight [20]. Adolescents may safely donate more autologous blood in a single setting, which may decrease the cost of autologous donation. Adolescents donating 20% of their circulating blood volume tolerated donation as well as those donating the traditional 10% of blood volume [19]. Because collection and storage of preoperative autologous blood donation increases the elective surgical expense, preoperative rHuEPO therapy to increase preoperative hematocrit (Hct) has also been studied [21,22]. In a retrospective review of the experience in all adolescent orthopedic surgery, preoperative rHuEPO resulted in higher preoperative Hct and less allogenic transfusions (4%) compared to those without (24%) preoperative rHuEPO [27].

However, the use of rHuEPO in children is associated with some concern. Stimulation by pharmacologic doses of rHuEPO commits iron to erythropoiesis, thereby limiting its availability to nonerythropoietic needs of the growing infant. There is at least a theoretical risk that combined administration of rHuEPO and iron can lead to oxidative injury and may increase the risk of retinopathy of prematurity [28]. Also, widespread systemic effects of rHuEPO have not been studied extensively to date. There is hence a lack of consensus on the use of rHuEPO in the pediatric population, although a trend towards its increased use, particularly in the critically ill child during the perioperative phase, is commonly seen.

Alternative strategies to the use of rHuEPO, including newer proteins such as novel erythropoiesis-stimulating protein (NESP), are currently under study in children, but have not yet been reported.

Autotransfusion strategies

Acute normovolemic hemodilution removes whole blood from the patient immediately before the surgical procedure and collects it in anticoagulant [29–34]. Depending on patient size, between 1 and 4 units of blood can be collected. During donation, circulating blood volume is maintained with acellular fluid (hetastarch or crystalloid) [31], and compensatory mechanisms, including increased preload, decreased afterload and increased heart rate, improve cardiac output (CO) and help maintain perfusion. Although most studies evaluating acute normovolemic hemodilution have been performed in adults, one controlled study of adolescent spine surgery showed that 79% of the nonhemodilution patients received transfusions, while 37% received transfusions in the hemodilution group [35]. An expert panel of the NIH recommends the use of ANH [33], while a Consensus Conference on Autologous Transfusion does not [36]. Many studies utilizing normovolemic hemodilution are flawed, utilizing historical controls or not clearly defining transfusion criteria. A meta-analysis of 24 prospective, randomized trials of normovolemic hemodilution in adults found a reduced likelihood of exposure to blood and exposure to a smaller number of units, but this finding did not hold up when analyzing the trials that employed strict transfusion criteria [37]. This meta-analysis excluded any studies treating children younger than 18 years. In children, plateletpheresis and plasmapheresis techniques have been reported to enhance the collection of clotting factors in normovolemic hemodilution techniques, but these methods have not been systematically studied [38]. Modification of hemodilution techniques by utilizing a hetastarch and balanced salt/lactate solution or a fluorocarbon emulsion shows promise for optimizing normovolemic hemodilution techniques in adults and could be studied in children [39–40].

Acute normovolemic hemodilution (ANH) has been studied extensively in adults, but its application in the pediatric population has been tempered due to several legitimate concerns. The ability of children to tolerate dilutional coagulopathy from ANH is more limited. In our own study on the application of ANH to six Jehovah's Witness children [41], all patients developed dilutional coagulopathy as evidenced by abnormal laboratory coagulation tests. However, whether this biochemical abnormality translates into increased bleeding is unclear. In one study that included pediatric patients undergoing cardiac surgery for cyanotic heart disease [42], extreme ANH was associated with marked abnormalities in various coagulation parameters; however, no significant increase in bleeding was noted. Another concern with ANH, especially pertinent to children, is the high fraction of Hb F resulting in a leftward shift of the oxyhemoglobin curve. There is hence a theoretical concern that hemodilution may significantly impair end-organ oxygen delivery. Lastly, while most studies on ANH in children have examined global physiological effects, specific organ function abnormalities have not been individually evaluated. A recent randomized study compared developmental outcomes in infants undergoing cardiopulmonary bypass (CPB) to an Hct of 21.5% or 27.8% [43]. Although neurological examinations and mental development index scores were comparable between the two groups, infants who underwent bypass at the lower Hct had significantly lower psychomotor developmental index scores. Hence, although ANH is a promising strategy for limiting transfusion in children, evidence supporting their routine use is still lacking.

Other autotransfusion strategies such as autologous blood donation have also been evaluated in children. Autologous donation results in decreased homologous blood use during spinal fusion in children and adolescents [44]. However, in very small children, the technique of autologous donation can be technically challenging and cumbersome.

The application of hemostatic agents

Blood loss is the most frequent indication for transfusion and hence strategies to limit blood loss are bound to significantly impact transfusion requirements. Following the advent of blood component fractionation, the use of acellular plasma, platelets or plasma coagulation factors such as cryoprecipitate to facilitate clotting has been widely accepted. Recently, several new nonplasma compounds have been introduced for facilitating coagulation. Antifibrinolytic agents, such as aminocaproic acid or tranexamic acid and aprotinin, are currently in widespread clinical use. Aminocaproic acid binds to plasminogen and prevents its breakdown to plasmin by tissue plasminogen activator, thereby stabilizing the clot. Similarly, aprotinin is a serine protease inhibitor that directly inhibits plasmin. Both agents have shown reductions in blood loss in many types of surgical patients [45] and should be studied more carefully in children. Desmopressin, a synthetic analog of the antidiuretic hormone, increases the release of von Willebrand factor from its storage sites on endothelial cells and enhances platelet function, thereby facilitating hemostasis. Conjugated estrogens have been used in children with uremia-related hemorrhage to induce clotting.

Recombinant activated factor VII (rFVIIa) is a synthetic protein derived from transfected hamster kidney cells that is increasingly gaining popularity amongst clinicians to treat reticent coagulopathy. Although its use has been approved only for hemophiliacs with antibodies against factors VIII and IX, several off-label indications are being reported. It has been used successfully in the adult population for trauma, hemorrhage associated with liver failure, spontaneous intracranial hemorrhage and for congenital factor VII deficiency. Recently, case reports have documented its safe and effective application in neonates with liver failure undergoing liver biopsy [46]. Given that rFVIIa acts by binding to activated platelets, its hemostatic effect is largely isolated to the site of active bleeding and is hence a very attractive therapeutic compound. Pilot studies have also evaluated the use of factor XIII in adult CPB and bone marrow transplant patients, though it is not currently approved for clinical use.

Perioperative approaches

Attention to perioperative factors and improved surgical technique can significantly decrease surgical blood losses [47–49]. Strategies for blood conservation include calculation of precise transfusion requirements, preoperative review of specific transfusion criteria for each patient, rehearsal of the operative procedure, shortening operative time and delaying the timing of transfusion as long as possible [48]. Development of specific instruments that minimize surgical blood loss is ongoing [49,50]. Evaluation of blood loss in endoscopic, compared to open, procedures has not been performed.

Controlled studies show that hypotensive anesthesia and cell-saving procedures are safe and decrease blood loss during pediatric orthopedic procedures [51], although there is a paucity of controlled studies in other pediatric surgical populations. The use of intraoperative cell salvage (ICS) in the pediatric population was hampered until recently by the lack of appropriate size devices. The introduction of small bowl sizes of cell-saver devices has increased the feasibility of cell salvage in very small children. Moderate to deep hypothermia can increase the amount of dissolved oxygen and decrease tissue oxygen demands during surgery, especially when hemodilution is being utilized. The use of hyperoxic ventilation strategy in one study offered an increased safety margin allowing for an extreme level of hemodilution to 3.0 g/dl [52].

Monitoring devices within central lines that perform in-line point-of-care blood testing can minimize blood loss pre-, intra- and postoperatively [53,54]. These devices have shown reliable results in small premature infants, with a decrease blood volume drawn (e.g. whole blood electrolytes and blood gas from 250 µl per test to < 25 µl). Studies have yet to show decreased transfusion requirements in patients with these in-line devices.

Physician awareness

The single most important contributing factor to the transfusion practice in any setting is the physician force. Several studies have documented marked variations in physician practice patterns resulting in dramatically different transfusion thresholds [55]. In one study, physicians in practice for longer had a lower knowledge base and were less likely to perceive shortages in blood supply than residents. In addition, the strongest impetus for transfusion by physicians-in-training was the influence of the attending physician [56].

A large body of evidence has now confirmed the safety of lower Hb levels even in critically ill infants. In fact, in one study, children who underwent RBC transfusion needed more resources than those who were not transfused [57]. The number of days of oxygen use, mechanical ventilation, vasoactive agent infusions and stay in the intensive care unit (ICU) and hospital were significantly higher in transfused children. Results such as these put traditional transfusion cutoff points and arbitrary single-point triggers under question. Physician awareness can thus increase the support for conservative transfusion practices and limit unnecessary transfusions.

Published literature has confirmed the role of focused physician education and practice audit as a transfusion-limiting strategy [58]. The most successful methods utilize a combination of education, real-time feedback, administrative control and pharmacological support. Although one-on-one teaching is a very effective mode of education, it is too cumbersome to be practical. However, educational programs aimed at specific physician groups can alter transfusion practices [59]. Further, studies have shown that hospitals tend to develop transfusion strategies that are ingrained within the institution and differ little between physicians at that center [60]. Hence, the institution of hospital-wide administrative tools has been evaluated and seems to improve adherence to transfusion guidelines.

Application of transfuison-limiting strategies to specific surgical situations

Neonatal surgery

The most common surgical emergency observed in premature infants is necrotizing enterocolitis (NEC) [61]. In NEC, anemia is common secondary to bleeding associated with thrombocytopenia and disseminated intravascular coagulation (DIC), as well as hemolytic anemia and iatrogenic blood loss [62–6]. The incidence of thrombocytopenia is 65–90% in NEC and 55–80% in any neonatal infection [67,68]. In severe infections and shock, the host defense system disturbs the equilibrium of the coagulation and fibrinolytic systems [68]. DIC, which occurs in 40% of premature infants with NEC and 17% of infants with sepsis, is generally treated with coagulation factors [64,65,67]. Infants with NEC therefore commonly require platelet concentrates, coagulation factors and erythrocytes [64,65,69]. Although blood loss from DIC and thrombocytopenia is so common in NEC or neonatal infections, a trial of rHuEPO in NEC has not been performed.

Premature neonates commonly undergo surgical procedures, and pediatric surgeons have long been pioneers in techniques that minimize blood loss and transfusions. Because allogenic transfusions are commonly given to premature neonates, the potential of autologous cord blood collection at delivery has been investigated. Although adequate volumes of autologous cord blood can be collected at delivery and stored for later transfusion [70–72], this practice has not been widely implemented secondary to technical and infectious concerns [73]. However, in neonates with prenatal diagnosis of surgical anomalies, collection and transfusion of cord blood for perioperative autologous transfusion has been reported and might warrant ongoing prospective, randomized investigation [74].

Cardiac surgery

Nearly all cardiac surgery procedures performed in neonatal and pediatric patients are those treating congenital heart defects. These children are commonly transfused perioperatively. In one study, the strongest predictor of transfusion in children undergoing open heart surgery was the patient's age [42]. Children less than 1 year received a mean transfusion number of 6, compared to 2 in those older than 1 year. Procedures to decrease blood exposure have been sought, including reducing duration or eliminating time spent on the CPB circuit [75]. Less invasive cardiac procedures would result in significant decreases in transfusion numbers. In recent years, development of transcatheter procedures treating neonatal heart disease has progressed, therefore eliminating, decreasing or delaying surgical cardiac procedures in neonates [76]. In addition to the classic balloon atrial septostomy, valvulotomies, balloon dilation of vessels (including coarctation of the aorta), stenting of vessels, coil embolization of vessels (including the patent ductus arteriosus), and biopsies have all been performed by catheter procedures in neonates [76]. Although not yet shown to reduce blood loss, video-assisted thoracoscopic ligation of the patent ductus arteriosus in premature infants as small as 500 g has resulted in less surgical trauma and faster recovery times [75]. Video-assisted thoracoscopic techniques have been utilized to divide vascular rings, treat chylothoraces and plicate the diaphragm in neonates [75].

One case report of cardiac surgery in a 10-year-old Jehovah's Witness described complete avoidance of transfusion [77]. Another report of a 5.3 kg, 14-week-old Jehovah's Witness infant described a cor triatriatum repair without need for transfusion [78]. This repair was accomplished by preoperative and postoperative rHuEPO therapy, bloodless priming of the bypass circuit, shortening of the tubing in the circuit, and hypothermic, hypotensive anesthesia [78]. A noncontrolled series of 14 Jehovah's Witness children, 6 years of age and older, reported congenital heart surgery repairs without blood exposure [16]. The lowest Hct during perfusion was 15% and lowest postoperative Hct was 16% [16]. In a retrospective description of children who were Jehovah's Witnesses, only 4 of 48 children less than 20 kg undergoing cardiac surgery received perioperative transfusion [17]. The authors employed bloodless total hemodilution of the bypass circuit and return of all patient's blood from the circuit immediately after bypass. Compared to historical controls whose bypass circuits were primed with blood, intubation time and ICU stay was similar. One prospective trial addressing bloodless cardiac surgery was found. A controlled study of pre- and postoperative rHuEPO therapy was performed in children undergoing cardiac surgery (mean age 5.5 years) expected to be placed on CPB [18]. All circuits were primed with crystalloid and all blood was returned to the patient immediately following bypass. All children receiving high-dose rHuEPO avoided transfusion, 91% of those with moderate-dose rHuEPO avoided transfusion and 69% of the controls (with oral iron only) avoided transfusion.

Utilization of blood salvaged from the extracorporeal membrane circuit after cardiac surgery may contribute a significant autologous transfusion volume to the pediatric patient postoperatively (50–150 ml of blood with an Hct of $52.7 \pm 9.7\%$) [79]. Additionally, use of an autotransfusion technique to replace postoperative blood loss through mediastinal drains has been utilized to decrease postoperative blood transfusions [80].

Orthopedic surgery

Much work has been done to minimize blood loss in pediatric orthopedic procedures and several retrospective descriptive reports were found [32]. One matched, controlled study was found that showed hypotensive anesthesia decreased blood loss and transfusion administration in spinal fusion procedures compared to control [81]. A well-designed study using closely matched historical controls showed that cell-saving procedures and autologous transfusion may also decrease blood loss and transfusion requirements [82]. It appears that ANH may be of most benefit during spinal fusion surgery in children. Although not thoroughly studied, techniques to minimize blood loss, used in combination with pre- and/or postoperative rHuEPO therapy, should work better than either strategy alone [32].

Craniosynostosis surgery

Craniosynostosis surgical procedures are associated with massive surgical blood losses. Because most craniosynostosis repairs occur in children less than 1 year of age, transfusion rates are commonly 100%. By careful attention to surgical blood loss, estimated red cell mass and transfusion criteria, precise control of transfusion volumes can be achieved [83]. One descriptive report utilized preoperative rHuEPO therapy, preoperative autologous blood donation, normovolemic hemodilution and ICS and achieved a 15% allogenic transfusion rate with craniosynostosis repairs [20]. We have performed a retrospective chart review of patients undergoing craniosynostosis repair by the same plastic surgeon at the Children's Hospital of Los Angeles between January 2002 and January 2003. A subgroup of patients (10/19) consented to the preoperative administration of rHuEPO. In addition, hemodilution techniques were used in eight of ten rHuEPO patients and none of the controls, while controlled hypotension was used in nine of ten and six of nine patients, respectively. The administration of rHuEPO resulted in a 28% increase in red cell mass over 4 weeks preoperatively. Transfusion requirements were lower in the rHuEPO group (4/10 vs. 9/9) as was the total volume of blood products transfused (154 cc vs. 421 cc, $p < 0.03$). Hct levels on the day of discharge was not significantly different between the two groups. The administration of rHuEPO significantly increased red blood cell mass allowing for the safer application of blood-conservation techniques including hypervolemic hemodilution, ANH and controlled hypotension.

Hepatic surgery

Blood loss during hepatic procedures can be extremely high. In an early report of blood transfusion in liver transplantation, there was a median of 11 transfusions given to 49 pediatric liver transplants [84]. In liver surgeries, hepatic inflow occlusion techniques are commonly employed to minimize blood loss. In hepatic inflow occlusion, the hepatic artery, portal vein and hepatic vein of the affected segment are ligated before the hepatic parenchyma is resected [85,86]. Although no controlled studies have been performed, blood loss with liver tumor resection in children has also been reported to be minimized with hypotensive, ANH anesthesia, with autotransfusion via cell saver [29]. Only three of eight children undergoing liver resections received any allogenic blood and those transfused received low (100–125 ml) volumes. Further, ultrasonically activated harmonic scalpels may improve hemostasis [87], but this has not undergone systematic study.

We have recently published our experience with bloodless live-donor liver transplantation (LDLT) in two Jehovah's Witness children, 6 months and 3 years of age [88]. Both children had end-stage liver disease secondary to biliary atresia. The first had undergone a Kasai procedure followed by rapidly deteriorating liver function and gastrointestinal (GI) bleeding. The second patient had previously received a live-donor liver at another institution that was lost to chronic rejection. Using rHuEPO preoperatively, their Hct levels were augmented to 37.1% and 31.5%, facilitating the removal of 170 cc and 250 cc of blood at the beginning of surgery for ANH. ICS recovered 90 cc and 40 cc of the blood loss. Intraoperative coagulopathy was managed by the use of aprotinin, desmopressin and rFVIIa. Despite an average operative duration of 9.25 h and estimated blood loss of 92 cc, the immediate postoperative Hct was 29% in both children. They recovered uneventfully, had an uncomplicated postoperative course and are well at $2\frac{1}{2}$ -year follow-up.

Burn surgery

Transfusions are common in burn patients. Pediatric patients (mean age 6.4 ± 1.2 years) with burns covering greater than 60% total body surface area commonly receive and tolerate massive (4.1 ± 1.7 units) transfusion of whole blood for near-total burn excision procedures [89]. Use of rHuEPO may decrease transfusion numbers in this population. Thermal injury is associated with lower serum EPO levels, such that rHuEPO should be effective at stimulating erythropoiesis [90]. Several case reports describe prevention of erythrocyte transfusions with rHuEPO therapy in burn patients

[24,25], including pediatric burn patients [26,91]. Additional strategies of decreasing blood loss in burn patients includes injection of adrenaline at donor site and excised wound, and utilization of tourniquets for limb procedures [92]. With these conservative techniques, transfusions can be decreased from 3.3 ± 3.1 units per case to 0.1 ± 0.3 units per case.

Trauma surgery

Based on the American Association for the Surgery of Trauma's Organ Injury Scaling System, strategies to decrease number of acute surgeries in trauma patients has been investigated [93]. As surgical blood losses are commonly massive, identification of the best surgical candidates can eliminate transfusions. A retrospective review of hemodynamically stable patients with blunt hepatic injury, including children, showed that a nonoperative strategy including intense observation resulted in less surgery, less abdominal infections, decreased hospital stays and less transfusions [94]. A pediatric series showed that of 27 patients, 22 qualified for nonoperative management of hepatic injury, while 5 received operative care [95]. Only 4.5% of the nonoperative group received transfusion while 60% of the operative group received transfusions. Nonoperative management of ruptured spleen secondary to blunt trauma has also been studied in children. In a Turkish study, 56 children met nonoperative criteria, while operative management was undertaken in 28 [96]. Only 57% of children in the nonoperative group required transfusion, while 100% of the operative group was transfused. An additional retrospective analysis of nonoperative management of ruptured spleen showed that 78 of 173 adult and pediatric patients met prospective criteria (lower severity score) and were monitored [97]. Only 2 of 78 required surgery and were failures. As many as 74% of the nonoperative patients avoided transfusions, while the operative patients averaged greater than 13 transfusions each.

Anemia of prematurity

Premature neonates are among the most frequently transfused group of hospitalized patients [98]. As in adults, Hb and Hct are imprecise measures of tissue oxygenation in neonates, but are commonly utilized to determine timing of erythrocyte transfusion in neonates [99]. In 1989, premature infants with birth weight under 1500 g received 8–10 transfusions during initial hospitalization, while currently two transfusions per infant are reported [100,101]. A lowering of the Hb or Hct values that trigger transfusions in premature infants has been observed [102]. Lower patient acuity scores, lower phlebotomy losses and delayed cord clamping at delivery have all been associated with reduced transfusion administration [103–4]. Advances in perinatal care have resulted in improved stability of premature neonates and are therefore associated with fewer transfusion numbers [101], but clinical transfusion practices vary widely [103,105]. The 1995 US Multicenter rHuEPO trial by Shannon *et al.* is noteworthy for both its use of rHuEPO and

Table 10.3 Neonatal transfusion guidelines

---

(1) Transfuse if hematocrit < 20% or hemoglobin < 7.0 g/dl and reticulocyte count < 100 000/mm^3 (or < 4%).

(2) Transfuse if hematocrit < 25% or hemoglobin < 8.0 g/dl and any of below present (other causes ruled out):
  (a) Increased severity of AB episodes:
    • more than ten episodes in 24 h or
    • more than two episodes requiring bag and mask over previous 24 h
  (b) Sustained tachycardia of > 180 bpm for 24 h or sustained tachypnea of > 80 bpm for 24 h by averaging monitor data
  (c) Cessation of previously adequate weight gain (> 10 g/day) over previous 4 days
  (d) Mild respiratory disease: infants on? − 1/4 L O$_2$/min nasal cannula or 0.25 to s FiO$_2$ by hood, NPCPAP or ventilator

(3) Transfuse if hematocrit < 30% or hemoglobin < 10.0 g/dl with moderate respiratory distress on < 1/4 L O$_2$/min nasal cannula or > 0.35 FiO$_2$ on hood, NPCPAP or ventilator

(4) Transfuse if hematocrit < 35% or hemoglobin < 12.0 g/dl in infants with 'severe' respiratory disease requiring mechanical ventilation and FiO$_2$ > 50%

(5) Acute blood loss with shock: blood replacement to reestablish adequate blood volume and hematocrit of 40%

(6) Transfuse if hematocrit < 30% and undergoing surgery [103]

Note: FiO$_2$, fraction of inspired oxygen.
NCPAP, nasal continuous positive airway pressure.
Source: [2,103,106,107].

its adherence to conservative consensus transfusion guidelines [103]. This study also reported guidelines for premature infants undergoing surgery [103]. After slight revision [2,106,107], many centers have adopted these conservative transfusion guidelines (see Table 10.3).

More than 40 studies treating anemia in premature infants with rHuEPO have been reported; however, a meta-analysis of controlled clinical trials of rHuEPO [12] found four highest quality studies [103,108–10] and concluded that rHuEPO reduced erythrocyte transfusion by 11.0 ml/kg per neonate [12]. Although not yet standard of care for all premature infants, rHuEPO therapy is used, especially in infants whose parents are practicing Jehovah's Witnesses [111,112].

Anemia of oncologic disease

rHuEPO has been used to treat anemia in children with hematopoietic malignancy and solid tumor [113–5]. Prospective, controlled rHuEPO trials in patients with solid tumors show higher Hb levels and either a significant decrease or a trend towards lower transfusion requirements with treatment [114,116]. Case reports of rHuEPO use in bone marrow or peripheral stem cell transplant resulted in avoidance of blood products in adult patients who are practicing Jehovah's Witnesses [117,118]. In prospective studies of rHuEPO in pediatric and adult bone marrow transplantation, rHuEPO accelerated erythrocyte recovery and decreased transfusion requirements after allogenic transplant, but not autologous bone marrow transplant [119–121].

Conclusion

Transfusion therapy has a unique application in children, both in terms of the narrow safety margin of anemia in this population and the need to tailor therapy with long-term outcomes in mind. Despite these differences, prospective studies that can translate into guidelines for the management of anemia in children are lacking, and much of our current understanding is extrapolation from studies performed on adults. However, evidence supports the application to the pediatric population of several approaches that have been shown to curtail blood loss and limit transfusion requirements in adults. Ongoing investigations at furthering our knowledge of the hematopoietic machinery and coagulation cascades will certainly strengthen efforts aimed at solidifying the practice of transfusion management in children.

Acknowledgements

We would like to acknowledge Jonathan Greenfield, MD, Arizona Pediatric Surgery LTD, for critical review and acknowledge funding by the Arizona Elks Major Projects. We would also like to acknowledge the kind permission given from NATA to reproduce parts of the following article: Kling PJ, Ohls. Transfusion alternatives in transfusion medicine. *NATA* 2002; **4**: 6–19.

References

1 NIH Consensus Development Panel. Perioperative red blood cell transfusion. *JAMA* 1988; **260**: 2700–3.
2 Simon TL, Alverson DC, AuBuchon J *et al.* Practice parameter for the use of red blood cell transfusions. *Arch Pathol Lab Med* 1998; **122**: 130–8.
3 Goodnough LT, Brecher ME, Kanter MH, AuBuchon JP. Transfusion medicine. *N Engl J Med* 1999; **340**: 438–47.
4 Carson JL, Chen AY. In search of the transfusion trigger. *Clin Ortho* 1998; **357**: 30–5.
5 Brooks SE, Marcus DM, Gillis D, Pirie E, Johnson MH, Bhatia J. The effect of blood transfusion protocol on retinopathy of prematurity: a prospective, randomized study. *Pediatrics* 1999; **104**: 514–18.
6 Brown MS, Phibbs RH, Garcia JF, Dallman PR. Postnatal changes in erythropoietin levels in untransfused premature infants. *J Pediatr* 1983; **103**: 612–17.
7 Ohls RK, Ehrenkranz RA, Wright LL *et al.* Effects of early erythropoietin therapy on the transfusion requirements of preterm infants below 1250 grams birth weight: a multicenter, randomized, controlled trial. *Pediatrics* 2001; **108**: 934–42.
8 Donato H, Vain N, Rendo P, Vivas N, Prudent L, Larguia M. Effect of early versus late administration of human recombinant erythropoietin on transfusion

requirements in premature infants: results of a randomized, placebo-controlled, multicenter trial. *Pediatrics* 2000; **105**: 1066–72.

9 Avent M, Cory BJ, Galpin J *et al*. A comparison of high versus low dose recombinant human erythropoietin versus blood transfusion in the management of anaemia of prematurity in a developing country. *J Trop Pediatr* 2002; **48**: 227–33.

10 Biesma DH, van de Wiel A, Beguin Y, Kraaijenhagen RJ, Marx JJM. Erythropoietic activity and iron metabolism in autologous blood donors during recombinant human erythropoietin therapy. *Eur J Clin Invest* 1994; **24**: 426–32.

11 Rutherford CJ, Schneider TJ, Dempsey H, Kirn DH, Brugnara C, Goldberg MA. Efficacy of different dosing regimens for recombinant human erythropoietin in a simulated perisurgical setting: the importance of iron availability in optimizing response. *Am J Med* 1994; **96**: 139–45.

12 Vamvakas EC, Strauss RG. Meta-analysis of controlled clinical trials studying the efficacy of rHuEPO in reducing blood transfusions in the anemia of prematurity. *Transfusion* 2001; **41**: 406–15.

13 Montini G, Zacchello G, Baraldi E *et al*. Benefits and risks of anemia correction with recombinant human erythropoietin in children maintained by hemodialysis. *J Pediatr* 1990; **117**: 556–60.

14 Bianchetti MG, Hammerli I, Roduit C, Neuhaus TJ, Leumann EP, Oetliker OH. Epoietin alfa in anaemic children or adolescents on regular dialysis. *Eur J Pediatr* 1991; **150**: 509–12.

15 Van Damme-Lombaerts R, Herman J. Erythropoietin treatment in children with renal failure. *Pediatr Nephrol* 1999; **13**: 148–52.

16 Chikada M, Furuse A, Kotsuka Y, Yagyu K. Open-heart surgery in Jehovah's Witness patients. *Cardiovasc Surg* 1996; **4**: 311–14.

17 Ashraf H, Subrmanian S. Bloodless cardiac surgery in children. *Saudi Heart Bull* 1990; **1**: 15–22.

18 Shimpo H, Mizumoto T, Onoda K, Yuasa H, Yada I. Erythropoietin in pediatric cardiac surgery. *Chest* 1997; **111**: 1565–70.

19 Erb T, Moller R, Christen P, Signer E, Frei FJ. Increased withdrawal volume per deposit for pre-opeartive autologous blood donation in adolescents. *Vox Sang* 2000; **78**: 231–4.

20 Velardi F, Di Chirico AD, Rocco CD *et al*. "No allogenic blood transfusion" protocol for the surgical correction of craniosynostoses. *Childs Nerv Syst* 1998; **14**: 732–9.

21 Rothstein P, Roye D, Verdisco L, Stern L. Preoperative use of erythropoietin in an adolescent Jehovah's Witness. *Anesthesiology* 1990; **73**: 568–70.

22 Polley JW, Berkowitz RA, McDonald TB, Cohen M, Figeroa A, Penney DW. Craniomaxillofacial surgery in the Jehovah's Witness patient. *Plast Reconstr Surg* 1994; **93**: 1258–63.

23 Atabek U, Alvarez R, Pello MJ, Alexander JB, Camishion RC, Curry C, Spence RK. Erythropoietin accelerates hematocrit recovery in post-surgical anemia. *Am Surgeon* 1995; **61**: 74–7.

24 Boshkov LK, Tredget EE, Janowska-Wieczorek A. Recombinant human erythropoietin for a Jehovah's Witness with anemia of thermal injury. *Am J Hematol* 1991; **37**: 53–4.

25 Moghtader JC, Edlich RF, Mintz PD, Zachmann GC, Himel HN. The use of recombinant human erythropoietin and cultured epithelial autografts in a Jehovah's Witness with a major thermal injury. *Burns* 1994; **20**: 176–7.

26 Deitch EA, Guillory D, Cruz N. Successful use of recombinant human erythropoietin in a Jehovah's Witness with a thermal injury. *J Burn Care Rehabil* 1994; **15**: 42–5.

27 Roye DP. Recombinant human erythropoietin and blood management in pediatric spine surgery. *Orthopedics* 1999; **22**: S158–S160.

28 Romagnoli C, Zecca E, Gallini F, Girlando P, Zuppa AA. Do recombinant human erythropoietin and iron supplementation increase the risk of retinopathy of prematurity? *Eur J Pediatr* 2000; **159**: 627–8.

29 Schaller RT, Schaller J, Furman EB. The advantages of hemodilution anesthesia for major liver resection in children. *J Pediatr Surg* 1984; **19**: 705–10.

30 Schaller RT, Schaller J, Morgan A, Furman EB. Hemodilution anesthesia: a valuable aid to major cancer surgery. *Am J Surg* 1983; **146**: 79–84.

31 Stehling L, Zauder HL. Acute normovolemic hemodilution. *Transfusion* 1991; **31**: 857–68.

32 Roye DP, Rothstein M, Rickert JB, Verdisco L, Farcy J-P. The use of preoperative erythropoietin in scoliosis surgery. *Spine* 1992; **17**: S204–S205.

33 NIH National Consensus Development Panel. Transfusion alert: use of autologous blood. *Transfusion* 1995; **35**: 703–11.

34 Goodnough LT, Monk TG, Brecher ME. Acute normovolemic hemodilution should replace preoperative autologous blood donation before elective surgery. *Transfusion* 1998; **38**: 473–6.

35 Copley LAB, Richards BS, Safavi FZ, Newton PO. Hemodilution as a method to reduce transfusion requirements in adolescent spine fusion surgery. *Spine* 1999; **24**: 219–24.

36 Consensus Conference on Autologous Transfusion. Final consensus statement. *Transfusion* 1996; **36**: 667.

37 Bryson GL. Does acute normovolemic hemodilution reduce perioperative allogenic transfusion? A meta-analysis. *Anesth Analg* 1997; **86**: 9–15.

38 Safwat AM, Reitan JA, Benson D. Management of Jehovah's Witness patients for scoliosis surgery: the use of platelet and plasmapheresis. *J Clin Anesth* 1997; **9**: 510–13.

39 Gan TJ, Bennett-Guerrero E, Phillips-Bute B *et al.* Hextend®, a physiologically balanced plasma expander for large volume use in major surgery: a randomized phase III clinical trial. *Anesth Analg* 1999; **88**: 992–8.

40 Spahn DR, van Brempt R, Theilmeier G *et al.* Perflubron emulsion delays blood transfusions in orthopedic surgery. *Anesthesiology* 1999; **91**: 1195–208.

41 Farlo, J. Management of hemostasis during extreme normovolemic hemodilution in pediatric Jehovah's Witness patients undergoing high-risk surgical procedures. *Anesthesiology* 2003; **99**: A1425.

42 Milam JD, Austin SF, Nihill MR, Keats AS, Cooley DA. Use of sufficient hemodilution to prevent coagulopathies following surgical correction of cyanotic heart disease. *J Thorac Cardiovasc Surg* 1985; **89**: 623–9.

43 Jonas RA, Wypij D, Roth SJ *et al.* The influence of hemodilution on outcome after hypothermic cardiopulmonary bypass: results of a randomized trial in infants. *J Thorac Cardiovasc Surg* 2003; **126**: 1765–74.

44 Murray DJ, Forbes RB, Titone MB, Weinstein SL. Transfusion management in pediatric and adolescent scoliosis surgery: efficacy of autologous blood. *Spine* 1997; **22**: 2735–40.

45 Dunn CJ, Goa KL. Tranexamic acid: a review of its use in surgery and other indications. *Drugs* 1999; **57**: 1005–32.

46 Sendensky A, Gutzwiller JP, Schneider-Frost J, Wuillemin WA, Graeni R, Beglinger C. Recombinant activated factor VII (NovoSeven) stops severe intra-abdominal bleeding after liver needle biopsy without surgery. *Blood Coag Fibrinolysis* 2004; **15**: 701–2.

47 Williams GD, Bratton SL, Ramamoorthy C. Factors associated with blood loss and blood product transfusions: a multivariate analysis in children after open-heart surgery. *Anesth Analg* 1999; **89**: 57–64.

48 Nelson CL, Fontenot HJ. Ten strategies to reduce blood loss in orthopedic surgery. *Am J Surg* 1995; **170**: 64S–68S.

49 Stauffer UG. The Shaw haemostatic scalpel in paediatric surgery: clinical report on 3000 operations. *Prog Pediatr Surg* 1990; **25**: 40–7.

50 Majeski J. Advances in general and vascular surgical care of Jehovah's Witnesses. *Int Surg* 2000; **85**: 257–65.

51 Tate DE, Friedman RJ. Blood conservation in spinal surgery. *Spine* 1992; **17**: 1450–6.

52 Fontana JL, Welborn L, Mongan PD, Sturm P, Martin G, Bunger R. Oxygen consumption and cardiovascular function in children during profound intraoperative normovolemic hemodilution. *Anesth Analg* 1995; **80**: 219–25.

53 Widness JA, Kulhavy JC, Johnson KJ, Cress GA, Kromer IJ, Acarregui MJ, Feld RD. Clinical performance of an in-line point-of-care monitor in neonates. *Pediatrics* 2000; **106**: 497–504.

54 Moya MP, Clark RH, Nicks J, Tanaka DT. The effects of bedside blood gas monitoring and blood loss and ventilator management. *Biol Neonate* 2001; **80**: 257–61.

55 Soumerai, SB, Salem-Schatz S, Avorn J, Cateris CS, Ross-Degnan D, Popovsky MA. A controlled tiral of educational outreach to improve blood transfusion practice. *JAMA* 1993; **270**: 961–6.

56 Salem-Schatz SR, Avorn J, Soumerai SB. Influence of clinical knowledge, organizational context, and practice style on transfusion decision-making: implications for practice change strategies. *JAMA* 1990; **264**: 476–83.

57 Goodman AM, Pollack MM, Patel KM, Luban NL. Pediatric red blood cell transfusions increase resource use. *J Pediatr* 2003; **142**: 123–7.

58 Toy P. The transfusion audit as an educational tool. *Transfus Sci* 1998; **19**: 91–6.

59 Morrison JC, Sumrall DD, Chevalier SP, Robinson SV, Morrison FS, Wiser WL. The effect of provider education on blood utilization practices. *Am J Obstet Gynecol* 1993; **169**: 1240–5.

60 Surgenor DM, Churchill WH, Wallace EL *et al*. The specific hospital significantly affects red cell and component transfusion practice in coronary artery bypass graft surgery: a study of five hospitals. *Transfusion* 1998; **38**: 122–34.

61 Ballance WA, Dahms BD, Shenker N, Kliegman RM. Pathology of neonatal necrotizing enterocolitis: a ten-year experience. *J Pediatr* 1990; **177**: S6–S13.

62 Kling PJ, Sullivan TM, Leftwich ME, Roe DJ. Score for neonatal acute physiology predicts erythrocyte transfusions in premature infants. *Arch Dis Pediatr Adolesc Med* 1997; **151**: 27–31.

63 Ringer SA, Richardson DK, Sacher RA, Keszler M, Churchill WH. Variations in transfusion practice in neonatal intensive care. *Pediatrics* 1998; **101**: 194–200.

64 Hutter JJ, Hathaway WE, Wayne ER. Hematologic abnormalities in severe neonatal necrotizing enterocolitis. *J Pediatr* 1976; **88**: 1026–31.

65 Patel C. Hematologic abnormalities in acute necrotizing enterocolitis. *Pediatr Clin N Am* 1977; **24**: 579–84.

66 Mehta P, Vasa R, Neumann L, Karpatkin M. Thrombocytopenia in the high-risk infant. *J Pediatr* 1980; **97**: 791–4.

67 Aronis S, Platokouki H, Photopoulos S, Eftychia A, Xanthou M. Indications of coagulation and/or fibrinolytic systems activation in healthy and sick very low birth weight neonates. *Biol Neonate* 1998; **74**: 337–44.

68 Tapper H, Herwald H. Modulation of hemostatic mechanisms in bacterial infectious diseases. *Blood* 2000; **96**: 2329–37.

69 Sola M, Vecchio A, Rimsza L. Evaluation and treatment of thrombocytopenia in the neonatal intensive care unit. *Neonatal Hematol* 2000; **27**: 655–79.

70 Ballin A, Arbel E, Kenet G, Berar M, Kohelet D, Tanay A, Zakut H, Meytes D. Autologous umbilical cord blood transfusion. *Arch Dis Child* 1995; **73**: F181–F183.

71 Beattie R, Stark JM, Wardrop CAJ, Holland BM, Kinmond S. Autologous umbilical cord blood transfusion. *Arch Dis Child* 1996; **74**: F221.

72 Eichler H, Schaible T, Richter E, Zieger W, Voller K, Leveringhaus A, Goldmann SF. Cord blood as a source of autologous RBCs for transfusion to preterm infants. *Transfusion* 2000; **40**: 1111–17.

73 Hume H. Red blood cell transfusions for preterm infants: the role of evidence-based medicine. *Sem Perinatol* 1997; **21**: 8–19.

74 Imura K, Kawahar H, Kitayama Y, Yoneda A, Yagi M, Suehara N. Usefulness of cord-blood harvesting for autologous transfusion in surgical newborns with ante-natal diagnosis of congenital anomalies. *J Pediatr Surg* 2001; **36**: 851–4.

75 Burke RP, Hannan RL. Reducing the trauma of congenital heart surgery. *Surg Clin N Am* 2000; **80**: 1593–605.

76 Kreutzer J. Transcatheter intervention in the neonate with congenital heart disease. *Clin Perinatol* 2001; **28**: 137–57.

77 Miyaji K, Furuse A, Takeda M, Chikada M, Ono M, Kawauchi M. Successful conduit repair using aortic homograft in a Jehovah's Witness child. *Ann Thorac Surg* 1996; **62**: 590–1.

78 Alexi-Meskishvili V, Ovroutski S, Dahnert I, Fischer T. Correction of cor triatriatum sinistrum in a Jehova's Witness infant. *Eur J Cardiothorac Surg* 2000; **18**: 724–6.

79 Calza G, Zannini L, Lerzo F, Nitti P, Mangraviti S, Perutelli P, Porlezza M. Quantitative and qualitative evaluation of blood salvaged after extracorporeal circulation in paediatric heart surgery. *Int J Artific Organs* 2000; **23**: 398–406.

80 Schaff HV, Hauer J, Gardner TJ, Donahoo JS, Watkins L, Gott VL, Brawley RK. Routine use of autotransfusion following cardiac surgery: experience in 700 patients. *Ann Thorac Surg* 1978; **27**: 493–9.

81 Malcolm-Smith NA, McMaster MJ. The use of induced hypotension to control bleeding during posterior fusion for scoliosis. *J Bone Joint Surg* 1983; **65-B**: 255–8.

82 Kruger LM, Colbert JM. Intraoperative autologous transfusion in children undergoing spinal surgery. *J Pediatr Orthoped* 1985; **5**: 330–2.

83 Kang JK, Lee SW, Baik MW, Son BC, Hong YK, Jung CK, Ryu KH. Perioperative specific management of blood volume loss in craniosynostosis surgery. *Childs Nerv Syst* 1998; **14**: 297–301.

84 Butler P, Israel L, Nusbacher J, Jenkins DE, Starzl TE. Blood transfusion in liver transplantation. *Transfusion* 1985; **25**: 120–3.

85 Kim YI, Ishii T, Aramaki M, Nakashima K, Yoshida T, Kobayashi M. The Pringle maneuver induces only partial ishcemia of the liver. *Hepato-Gastroenterol* 1995; **42**: 169–71.

86 Quan D, Wall W. The safety of continuous hepatic inflow occlusion during major liver resection. *Liver Transpl Surg* 1996; **2**: 99–104.

87 Gertsch P, Pelloni A, Guerra A, Krpo A. Initial experience with the harmonic scalpel in liver surgery. *Hepato-Gastroenterol* 2000; **47**: 763–6.

88 Jabbour N, Gagandeep S, Thomas D, Stapher M, Mateo, R, Sher L, Selby R, Genyk Y. Transfusion-free techniques in pediatric live donor liver transplantation. *J Pediatr Gastroenterol Nutr* 2005; **40**(4): 521–3.

89 Barret JP, Desai MH, Herndon DN. Massive transfusion of reconstituted whole blood is well tolerated in pediatric burn surgery. *J Trauma Inj Infect Crit Care* 1999; **47**: 526–8.

90 Deitch EA, Sitting KM. A serial study of the erythropoietic response to thermal injury. *Ann Surg* 1993; **217**: 293–9.

91 Law EJ, Still JM, Gattis CS. The use of erythropoietin in two burned patients who are Jehovah's Witnesses. *Burns* 1991; **1991**: 75–7.

92 Cartotto R, Musgrave MA, Beveridge M, Fish J, Gomez M. Minimizing blood loss in burn surgery. *J Trauma* 2000; **49**: 1034–9.

93 Moore E, Shackford SR, Pachter HL *et al*. Organ injury scaling: spleen, liver and kidney. *J Trauma* 1989; **1989**: 1664–6.

94 Malhotra AK, Fabian TC, Croce MA *et al*. Blunt hepatic injury: a paradigm shift from operative to non-operative management in the 1990s. *Ann Surg* 2000; **231**: 804–13.

95 Leone RJ, Hammond JS. Nonoperative management of pediatric blunt hepatic trauma. *Am Surgeon* 2001; **67**: 138–42.

96 Kilic N, Gurpinar A, Kiristioglu I, O A, Balkan E, Dogruyol H. Ruptured spleen due to blunt trauma in children: analysis of blood transfusion requirements. *Eur J Emerg Med* 1999; **6**: 135–9.

97 Smith JS, Cooney RN, Mucha P. Non-operative management of the ruptured spleen: a revalidation of criteria. *Surgery* 1996; **120**: 745–51.

98 Sacher RA, Luban NLC, Strauss RG. Current practice and guidelines for the transfusion of cellular blood components in the newborn. *Trans Med Rev* 1989; **3**: 39–54.

99 Jones JG, Holland BM, Hudson IRB, Wardrop CAJ. Total circulating red cells versus haematocrit as the primary descriptor of oxygen transport by the blood. *Br J Haematol* 1990; **1990**: 288–94.

100 Strauss RG. Transfusion therapy in neonates. *Am J Dis Child* 1991; **145**: 904–11.

101 Widness JA, Seward VJ, Kromer IJ, Burmeister LF, Bell EF, Strauss RG. Changing patterns of red blood cell transfusion in very low birth weight infants. *J Pediatr* 1996; **129**: 680–7.

102 Maier RF, Sonntag J, Walka MM, Liu G, Metze BC, Obladen M. Changing practices of red blood cell transfusions in infants with birth weights less than 1000 g. *J Pediatr* 2000; **136**: 220–4.

103 Shannon KM, Keith JM, Mentzer WC *et al*. Recombinant human erythropoietin stimulates erythropoiesis and reduces erythrocyte transfusions in very low birth weight preterm infants. *Pediatrics* 1995; **95**: 1–10.

104 Kinmond S, Aitchison TC, Holland BM, Jones JG, Turner TL, Wardrop CAJ. Umbilical cord clamping and preterm infants: a randomised trial. *Br Med J* 1993; **306**: 172–5.

105 Bednarek FJ, Weisberger S, Richardson DK, Frantz ID, Shah B, Rubin L. Variations in blood transfusions among newborn intensive care units. *J Pediatr* 1998; **133**: 601–7.

106 Ohls RK. Erythropoietin to prevent and treat the anemia of prematurity. *Curr Opin Pediatr* 1999; **11**: 108–14.

107 Ohls RK, Ehrenkranz RA, Wright LL *et al*. The effects of early erythropoietin therapy on the transfusion requirements of preterm infants below 1250 g birthweight: a multicenter, randomized controlled trial. *Pediatrics* 2001; **108**: 934–42.

108 Kumar P, Shankaran S, Krishnan RG. Recombinant human erythropoietin therapy for treatment of anemia of prematurity in very low birth weight infants: a randomized, double-blind, placebo-controlled trial. *J Perinatol* 1998; **18**: 173–7.

109 Ohls RK, Harcum J, Schibler KR, Christensen RD. The effect of erythropoietin on the transfusion requirements of preterm infants weighing 750 g or less: a randomized, double-blind, placebo-controlled study. *J Pediatr* 1997; **131**: 661–5.

110 Ohls RK, Ehrenkranz RA, Lemons JA *et al*. A multicenter randomized double-masked placebo-controlled trial of early erythropoietin and iron administration to preterm infants. *Pediatr Res* 1999; **45**: 216A.

111 Bausch LC. Blood transfusions and the Jehovah's Witness: neonatal perspectives. *Nebr Med J* 1991; **76**: 283–4.

112 Davis P, Herbert M, Davies DP, Verrier-Jones ER. Case study: erythropoietin for anemia in a preterm Jehovah's Witness. *Early Hum Develop* 1992; **28**: 279–83.

113 Beck MN, Beck D. Recombinant erythropoietin in acute chemotherapy-induced anemia of children with cancer. *Med Pediatr Oncol* 1995; **25**: 17–21.

114 Leon P, Jimenez M, Barona P, Sierraseumaga L. Recombinant human erythropoietin for the treatment of anemia in children with solid malignant tumors. *Med Pediatr Oncol* 1998; **30**: 110–16.

115 Bolonaki I, Stiakaki E, Lydaki E, Dimitriou H, Kambourakis A, Kalmantis T, Kalmanti M. Treatment with recombinant human erythropoietin in children with malignancies. *Pediatr Hematol Oncol* 1998; **13**: 111–21.

116 Csaki C, Ferencz T, Schuler D, Borsi JD. Recombinant human erythropoietin in the prevention of chemotherapy-induced anaemia in children with malignant solid tumors. *Eur J Cancer* 1998; **34**: 364–7.

117 Ballen KK, Ford PA, Witkus H, Emmons RVB, Levy W, Doyle P, Stewart FM, Quesenberry PJ, Becker PS. Successful autologous bone marrow transplant without use of blood product support. *Bone Marrow Transpl* 2000; **26**: 227–9.

118 Estrin JT, Ford PA, Henry DH, Stradden AP, Mason BA. Erythropoietin permits high-dose chemotherapy with peripheral blood stem-cell transplant for a Jehovah's Witness. *Am J Hematol* 1997; **55**: 51–2.

119 Beguin Y, Oris R, Fillet G. Dynamics of erythropoietic recovery following bone marrow transplantation: role of marrow proliferative capacity and erythropoietin production in autologous versus allogenic transplants. *Bone Marrow Transpl* 1993; **11**: 285–92.

120 Locatelli F, Zecca M, Pedrazzoli P, Prete L, Quaglini S, Comoli P, DeStefano P, Beguin Y, Robustelli della Cuna G, Severi F *et al*. Use of recombinant human erythropoietin after bone marrow transplantation in pediatric patients with acute leukemia: effect on erythroid repopulation in autologous verus allogenic transplants. *Bone Marrow Transpl* 1994; **13**: 403–10.

121 Biggs JC, Atkinson SA, Booker V, Concannon A, Dart DW, Dodds A, Downs A, Szer J, Turner J, Worthington R. Prospective randomised double-blind trial of the in vivo use of recombinant human erythrpoietin in bone marrow transplantation from HLA-identical sibling donors. *Bone Marrow Transpl* 1995; **15**: 129–34.

CHAPTER 11

The Cost of Blood Product Transfusion

Gary Zeger, Nicolas Jabbour

This chapter will address the cost of blood in the USA. We will see what these costs are, how they are calculated and why they are so high. We will show how blood collected from unpaid volunteer donors costs the health care system multiple billions of dollars.

Where blood comes from: volunteer donor to patient

A schematic of how blood is drawn from an unpaid volunteer donor is represented in (Figure 11.1).

The donor room

Whole blood and apheresis platelets are, by far, the most common components collected in the donor room. Blood and platelets are collected from volunteer donors under the supervision of highly trained, licensed professionals. Approximately 93% of the US blood supply is collected by centers affiliated with the American Red Cross and America's Blood Centers [1]. Many of the large blood collection agencies, the largest of which is the American Red Cross, may have one or more regional headquarters, which also serve as manufacturing centers. Headquarters may contain a donor room and there is often a network of smaller satellite donor rooms that serve to collect blood, which is then sent to the manufacturing center for further processing. Blood centers often run mobile operations that send collection teams out to set up blood drives sponsored by institutions such as schools, churches, businesses, hospitals and the military. Organization and recruitment are usually a significant expense.

The remaining 7% of collected blood comes from independent hospital-affiliated donor centers [1]; however, the increasingly complicated regulatory requirement and more expensive and sophisticated infectious disease testing make these more difficult to set up and maintain. The advent of nucleic acid testing (NAT) for infectious disease has made it necessary for many of these independent donor rooms to rely on outside sources for infectious disease testing.

Collection standards are rigorous, numerous and constantly changing, often in response to threats posed by infectious diseases and medications

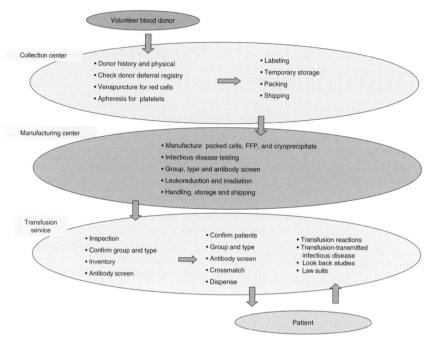

Figure 11.1 Volunteer blood donor to patient.

that might prove harmful to blood recipients [2]. The donor must answer a long questionnaire with emphasis on potential personal lifestyle problems, which would put the recipient at risk for transfusion-transmissible infectious diseases. More and more donors are also being deferred for certain prescription medications, body piercings, tattoos, medical problems and travel to areas where exposure to malaria or new variant Creutzfeldt–Jakob disease is considered a risk factor [3,4]. A very significant percentage of donors will be deferred for any of these reasons, which wastes resources and decreases the blood supply [5].

Donors must undergo a simple physical exam consisting of blood pressure, hematocrit (Hct), pulse, temperature and examination of veins for suitability of venapunture and absence of signs of illicit intravenous (IV) drug use. Many women, in particular, are deferred for low Hct. These deferrals also use up resources and diminish the number of potential blood donors [5].

When a suitable donor is identified, whole blood is collected by simple venapuncture into a sterile bag containing anticoagulant. Currently, however, platelets are often collected on sophisticated automated apheresis machines that require specially trained operators and expensive software [6]. Once collected, the blood and platelets must be properly labeled, stored and transported, under strict conditions, to a manufacturing center.

Imported blood

Until recently, much of the blood coming to parts of the east coast was imported from Europe. Even in 2001, 25% of New York City's blood supply was imported from a number of European countries [7]. The ban on blood donors from countries with populations at risk for Creutzfeld–Jakob disease has dried up this supply, putting more pressure on the blood system [4]. Blood for transfusion is no longer imported into the USA.

The manufacturing center

This is often central headquarters and the hub of the blood collection system where whole blood is separated into packed cells and fresh frozen plasma (FFP) by centrifugation. With further centrifugation, a unit of random-donor platelets can be further extracted from the plasma, although the trend has been towards single-donor platelets collected by apheresis technology [6]. Infectious disease testing is performed (Table 11.1) and the ABO and Rh types are determined. The blood is also tested for unexpected anti–red blood cell (RBC) antibodies (the antibody screen). Leukoreduction is done on most RBC units and all platelets that are stored at room temperature, and are recently cultured for bacteria [8]. Units are labeled with unique identifiers so that any unit of blood can later be tracked from the donor to the patient.

Blood, platelets and plasma must be stored under specific, closely monitored temperatures and conditions. It is important to note that all blood components have an expiration date after which they generally should not be used. Whole blood can survive, refrigerated, for up to 42 days and even longer if frozen. Platelets are only good for 5 days at room temperature and FFP is good for 1 year if frozen to -18°C [9]. These expiration times, particularly on platelets, add to wastage, which increases the overall cost of the blood system.

A distribution department with a fleet of delivery vehicles must be available to ship blood to the many client transfusion services, often on short notice and emergency basis, at any hour of the day or night.

Table 11.1 Infectious disease testing of blood for transfusion.

- Human immunodeficiency virus I/II – antibodies
- Human immunodeficiency virus I – nucleic acid testing
- Hepatitis B virus – antibody to core antigen
- Hepatitis B virus – surface antigen
- Hepatitis C virus – antibodies
- Hepatitis C virus – nucleic acid testing
- Human T-cell lymphotropic virus I/II – antibodies
- West Nile virus – nucleic acid testing
- Syphilis - antibody screening

Source: Based on infectious disease testing at the HemaCare Corporation, Sherman Oaks, California, November 2004.

The transfusion service

The transfusion service is where blood is stored, processed and prepared for transfusion to a particular patient. Transfusion services are often part of a hospital-based clinical laboratory serving the needs of medical and surgical services and occasionally a trauma center. Transfusion services may serve outpatient day hospitals, often clinics of cancer hospitals, which attend to patients' needs for chemotherapy and related transfusion support. For smaller operations, where a full transfusion service is not feasible or necessary, such as a dialysis center, blood centers will often provide small numbers of units specifically crossmatched for an individual patient, at an additional cost.

At the transfusion service, licensed technologists must perform a number of additional steps. The blood must first be inspected for proper temperature, leakage, breakage, contamination or any other possible deficiency. The units are then entered into inventory, often through a computer. RBCs are retested to confirm the blood type. Blood from the intended patients must also be tested, often more than once, to determine and confirm the patient's blood type. The patient's serum is also screened for unexpected anti-RBC antibodies. Any antibodies that are detected must be identified and RBC units must be phenotyped to find compatible units. For difficult cases, which are not at all uncommon, a specialized regional reference laboratory, often located in the blood centers' manufacturing headquarters, must be utilized to identify the antibody and find compatible blood.

Meticulous and rigorous safety checks are performed before units can leave the transfusion service for the patient's bedside and again prior to transfusion. Transfusion itself is performed under stringent conditions with close observation for adverse reactions, which are not uncommon [10]. The more serious reactions are evaluated by the transfusion service through a number of additional tests, often with physician participation. Even minor allergic reactions often result in disposal of any remaining untransfused blood, which results in further expense of wastage and supplying a replacement unit. Reactions may also be severe, causing significant morbidity and even mortality [11].

Patients not experiencing immediate reactions may later develop delayed reactions where exposure to previously transfused blood results in a patient forming anti-RBC antibodies, which will significantly complicate further transfusions [12]. Transfusion-transmitted infectious disease, even when only suspected, requires extensive investigation. For the patient contracting a transfusion-transmitted disease, although rare, the morbidity and the expense of diagnosis and treatment may be extreme [10].

When all of these factors are taken into account, it becomes apparent how unpaid blood donations result in the extreme cost of blood transfusion.

Some difficulties in estimating cost

The price of blood from the blood center is fairly straightforward in the sense that blood centers generally have contracted fee schedules with client transfusion services. These prices, however, vary significantly in different parts of the country, influenced, in part, by local costs for labor, transportation, taxation and real estate. Blood is sold to transfusion services that are often hospital-based. Negotiated contract prices may depend on a number of factors and may vary significantly. Hospital chains may bargain for volume discounts and individual hospitals may also receive more favorable rates for larger contracted volumes. Exclusivity with a single vendor may also be rewarded by lower prices. Return policies for unused units may factor into the equation, particularly for smaller services, which might otherwise have to waste unused blood if not used by other patients before the blood expires. The conditions and pricing of blood transportation are often a negotiating point, as blood is often needed unexpectedly and for emergency situations, particularly at trauma centers. Some blood centers may request permission and assistance in organizing blood drives at the client hospital and these hospitals, likewise, may request such services. The numbers often involve hundreds of thousands of dollars and the sales tactics between local vendors can be highly competitive, and often cutthroat. Independent hospital-based donor centers have their own accounting methods, which vary from center to center.

The remarkable complexity and confusion about the cost of blood comes not from what a transfusion center is charged, but when considering what a payer, often Medicare, Medicaid or a private insurer, will reimburse a hospital or transfusion center. The rules and regulations are so complex that recently Medicare reported that fewer than half of all hospitals bill for blood transfused in an inpatient setting [13,14]. Although a detailed discussion of reimbursement is outside of the scope of this chapter, it has been estimated that hospitals have been underbilling for blood transfusions, and any accurate estimate of how much hospitals are reimbursed will be somewhat theoretical at this point [1]. The diagnosis-related group (DRG) method of payments has significantly added to the confusion of the cost of blood as this system pays the health care provider on the basis of a specific diagnosis code [13]. The cost of blood transfusion may have little to do with the amount paid to the hospital. Due to the difficult financial situation that many hospitals find themselves in, there has been a concerted effort to understand and accurately bill for blood transfusion.

There are some factors relating to the cost of transfusion that this chapter will not cover in any depth but should be mentioned. Not covered here are the actual costs of transfusing the blood. These can be calculated in many ways that may factor in required the credentials of the persons performing the transfusions, the time required and supplies needed. Once again, in a DRG payment system, none of this may matter, as there will be a single fixed payment for the medical care no matter how individual costs are calculated.

Another set of costs relates to posttransfusion sequelae, which include the morbidity and mortality of transfusion reactions and transfusion-transmitted disease. Although these costs are significant, they are not easily estimable and should be kept in mind as significant additional expenses [15].

The bottom line is that calculating the cost of blood transfusion is imprecise and problematic. Figures used in the chapter are based on what transfusion might cost in a 250-bed hospital. The charges to hospitals are based on a local Red Cross price schedule and are fairly straightforward. These figures are included to provide the reader with a sense of the magnitude of the sums involved. The section on how a hospital might charge a patient for blood transfusion is modeled after the same type of hospital. It reflects how the hospital bills patients but does not make assumptions about what the hospital will actually collect.

The numbers here apply to the USA; however, it is likely that the factors responsible for the high costs, such as increasing donor restrictions, more extensive infectious disease testing and shortage of trained personnel, will be reflected in the cost of blood transfusions in other parts of the world. It is estimated that the cost of blood transfusion will increase by about 6% per year [16]. New agents of potentially transfusion-transmissible diseases and elaborate screening and testing methodologies may cause prices to rise much faster than anticipated.

Why blood from volunteer donors costs over $4 billion

Blood is free in the sense that it must be collected from unpaid volunteer donors. Paid donors are not acceptable in the USA for blood or platelets that are to be used for human transfusion. Only donors for plasma collected for nonhuman use can be paid. Incentives for donation are limited to gifts of no intrinsic monetary value; usually T-shirts, coffee mugs, or gift certificates to movies or restaurants [17]. Yet in 2001, 14 million units, at the cost of approximately $225 per unit, had an initial cost of over $3 billion [17]. An additional 15 million blood components were transfused that year [17]. Extrapolating percentages of components collected from the blood collection statistics listed in the United Blood Systems (UBS) web site annual report [18], approximately 10% of these components, 1.4 million units, may be apheresis platelets, which are sold for approximately $500 per unit, or a cost of $700 million. If the remaining 12.6 million components are random-donor platelets, FFP and cryoprecipitate, which would sell for approximately $50 a unit, there is an additional $630 million. The grand total amounts to over $4 billion (Table 11.2). Costs not included are hospital charges to patients, the cost of the actual act of transfusion, blood filters, transfusion reactions, transfusion-transmitted disease, medical-legal costs and regulatory require- ments. Some of the factors contributing to the high cost of transfusion are listed in Table 11.3.

How does blood collected from unpaid volunteer donors eventually cost more than $4 billion? This is because the cost of a blood transfusion is usually not considered as the cost of the blood itself but rather the cost of a process comprising multiple services, which eventually result in a blood transfusion [13]. It should be noted that some blood sources, particularly hospital donor

Table 11.2 An estimate of blood charges to US hospitals in 2001.

	Unit numbers	Price/unit ($)	Total ($)
Red blood cells	14 000 000	225	3 150 000 000
Platelets, pheresis	1 400 000	500	700 000 000
CRYO, FFP, and RDPs	12 600 000	50	630 000 000
Total			4 480 000 000

Table 11.3 Costs incurred in the provision of blood.

Recruitment and collections
Infectious disease testing
Manufacturing, shipping, handling, labeling
Pre-transfusion testing
Transfusion costs
Posttransfusion sequellae
Regulatory and legal costs

rooms, may charge for blood as a product, not a process, but they are by far in the minority [13]. This may have also been true in the days of the paid donor, who no longer exists. This chapter will focus on the process of providing blood for transfusion, what those services are, and why they are so expensive.

Why blood is usually a service, and not a product

Blood is inherently unsafe and could never meet standards as applied to strict product liability laws. Transfusion reactions, both idiopathic and due to human error, are not uncommon, and the result may be serious morbidity and mortality. Transfusion-transmitted disease, however, is possibly the most feared complication of blood transfusion. Although human immunodeficiency virus (HIV), hepatitis B virus (HBV) and hepatitis C virus (HCV) are relatively under control [19], on an alarmingly regular basis we are learning of new infectious agents with the potential transmission through blood transfusion. The latest concerns include West Nile virus (WNV) [20], SARS [21], mad cow disease [10], postvaccination small pox [22] and monkey pox [23]. With increasing globalization, more people are traveling long distances and carrying their potentially transfusion-transmissible diseases with them [10]. WNV has already had deadly impact.

Blood, therefore, is never legally considered a 'product'. In fact, most states now have 'blood shield laws' that limit the liability of blood collection centers and transfusion facilities to issues of the improper provision of blood, not in the safety of the blood itself [24,25].

Provision of blood, therefore, might be considered a process – the result of a series of many services. The cost of blood is the cost of all these services, which are meticulously developed, scrupulously performed and rigorously inspected.

An intense but thorough regulatory environment

An important reason for the high cost of blood is the intense regulatory system placed on the blood banking industry as a result of lessons learned from transfusion-transmitted diseases [26]. Blood transfusions in the 1960s and 1970s were associated with significant risk of transfusion-transmitted disease, especially hepatitis. This was due to inadequate screening and the acceptance of paid blood donors who may have been desperate for money to feed a drug or alcohol habit. The incidence of viral transmitted diseases, particularly hepatitis B, was very high [27–29].

Termination of the paid donor system plus more careful donor screening and improved infectious disease testing contributed to transfusion safety [30,31]. Even so, the incidence of transfusion-transmitted hepatitis C (then called non-A, non-B hepatitis) still remained at approximately 10% of patients transfused [27,32,33] until 1989. Although this is a staggeringly high percentage compared to today's standards, the blood banking industry was aggressively working on the problem and the public was not highly focused on transfusion safety issues.

In the early 1980s HIV was still poorly understood by the medical community but not yet in the public eye. Soon, however, the sheer number of cases and the many high-profile victims had attained widespread media coverage. It became evident that HIV was transmitted by blood transfusion [34,35]. In areas with high-risk donor populations, such as New York, Los Angeles, and San Francisco, the risk for transfusion-transmitted HIV could be as high as 1 per 1000 units [36]. Media attention was extreme and many patients feared blood transfusion.

There is still controversy over early management of HIV in the blood supply. Overall, blood industry and the Food and Drug Administration (FDA) received a good deal of negative publicity, whether deserved or not. The result has been a very intense regulatory environment to insure that there will never be another transfusion-transmitted HIV-type tragedy.

Blood banks are amongst the most highly regulated and carefully inspected US institutions. Blood banks and transfusion services are often inspected by three different accreditation services including the FDA, the American Association of Blood Banks, and additional professional and local authorities. Any of these inspections can take full days and even weeks to complete. A no-fault-tolerance attitude toward any sort of error is generally accepted. Regulations change frequently and most blood centers now have at least one full-time compliance officer whose basic responsibility is to learn and enforce the many new laws and regulations as they appear.

This is complicated by new and often poorly understood threats to the blood supply, which often require new, complicated and constantly changing donor deferral criteria and new infectious disease testing strategies. Recent requirements for bacterial testing of platelets have led to more complications and expenses [8].

Blood collections require rigid collection, transportation, storage, labeling, processing and testing procedures, all of which allow no room for error. Blood is now tested for HIV, HBV, HCV, human T-lymphotropic virus (HTLV), WNV and syphilis. New and improved testing technologies such as NAT have become standard and are significantly more expensive [37,38].

Today, the blood industry generally uses no-fault-tolerance with extensive systems to help guarantee that blood for transfusion is of the highest quality possible [39]. The result is safer and much more expensive blood transfusion.

Current costs

Hospital costs

The costs of blood transfusion are immense. Table 11.4 illustrates a partial fee schedule with prices similar to those that might be provided to a moderate-sized hospital by the American Red Cross of Southern California, the major blood provider in Los Angeles County [40]. Only the more commonly used components are listed. The prices are similar to what other hospitals in the region might pay and not grossly dissimilar to those found in other regions of the country.

Table 11.4 Red Cross fee schedule (fiscal year 2005).

Blood component	Price ($)
Red blood cells packed leukoreduced	276
Red blood cells washed and leukoreduced	450
Red blood cells frozen	511
Red blood cells deglycerolized	686
Whole blood	331
Platelets pheresis leukoreduced	494
Platelets from concentrate	69
Fresh frozen plasma	53
Fresh frozen plasma jumbo > 400 ml	106
Fresh frozen plasma cryoprecipitate-reduced	80
Cryoprecipitate	52
Leukofiltration surcharge	15
Irradiation surcharge	40
CMV negative surcharge	40
Autologous blood surcharge	125
Directed donor surcharge	125

There are many additional fees that can add significantly to the price of a blood component. Some of these costs are discussed below.

Leukoreduction

Leukoreduction is the removal of white blood cells (WBCs) from a blood component. For RBCs, this usually implies filtration technology. Pheresis platelets are generally collected on machines that minimize WBC contamination at the time of collection. Leukoreduced blood components are now offered exclusively by many blood centers including the American Red Cross Blood Services, Southern California Region, which is the major blood provider in Southern California. Leukoreduction decreases the incidence of febrile nonhemolytic transfusion reactions and cytomegalovirus (CMV) transmission [41]. There is also literature that attributes leukoreduction to improved immune function compared to nonleukoreduced transfusion evidenced by decreased postoperative infections, less tumor metastasis and fewer inpatient hospital days [42]. The need for universal leucoreduction is still controversial and not yet generally agreed upon. Leukoreduction adds $15 to the price of a unit of packed cells.

Washing

Washing is the removal of plasma from a packed RBC unit. This is done by repeatedly washing the cell with saline until very little of the original plasma is left. This is often done on an apparatus called a cell washer. Washed RBCs are used for patients who have significant allergic reactions to foreign plasma proteins, particularly IgA [43]. Washed cells are available for $450, an additional $174 to a nonwashed leukoreduced RBC unit. Washed cells have a 24-h expiration from the time of washing, which makes wastage a serious problem when the transfusion is delayed. At one time there was a trend for use of washed cells as a superior RBC product compared to nonwashed RBCs; however, this trend did not catch on, excessive cost being one of the reasons.

Freezing and deglycerolizing

RBCs are sometimes frozen to delay expiration time [44]. This involves adding glycerol to the cells to avoid perforation by ice crystals. The glycerol must be removed upon thawing, prior to transfusion. This is generally done by a cell washer and requires skilled technical support. Often only rare blood types are frozen for specific patient needs; however, in times of severe shortage, frozen cells are used for general transfusion purposes. A deglycerolized unit of blood costs $686 and has a 24-h expiration time leading to the same wastage problems seen with washed blood.

Irradiation

Irradiation of blood components inhibits lymphocytes from replicating. It is used to stop graft-versus-host disease (GVHD) in situations where this might be a problem [45]. The surcharge for irradiation is $40.

Cryoprecipitate-reduced fresh frozen plasma

This component is used as a plasma replacement for patients receiving plasmapheresis for thrombotic thrombocytopenic purpura [46]. The cost is $80 per unit and it is often given in multiple treatments, which require 10–15 units per treatment depending on many clinical conditions including the patient's blood volume and the physician's judgment.

Cytomegalovirus-negative components

An additional $40 is charged if the component is tested and found negative for antibodies to the CMV. This may be important for immunosuppressed patients [47].

Autologous and directed units

Patients may be able to donate blood for themselves (autologous donation) or have others specifically donate for them (directed donation). In California, the right to autologous and directed donation is guaranteed by the Paul Gann Blood Safety Act [48]. The surcharge is $125 per unit.

Pediatric units

There is an additional fee charged to divide a normal-sized unit of blood into smaller pediatric units.

Hospital charges

Once a unit of blood arrives at the transfusion facility, often a hospital transfusion service, a number of other substantial fees are attached to the blood component (Table 11.5).

For RBCs, the ABO group and Rh type must be confirmed before the unit can be transfused. The patient's group and type must also be confirmed in duplicate prior to transfusion. An antibody screen must be done on the

Table 11.5 Hospital charges for blood transfusion.

Service	Price ($)
Blood type ABO	156
Blood type Rh	85
Antibody screen	182
Crossmatch, immediate spin	350
Crossmatch, antiglobulin (Coombs phase)	391
Red blood cell antigen screening (per antigen)	108
Fresh frozen plasma thawing	156
Cryoprecipitate pooling (per pool)	43
Antigen phenotyping	108
Handling and other	86
Surcharge	15%

Table 11.6 Additional charges to patient ($).

Product	Base price	15% surcharge	Handling and other	Crossmatch	Thawing	Pooling	Total
Red blood cells	276.00	41.40	86.00	350.00			753.40
Platelets	500.00	75.00	86.00				661.00
FFP	53.00	7.95	86.00		156.00		302.95
10 CRYO pool	520.00	78.00	860.00			43.00	1 501.00

patient's plasma to determine if there are any clinically significant anti-RBC antibodies capable of causing hemolytic transfusion reactions. If any antibodies are discovered, they must be identified with an antibody detection panel and compatible units must be phenotyped to make sure the offending antigen is not present. This can often be done in the transfusion service; however, for difficult cases phenotyped units must be ordered from the local blood center reference laboratory. Individual RBC units must be crossmatched to help assure compatibility with the donor. If unexpected anti-RBC antibodies are detected, an extended Coombs phase crossmatch must be performed for an additional fee [49].

Hospitals may also charge additional fees to cover handling, wastage, transportation and transfusion [13]. Examples of how additional charges may increase the amount billed to a patient are illustrated in Table 11.6.

Case studies

To illustrate how multiple costs of blood transfusion add up, two case studies are presented. Although the numbers are hypothetical, they are not atypical of what might be found in many hospitals.

The first is a fairly uncomplicated case of open heart surgery in an adult (Table 11.7). A description of the hospital fees is listed above. Fees for RBCs include $350 per unit for an immediate spin (abbreviated) crossmatch and a

Table 11.7 Case study 1: Adult open heart surgery.

Product	Number	Product fee/unit ($)	Hospital fee/unit ($)	Total ($)
Red blood cells	6	276	477	4520
FFP	5	53	250	1515
Platelets	1	500	200	1400
Pt ABO type	1		156	185
Pt Rh type	1		85	85
Pt antibody screen	1		182	182
Total				7887

Table 11.8 Case study 2: Liver transplant with alloantibodies and directed donors.

Product	Number	Product fee ($)	Hospital fee ($)	Total ($)
Red blood cells	5	276	518	3970
Red blood cells directed	3	401	537	2814
Pt ABO type	1		156	156
Pt Rh type	1		85	85
Pt antibody screen	1		182	182
Antibody ID	1		465	465
Phenotype patient	1		108	108
Phenotyping units (3 ags each)	24		108	2592
FFP	4	53	250	1212
Platelets	2	500	200	1400
Cryoprecipitate	10	52	1833	2353
Total				15337

$250 fee for dispensing. An extra $86 is added for 'handling and other', which is to cover storage and wastage.

Case 2 illustrates what might occur in a liver transplant in which three unexpected anti-RBC antibodies are identified and phenotyped compatible units provided (Table 11.8). In this hypothetical, though not atypical case, not only are 5 allogeneic (ordinary volunteer) RBC units used but 3 directed donor units (from friends or relatives) are also transfused. Each directed unit has an additional $125 fee attached. This patient has three unexpected anti-RBC alloantibodies, which must be identified for $465. As part of the workup, the patient's own RBCs must be tested for the three antigens, which correspond to the three alloantibodies for a single charge of $108. This is done to further confirm the antibody identities. Each unit of RBCs must also be phenotyped for each of these antigens to help guarantee compatibility for $108 for each of three antigens on 8 different units ($24 \times \$108$). Because there is an alloantibody, each unit must receive a full crossmatch for $391.

Artificial blood and pharmacologic agents

Although there have been multiple and ongoing attempts to create artificial blood, at the time of this writing, there are no approved blood substitutes [50]. There are a number of fairly well known agents that function to reduce surgical bleeding; however, they cannot replace blood transfusion in many cases and they have their own limitations and side-effects [51]. These agents also tend to be expensive and their cost-effectiveness has yet to be proven [52]. Table 11.9 summarizes the average coast of some of these products used as a means to conserve blood.

Table 11.9 Pharmacologic agents commonly used to conserve blood.

Product name	Average wholesale price (awp) ($)	Therapeutic dose	Average cost per dose ($)
Erythropoietin (Procrit®)	2350.00 (40 000 units × 4 vials)	40 000 units SC/IV	587.50
Darbepoetin (Aranesp®)	528.76 (25µg × 4 vials)	25µg SC/IV	132.19
Aminocaproic acid (Amicar®)	17.70 (5 g)	5 g load; then 1 g/h × 8 h	46.02
Aprotinin (Trasylol®)	539.06 (200 ml)	200 ml load; then 50 ml/h	
Desmopressin (DDAVP®)	288.40 (4µg × 4 amps)	0.3µg/kgIV	144.20
Tranexamic acid (Cyklokapron®)	361.60 (1000 mg × 10 amps)	1000 mg IV × 2	72.32
Factor VIIa (NovoSeven®)	1764.00 (1.2 mg vial)	4.8 mg IV	7056.00
Factor VIII (Monarc-M®)	1.10/I.U.	2160 IU AHF	2376.00
Factor VIII/vWF (Humate-P®)	1.00/I.U.	Variabe	
Factor IX (AlphaNine®)	1.18/I.U.	Variable	

Conclusion

Blood transfusion is now enormously expensive and will only become more so. We are continuously discovering new agents of transfusion-transmitted disease and taking precautions against agents suspected of causing transfusion-transmitted disease. We can expect new, more sensitive, NAT technologies, which may minimally increase transfusion safety but significantly increase the cost of transfusion. New technologies for detection or prion-related disease are currently under development and may be brought on-line in the near future at additional expense [53,54]. Increasingly, strict donor restrictions for everything including tattoos, medications and vaccinations, and geographical restrictions due to infectious agents such as WNV and CJD can be expected to significantly decrease donor numbers. A decrease in the number of donors will result in a decreased blood supply, which will likely drive prices up. New blood-utilizing surgical technologies, such as organ transplantation, may serve to increase the demand. Artificial blood is not an option at this time and pharmaceutical agents are expensive and do not replace the need for transfusion.

All things considered, we can only expect the cost of transfusion to increase as the blood supply decreases. Blood-sparing technologies and pharmaceutical agents may reduce the demand for blood components, but not necessarily the price. Until affordable artificial blood is a reality, the best hope may be to improve the existing blood procurement systems and develop blood conservation programs.

References

1 The Lewin Group, Goodman C, Chan S, Collins T, Haught R, Chen Y, Wolenski A. Ensuring blood safety and availability in the US: technology advances, costs, and challenges to payment. Final report prepared for Advanced Medical Technology Association, September 2002.

2 American Association of Blood Banks web site, Medication Deferral List, November 2004, http://www.aabb.org/pressroom/in_the_news/udhqmeddef04.pdf.

3 Zoon K. Recommendations for deferral of donors for malaria risk: memorandum to all registered blood establishments. Washington, DC: Department of Health and Human Services, Food and Drug Administrations, 26 July 1994.

4 Murphy EL, Connor DJ, McEvoy P, Hirschler N, Busch MP, Roberts P, Nguyen KA, Reich P. Estimating blood donor loss due to the variant CJD travel deferral. *Transfusion* 2004; **44**: 645–50.

5 Custer B, Johnson ES, Sullivan SD, Hazlet TK, Ramsey SD, Hirschler NV, Murphy EL, Busch MP. Quantifying losses to the donated blood supply due to donor deferral and miscollection. *Transfusion* 2004; **44**: 1417–26.

6 Vassallo RR Jr, Wahab F, Giordano K, Murphy S. Improving technology for collecting platelets by apheresis: five-year experience in one blood center. *Transfus Med Rev* 2004; **18**: 257–66.

7 Orfinger B. ''Mad Cow'' fears prompt advisory committee to recommend tighter blood donor restrictions. From the American Red Cross web site, November 2004, http://www.redcross.org/news/bm/tse/010628madcow.html

8 Standards, The American Association of Blood Banks (March 2003): 5.1.5.1, 5.1.5.1.1.

9 AABB Technical Manual, 14th edn. In: Brecher ME, ed. Chapter 8, *Components from Whole Blood Donations*. Maryland: American Association of Blood Banks, 2002.

10 Goodnough L. Risks of blood transfusion. *Crit Care Med* 2003; **31**(Suppl.): S678–S686.

11 Dabrow MB, Wilkins JC. Hematologic emergencies: management of transfusion reactions and crises in sickle cell disease. *Postgrad Med* 1993; **93**: 183–90.

12 Howard PL. Delayed hemolytic transfusion reactions. *Ann Clin Lab Sci* 1973; **3**: 13–16.

13 AABB REIMBURSEMENT GUIDE FOR BLOOD PRODUCTS AND SERVICES, May 2004, From AABB web site, www.aabb.org

14 67 *Federal Register* 31441

15 van Hulst M, de Wolf JT, Staginnus U, Ruitenberg EJ, Postma MJ. Pharmacoeconomics of blood transfusion safety: review of the available evidence. *Vox Sang* 2002; **83**: 146–55.

16 National Blood Data Resource Center web site, October 2004, http://www.nbdrc.org/faqs.htm

17 http://www.fda.gov/ora/compliance_ref/cpg/cpgbio/cpg230-150final.htm

18 United Blood Services web site, Annual Report, http://www.unitedbloodservices.org/pdfs/backup/Annualrpt02.pdf

19 Pomper GJ, Wu Y, Snyder FL. Risks of transfusion-transmitted infections. *Curr Opin Hematol* 2003; **10**: 412–18.

20 Centers for Disease Control and Prevention (CDC). Transfusion-associated transmission of West Nile Virus – Arizona, MMWR. *Morb Mort Weekly Rep* 2004; **53**: 842–4.

21 Schmidt M, Brixner V, Ruster B, Hourfar MK, Drosten C, Preiser W, Seifried E, Roth WK. NAT screening of blood donors for severe acute respiratory syndrome: Coronavirus can potentially prevent transfusion-associated transmissions. *Transfusion* 2004; **44**: 470–5.

22 American Red Cross web site, Blood Donation Eligibility Guidelines, October 2004, http://www.redcross.org/services/biomed/0,1082,0_557_,00.html

23 Reed KD, Melski JW, Graham MB, Regnery RL, Sotir MJ, Wegner MV, Kazmierczak JJ, Stratman FJ, Li Y, Fairley JA, Swain GR, Olson VA, Sargent EK, Kehl SC, Frace MA, Kline R, Flody SL, Davis JP, Damon IK. The detection of monkeypox in humans in the western hemispheres. *N Engl J Med* 2004; **350**: 342–50.

24 Rueda A. Rethinking blood shield statutes in view of the hepatitis C pandemic and other emerging threats to the blood supply. *J Health Law* 2001; **34**: 419–58.

25 Baker AF. Liability without fault and the AIDS plague compel a new approach to cases of transfusion-transmitted disease. *Specialty Law Digest – Health Care* 1991; August: 7–40.

26 Solomon JM. The evolution of the current blood banking regulatory climate. *Transfusion* 1994; **34**: 272–7.

27 Screening Donors of Blood, Plasma, Organs, Tissues, and Semen for Evidence of Hepatitis B and Hepatitis C. Occupational Exposure web site, October 2004, http://www.hivpositive.com/f-OccExposure/OccExpHepatitis/v40rr4.htm

28 Prince AM, Brotman B, Grady GF *et al.* Long-incubation post-transfusion hepatitis without serological evidence of exposure to hepatitis B virus. *Lancet* 1974; **2**: 241–6.

29 Koretz RL, Gitnick GL. Prevention of post-transfusion hepatitis: role of sensitive hepatitis B antigen screening tests, source of blood and volume of transfusion. *Am J Med* 1975; **59**: 754–60.

30 Daytona Beach Red Cross web site, Significant dates in American Red Cross blood services history, November 2004, *http://www.daytonaredcross.org/make_a_commitment_to_donate_bloo.htm*

31 KTTC-TV web site, November 2004, http://msnbc.msn.com/id/6242350/

32 Aach RD, Lander JJ, Sherman LA *et al.* Transfusion-transmitted viruses: interim analysis of hepatitis among transfused and nontransfused patients. In: Vyas GN, Cohen SN, Schmid R, eds. *Viral Hepatitis*. Philadelphia: Franklin Institute Press, 1978: 383–96.

33 Alter HJ, Purcell RH, Feinstone SM, Holland PV, Morrow AG. Non-A, non-B hepatitis: a review and interim report of an ongoing prospective study. In: Vyas GN, Cohen SN, Schmid R, eds. *Viral Hepatitis*. Philadelphia: Franklin Institute Press, 1978: 359–69.

34 Levy J. *HIV and the Pathogenesis of AIDS*, 2nd edn. Washington, DC: ASM Press, 1998.

35 Curran JW, Lawrence DN, Jaffe H *et al.* Acquired immunodeficiency syndrome (AIDS) associated with transfusions. *N Engl J Med* 1984; **310**: 69–75.

36 Joint United Nations Programme on HIV/AIDS. AIDS epidemic update: December 2000. Geneva, Switzerland: UNAIDS, 2000.

37 Stramer SL, Glynn SA, Kleinman SH, Strong DM, Sally C, Wright DJ, Dodd RY, Busch MP; National Heart, Lung, and Blood Institute Nucleic Acid Test Study Group. Detection of HIV-1 and HCV infections among antibody-negative blood donors by nucleic acid-amplification testing. *N Engl J Med* 2004; **351**: 819–22.

38 Candotti D, Temple J, Owusu-Ofori S, Allain JP. Multiplex real-time quantitative RT-PCR assay for hepatitis B virus, hepatitis C virus, and human immunodeficiency virus type 1. *J Virol Methods* 2004; **118**: 39–47.

39 AABB Technical Manual, 14th edn. In: Brecher ME, ed. Chapter 1, *Quality Systems*. Maryland: American Association of Blood Banks, 2002: 1–36.

40 Taken from a Representative Fee Schedule for The American Red Cross Blood Services, Southern California Region, 2004.

41 Pruss A, Kalus U, Radtke H, Koscielny J, Baumann-Baretti B, Balzar D, Dorner T, Salama A, Kiesewetter H. Universal leukodepletion of blood components results in significant reduction of febrile non-hemolytic but not allergic transfusion reactions. *Transfus Apheresis Sci* 2004; **30**: 41–6.

42 Ross WB, Blumberg N, Heal JM, Busch ORC, Marquet RL, Hop WCJ, Jeekel J. Blood transfusions and prognosis in colorectal cancer. *N Engl J Med* 1993; **329**: 1354–6.

43 Popovsky MA. Frozen and washed red blood cells: new approaches and applications. *Transfus Apheresis Sci* 2001; **25**: 193–4.

44 AABB Technical Manual, 14th edn. In: Brecher ME, ed. Chapter 8, *Components from Whole Blood Donations*. Maryland: American Association of Blood Banks, 2002: 177–9.

45 Przepiorka D, LeParc GF, Stovall MA *et al*. Use of irradiated blood components: practice parameter. *Am J Clin Pathol* 1996; **106**: 6–11.

46 Owens MR, Sweeney JD, Tahhan RH *et al*. Influence of type of exchange fluid on survival in therapeutic apheresis for thrombotic thrombocytopenic purpura. *J Clin Apheresis* 1995; **10**: 178.

47 Preiksaitis JK. The cytomegalovirus ''safe'' blood product: is leukoreduction equivalent to antibody screening? *Transfus Med Rev* 2000; **14**: 112–36.

48 Carey JS, Cukingnan RA, Carson E. Transfusion therapy in cardiac surgery: impact of the Paul Gann Blood Safety Act in California. *Am Surg* 1991; **57**: 830–5.

49 Technical Manual, 14th edn. In: Brecher ME, ed. Chapter 18, *Pretransfusion Testing*. Maryland: American Association of Blood Banks.

50 Winslow RM. Current status of blood substitute research: towards a new paradigm. *J Intern Med* 2003; **253**: 508–17.

51 Hardy JF. Pharmacological strategies for blood conservation in cardiac surgery: erythropoietin and antifibrinolytics. *Can J Anaesth* 2001; **48**(Suppl.): S24–S31.

52 Gleason DH, Leone BJ. Cost effectiveness of blood transfusions: risk and benefit. *CRNA* 1997; **8**: 69–76.

53 Kubler E, Oesch B, Raeber AJ. Diagnosis of prion diseases. *Br Med Bull* 2003; **66**: 267–79.

54 Minor PD. Technical aspects of the development and validation of tests for variant Creutzfeldt–Jakob disease in blood transfusion. *Vox Sang* 2004; **86**: 164–70.

CHAPTER 12

Oxygen Therapeutics – The Quest for Artificial Blood

Robert Bartlett

The need

The quest for blood substitutes has spanned half a century. Some of the established limitations to the use of banked blood include (1) a limited shelf life of 42 days; (2) the time-consuming process of crossmatching; (3) the risk of viral and bacterial transmission; and (4) the limited oxygen-transport capacity of banked blood during the initial hours following transfusion.

Additional concerns surrounding transfusion encompass the known transmissible diseases as well as those yet to be discovered. Transfusion science has been humbled sufficiently in recent history, to regard blood as an 'ever-present vector' for disease transmission. In addition, the case for immune suppression is well established. The clinical significance of this suppression has been verified with increased infection rates and tumor recurrence. There is now evidence that links transfusion to multiorgan failure syndrome in the setting of trauma resuscitation [1]. Many of these adverse side-effects have been linked to the presence of residual leukocytes. With this in mind, most blood banks have switched to leukodepletion, which has added to the cost of blood. This at a time when reserves are running dangerously low. Although leukodepletion appears to offer benefits, there is growing evidence that it will not completely eliminate transfusion-mediated immune depression, bone marrow depression or the multiorgan failure syndrome [2,3].

With each passing decade, the need for a solution with gas-transporting properties similar to blood has increased. The ideal blood substitute should not require cross matching or refrigeration, which would permit ease of use in prehospital care. More importantly, it should also have a long shelf life and be disease-free. Although the term 'blood substitutes' has been popularized in the literature, it is a technical misnomer given the variety of functions carried out by this 'liquid organ' blood. With oxygen delivery (DO_2) as the singular goal of these man-made solutions, a more appropriate term is red cell substitutes or the more generic term 'oxygen therapeutics'. Oxygen therapeutics offers features not found in natural red blood cells (RBCs). The most important feature may be their ability to penetrate into compromizsed capillary beds, which cannot be reached by an RBC with its 7-μm diameter.

There are four broad categories of oxygen therapeutics to consider:

1 Hemoglobin-based oxygen carriers (HBOCs), which are chemically modified derivatives of Hb or recombinant DNA derivatives of Hb. Here the base Hb is either human or bovine.
2 Perfluorocarbons, which have a high solubility coefficient for oxygen.
3 Synthetic allosteric modifiers, which shift the oxyhemoglobin dissociation curve to the right, producing a greater release of oxygen in the capillary beds.
4 Hyperbaric oxygen (HBO), which makes use of the natural gas laws to dissolve large volumes of oxygen in plasma.

The hemoglobin-based oxygen carriers

Physiological challenges

In the 1930s and 1940s it was learned that removal of the RBC membrane eliminated the antigenicity associated with blood types and the need for crossmatching. Such 'stroma-free' Hb also had a relatively long shelf life. Experiments with lactated Ringer's solution containing Hb demonstrated that animals could undergo a complete exchange transfusion. However, several significant problems are associated with the use of simple Hb solutions. These include a very high affinity for oxygen, high oncotic pressures, methemoglobin (MetHb) formation, renal and neurotoxicity, and short intravascular half-lives. To produce a viable carrier these problems need to be addressed through some form of chemical modification of Hb.

Oxygen affinity

RBCs are more than membrane envelopes for Hb. The cytosol of the RBC is designed to protect and regulate HB. The high intracellular concentrations of adenosine triphosphate (ATP) and 2,3-diphosphoglycerate (2,3-DPG) decrease the oxygen affinity of Hb. Typically the P_{50} for Hb inside an RBC is ~26 mmHg. The P_{50} represents the oxygen pressure at which 50% of the Hb is carrying oxygen. In contrast, the P_{50} for Hb outside the RBC is ~12 mmHg. In the absence of intracellular ATP and 2,3-DPG, stroma-free Hb exhibits a very high affinity for oxygen that interferes with 'appropriate' oxygen release within the tissue beds. Several different strategies have been used to readjust the affinity of extracellular Hb. One method is to chemically bind organic phosphate to serve the function of 2,3-DPG and ATP. The most common approach is to cross-link the dimers into tetramers.

Oncotic properties

The presence of the RBC membrane maintains an osmotic balance between the high concentration of Hb inside and the plasma outside. In the absence of the RBC membrane, a solution of free Hb exerts a significant oncotic force.

Fortunately stroma-free Hb is commonly cross-linked and polymerized to improve intravascular retention. This has the added advantage of lowering the oncotic pressure by reducing the overall number of molecules. Current solutions consist of a mix of 2-, 3- and 4-hemoglobin molecule polymers. Solutions of cross-linked tetramers must be diluted to reduce the oncotic pressure and therefore have a lower concentration than an equivalent volume of blood. These solutions generally have a lower viscosity than blood, which is thought to be a desirable trade-off.

Half-life

Within the RBC, Hb normally exists as a tetramer composed of 2 beta units complexed with 2 alpha units. Following membrane lysis, Hb rapidly dissociates from the tetrameric form into smaller alpha–beta dimers and monomers that are readily filtered by the kidney. The intravascular half-life of these lower–molecular weight subunits is 2–4 h. Increasing the molecular size by polymerizing the subunits prolongs the half-life. They appear to saturate the endothelial system early and then follow a zero-order pattern of clearance that ranges from 12 to 24 h.

The 'effective' half-life of stroma-free Hb is also a function of heme oxidation from the ferrous (Fe^{2+}) to the ferric (Fe^{3+}), which is MetHb. This oxidized form of Hb does not transport oxygen. RBCs contain MetHb reductase that reduces MetHb back to Hb; however, this enzyme is lost with the removal of the RBC membrane. At the time of infusion, the MetHb content of HBOCs is ~5% and increases rapidly in the circulation [45]. If this were not cleared by the reticuloendothelial system, it would become a problem. Clinically, it has not been determined whether there is a maximum cumulative dosing that would overload the reticuloendothelial system.

Hypertension and smooth muscle effects

One of the formidable problems associated with HBOCs is vasoconstriction and hypertension. Several mechanisms have been considered [6]. The predominate mechanism is most likely the result of heme-mediated absorption of nitric oxide (NO), also known as endothelial-derived relaxing factor (EDRF), which relaxes vascular smooth muscle and lowers blood pressure [7]. When Hb is enclosed within the RBC membrane, there is a controlled absorption and dissemination of NO that may actually facilitate the delivery of oxygen by producing local vasodilatation [8]. When Hb is deprived of a regulatory membrane, it becomes an unregulated scavenger of NO, resulting in hypertension.

In human trials with HBOCs, gastrointestinal (GI) side-effects are common. The symptoms include generalized pain, heart burn, dysphagia, nausea, vomiting and diarrhea, although they rarely require treatment. These symptoms are believed to be related to NO binding, causing GI smooth muscle contraction [9].

Initially the vasoconstrictive effect of HBOCs was attributed to the binding of intravascular NO. Later investigations revealed that much of the hypertensive effect was due to scavenging of NO in the extravascular space by small nonpolymerized 64 kDA tetramers, which easily diffuse out of the blood vessels. The production of polymerized Hb requires several steps designed to provide a pure, fully polymerized end product. Nonetheless, some small nonpolymerized Hb tetramers are found in the final product. The HBOCs that have the lowest number of tetramers are also associated with the least amount of extravasation and hypertension.

Working on the theory that vasoconstriction is solely a result of NO binding by Hb, Baxter Healthcare developed a recombinant form of Hb with almost no affinity for NO. Although there was a significant reduction in hypertension, it was not eliminated. This study and others suggested that mechanisms other than NO regulation were at play [10].

The hypertensive effect of oxygen therapeutics is also attributed to delivering excess oxygen to terminal arterioles, thus triggering vasoconstriction [11]. Intaglietta developed a method for the measurement of PO_2 in the microcirculation and showed that it drops continuously as blood passes from systemic vessels into progressively smaller vessels until it reaches tissue capillaries, after which PO_2 rises again [12]. This observation confirms the concept that significant amounts of oxygen exit the circulation from precapillary vessels. Within this zone of circulation the precapillary arterioles exert a regulatory role, which is believed to be governed in part by PO_2 [13,14]. This form of control is referred to as the autoregulation theory of blood flow. Facilitation of oxygen diffusion by oxygen carriers (Hb, myoglobin) was demonstrated many years ago by Scholander [15]. Since that time, other investigators have shown that cell-free Hb augments both the uptake and release of oxygen.

Free radicals

Heme and free iron can contribute to the generation of oxygen-free radicals in tissue. The ferrous iron (Fe^{2+}) center frequently loses an electron to oxygen, resulting in superoxide (O_2^-) and the ferric (Fe^{3+}) iron state of MetHb. Normally, if this is occurring within the RBC membrane, the superoxide radical is neutralized by MetHb reductase present in the cytosol of the RBC. In the absence of MetHb reductase, O_2^- can react with NO to produce peroxynitrite ($ONOO^-$), which readily decays to yield hydroxyl radicals (OH^-) that are highly reactive and denature proteins. In addition this process consumes NO and exacerbates vasoconstriction. Additional protection is provided by superoxide dismutase and catalase that are present in the cytosol and convert superoxide into hydrogen peroxide, which in turn is converted into water and oxygen.

Types of hemoglobin-based oxygen carriers

Human hemoglobin

Human Hb solutions have the advantage of being derived from a naturally occurring product that has been extensively studied. The primary disadvantage relates to limitations in the availability of outdated RBCs. Currently, only 5–15% of the 14 million units of blood donated in the USA each year is discarded.

Bovine hemoglobin

Animal Hb as a substrate is potentially inexpensive and widely available. Bovine-derived Hb has a P_{50} of 30 mmHg, which is remarkably close to that of human RBCs (P_{50} of 26.5 mmHg) [16]. In addition there is a more pronounced Bohr effect (the rightward shift in the oxygen dissociation curve in the presence of carbon dioxide) of bovine Hb, providing for better oxygen unloading in an acidic environment. In its natural state, the concentration of chloride ions in solution controls the oxygen dissociation curve of bovine Hb. Thus, bovine Hb does not shift to the left (increasing its oxygen affinity) with a drop in pH to the degree that human Hb does. There remains a level of uncertainty regarding animal pathogens (e.g. bovine spongiform encephalitis) that may require purification. If bovine Hb were used as the substrate, a herd of about 150 000 cows could generate enough Hb to make the equivalent of 6 million units per year.

Recombinant hemoglobin

Utilizing recombinant DNA technology, the human gene for Hb has been inserted into the DNA of *Escherichia coli* bacteria, which in turn produce the final Hb protein [17]. Recombinant Hb (rHb) has as its primary limitations the cost of the technical facilities required to produce the enormous volumes of bacterial culture, and the need for stringent purification methods. The obvious potential benefit of rHb is the product source, theoretically devoid of the microbiologic contamination of human or animal sources. Furthermore, genetic control over the product source allows for future adjustments or improvements to the current generation of products to be simply written into the code. Indeed, since the initial creation of genetic rHb1.1, a new form rHb2.0 has been created by Somatogen, Inc. (Boulder, Colorado) [18]. The first-generation rHb had an NO scavenging rate similar to that of native human Hb and produced the undesirable side-effects of inappropriate vasoconstriction. A second-generation Hb, rHb2.0, has an NO scavenging rate 20- to 30-fold lower than that of rHb1.1 [18]. Like rHb1.1, rHb2.0 is expressed in E. coli and the alpha chains are fused to prevent dissociation. Amino acid substitutions were made in the distal heme pocket by site-directed mutagenesis to reduce the rate of NO scavenging. rHb2.0 is also polyethylene glycol-polymerized and is formulated at a concentration of 10.0 g/dl in a gluconated electrolyte solution. At this Hb concentration, rHb2.0 has a viscosity of 2.3 cP, a colloid osmotic pressure of 62 torr and a P_{50} of 34 torr.

Encapsulated hemoglobin

Liposome-encapsulated Hb (HbV) is created from stroma-free Hb, which is then emulsed or encapsulated within double phospholipid membranes coated with polyethylene glycol [19]. The encapsulation of Hb prolongs the circulation time in the organism and prevents direct contact of Hb with the endothelial lining, thus suppressing vasoconstriction due to NO scavenging, which has been attributed to chemically modified Hb. Another major advantage of the HbV is that oxygen affinity may easily be adapted to the needs of the tissue by supplementing the appropriate amount of coencapsulated allosteric effector (pyridoxal 5'-phosphate). The size of the vesicles averages 250 nm. The oxygen-carrying capacity of a typical solution is $9 \, mlO_2/100 \, ml$ (blood is $\sim 20 \, ml \, O_2/100 \, ml$) with an oncotic pressure that is about twice that of blood. HbV has not been produced on a scale that would permit human testing, but small animal studies indicate that it is well tolerated. Encapsulated Hb, also known as Hb vesicle, has been associated with stimulation of the reticuloendothelium system. Experiments in rats show that repeated dosing with HbV doubles the weight of the liver and spleen, and its use is therefore still restricted to preclinical work [20].

Arenicola hemoglobin
The discovery of this Hb occurred just recently. This Hb is found in a common marine worm, *Arenicola marina*, and does not appear to be associated with any of the complications of vertebrate-derived Hb when administered to mice [21]. The molecule's large size and natural cross-linking make it an ideal oxygen carrier with limited extravasation. According to biologist Franck Zal of the Université Pierre et Marie Curie in Paris, 'We don't have to modify anything, only collect it and purify it' [22]. At present, this Hb is undergoing further animal evaluation.

Allosteric modifiers
Allostery is a branch of biochemistry, which focuses on influencing protein activity by changing protein conformation by other molecules or proteins. The oxygen dissociation curve for Hb demonstrates such allosteric phenomenon in the presence of 2,3-DPG. Oxygen affinity will decrease in physiologic conditions characterized by oxygen deprivation; however, this compensatory change takes several days to occur. The use of an intravenous (IV) 'synthetic allosteric modifier', which could instantly reduce the oxygen affinity of Hb, would increase delivery, especially if the patient were to breathe supplemental oxygen to ensure complete 'oxygen loading' of the RBCs.

Perfluorocarbons
Fluorocarbons are carbon fluorine compounds characterized by a high gas-dissolving capacity (oxygen and carbon dioxide), low viscosity, and chemical and biological inertness. The oxygen transport characteristics of modified Hb solutions and fluorocarbon emulsions are fundamentally different. HBOCs exhibit a sigmoid oxygen dissociation curve similar to blood. In contrast, the fluorocarbon emulsions are characterized by a linear relationship between

oxygen partial pressure and oxygen content. The content of oxygen in arterial plasma is directly proportional to the partial pressure of oxygen in the lungs. Consequently, supplemental oxygen must be provided to maintain relatively high arterial oxygen partial pressures, which are necessary to maximize the oxygen transport capacity of fluorocarbon emulsions. Despite these fundamental differences, the efficiency of both groups of artificial oxygen carriers has been demonstrated experimentally and clinically.

The only blood substitute that was approved in the USA was a perfluorocarbon, Fluosol 20. This first-generation product, which is no longer available, may soon be replaced by a second-generation version known as perflubron (Oxygent), produced by Alliance Pharmaceuticals. This newer formulation is easier to handle, has few side-effects and dissolves more oxygen per unit volume. It is administered as an emulsion containing particles with a diameter of $\sim 0.2\,\mu m$ and is eliminated unchanged by the lungs.

The amount of oxygen dissolved into the perfluorocarbon is linearly related to the PaO_2. Intravascular perfluorocarbon solutions loaded with oxygen at a PaO_2 of 200 mmHg can deliver 5 vol% of oxygen per deciliter of perfluorocarbon. Because perfluorocarbons release 80% of their carried oxygen, it can deliver approximately four times the oxygen that would be delivered by the same volume of Hb. Giving 120 ml of Oxygent to a 70-kg patient is equivalent to 500 ml transfusion of whole blood.

Products currently under clinical investigation

Hemoglobin-based oxygen carriers

The first studies demonstrating the *in vivo* ability of Hb solutions to transport oxygen in mammals was reported in 1933 [23]. From these early investigations they proceeded to use lysed RBC solutions in 14 patients, documenting the ability of free Hb to transport oxygen and reporting its nephrotoxic side-effect [24]. In the 1960s the US military started a formalized research program to develop a stroma-free Hb under the belief that the RBC membrane was responsible for many of the side-effects of lysed RBC solutions. By the late 1970s it was determined that highly purified Hb still had side-effects that were attributed to the dissociation of the Hb tetramer into dimers and monomers. In the 1980s private industry pioneered a variety of cross-linking methods to stabilize and polymerize Hb. There are currently three companies with chemically modified HBOCs that have completed phase III studies: Northfield Laboratories' product PolyHeme, which is a glutaraldehyde cross-linked human Hb; Hemosol's product Hemolink (o-raffinose polymerized Hb); and Biopure's product Hemopure, which is a glutaraldehyde cross-linked bovine Hb. Biopure has received US approval for its veterinary product Oxyglobin and South African approval for its human product Hemopure. The design of such studies is difficult, given the absence of agreement on transfusion triggers as previously discussed (Chapter 3).

PolyHeme – Northfield laboratories

PolyHeme is now in phase III (efficacy) trials and appears to lack the vaso-pressor effect of some of the other blood substitutes. Northfield completed the first randomized clinical trial comparing PolyHeme with blood in trauma patients [25], where 44 patients with severe injury (mean injury severity score of 21) were randomized to receive RBCs or up to 6 units of PolyHeme. The PolyHeme group experienced no adverse events and reduced the initial use of allogeneic blood. There were no differences in circulating Hb levels, but the mean number of allogeneic RBC transfusions within the first 24 h was only 7.8 units in the PolyHeme group, while controls received 10.4 units ($p < 0.05$).

Favorable outcomes were found in a recent prospective cohort study com-paring the 30-day mortality of trauma patients given PolyHeme versus a historical control of 300 patients who abstained from blood due to religious grounds. Rapid infusions of 1–20 units of PolyHeme were given to 171 patients as the initial management for trauma and urgent surgery, and 40 of the patients had nadir RBC Hb $\leq$ 3 g/dl. The 30-day mortality was 25% compared with 64% in the control group [26].

Beyond the reduction in allogeneic blood use, a secondary benefit may be the risk reduction for multiorgan failure syndrome, which appears to be partially linked to allogeneic blood transfusions. It is now clear that a number of mediators present in stored packed RBCs have the potential to contribute to multiple organ failure through priming of circulating neutrophils. Poly-Heme is devoid of such natural priming agents and should attenuate neutro-phil priming during resuscitation. In a prospective study of trauma patients resuscitated with either PolyHeme or packed RBCs, no PMN priming occurred when PolyHeme was used.

Hemosol – Hemosol Inc.

The o-raffinose cross-linked human Hb is prepared from outdated human RBCs obtained from the Canadian Red Cross Blood Transfusion Service. The cells are washed to remove plasma proteins and lysed by gentle osmotic shock. The crude Hb is separated from RBC ghosts by filtration and then pasteurized for 10 h at 62°C. The pasteurized Hb is purified by a combination of anion and cation exchange chromatography that yields a preparation of Hb A0, which is > 99% pure. Hemolink is prepared by reacting purified deoxy-genated Hb A0 with o-raffinose to covalently link the alpha–beta dimers. The chemically modified, cross-linked Hb is mixed with lactated Ringer's solution to give a final concentration of 10 g/dl. The product is then frozen and stored at −80°C.

Hemolink was evaluated in a phase III clinical trial in Canada and the UK. This trial involved 299 patients undergoing coronary artery bypass grafting in conjunction with autologous normovolemic hemodilution (ANH). The Hemolink group had a higher rate of complete transfusion avoidance (83%)

and fewer units of blood transfused. There was no difference in the adverse events profile between the two groups. However, Hemosol recently suspended enrollment of patients into its HLK 213 trial of Hemolink for coronary artery bypass graft patients due to an imbalance in the number of myocardial infarctions occurring in the Hemolink group. The matter is currently under review.

Hemopure – Biopure Inc.

Hemopure is ultrapurified, glutaraldehyde-polymerized, bovine Hb in a balanced electrolyte solution. It has a lower oxygen affinity than human Hb ($P_{50} = 38$ mmHg compared with 26 mmHg for human Hb), which facilitates the unloading of oxygen. It also has a markedly reduced viscosity of 1.3 cP (similar to crystalloid solutions and about one-third that of blood). Hemopure does not require refrigeration and is stable at room temperature for 2 years. Hemopure has been in 22 clinical trials involving more than 800 subjects and completed phase III studies in both Europe and the USA where it has been shown to reduce transfusion requirements in 35–40% of patients [27]. The *New England Journal of Medicine* featured a dramatic case report of a patient with a hemolytic anemia who was supported for several days with Hemopure and ultimately recovered from her hemolytic process [28]. Hemopure has been approved in South Africa for the treatment of adult surgical patients who are acutely anemic and for the purpose of eliminating, delaying or reducing the need for allogeneic (donated) RBCs. Biopure filed an application for clinical use with the Food and Drug Administration (FDA) in October 2003.

The next generation of hemoglobin-based oxygen therapeutics

Capitalizing on past experience, developers are engineering the next generation of oxygen therapeutics [30]. To offset the problems of NO binding, a new form of human rHb has been developed that has less affinity for NO. This new tetrameric rHb does not cause vasoconstriction when infused into animals. However, there was a change in the oxygen release characteristics (lower P_{50}), which was corrected through further genetic changes that replaced the distal histidine with glutamine resulting in a normal oxygen release curve.

Superoxide dismutase and catalase are normal constituents of RBCs where they convert superoxide into hydrogen peroxide, which is, in turn, converted into water and oxygen. This activity may be especially important in the presence of reperfusion injuries with damaged tissue such as stroke, heart attacks and resuscitation from hemorrhagic shock. Steps are underway to cross-link superoxide dismutase and catalase enzymes to polymerized Hb [30].

Small Hb-filled spheres are created using biodegradable polymers such as polylactides or polyglycolides, which are commonly used in absorbable sutures [31]. These capsules have the long half-life and limited NO-scavenging advantages of HbV without reticuloendothelial system engorgement. The diameter of these 'artificial cells' ranges from 80 nm to 200 nm, which is quite small compared to an RBC diameter of 7500 nm. Polylactide is first degraded into lactic acid and then into water and carbon dioxide. For a 500 ml suspension, the total lactic acid produced is 83 mEq. This is only a small fraction of the normal human lactic acid production (1000–1400 mEq/day).

Winslow has advanced a new paradigm for the design characteristics of second-generation products. It was originally believed that a low viscosity (1 cP) was desirable; however, the new paradigm espouses a viscosity closer to blood (4 cP) in order to preserve sheer forces [32]. The osmotic pressure should be higher to maintain vascular volume. Oxygen affinity should also be higher than normal Hb. This characteristic is based on the concept that vasoconstriction is mediated in part by high precapillary PO_2 values. This occurs through premature release of oxygen or increased diffusion of oxygen. Because of their small size, these agents easily move into the extravascular space where they facilitate the diffusion of oxygen from the bloodstream.

Sangart Inc. (San Diego, California) has formulated a new Hb derivative based on the new paradigm [33]. This product (MP4) is formulated by taking the basic Hb tetramer and attaching 6 molecules of polyethylene glycol to produce a larger molecule, which does not easily move into the extravascular space. MP4 has been shown to be free of vasoconstriction in the hamster microcirculation [34]. In a phase I trial in Sweden there were none of the customary side-effects of hypertension and GI distress. The second novel characteristic of MP4 is its high oxygen affinity – a P_{50} of 7 mmHg. Research with this product in hamster shock model has shown that it is very effective in oxygenating hypoxic tissue as a result of this high oxygen affinity.

Researchers at the University of Maryland recently reported their experience with their new Hb derivative called zero-linked Hb. This product is created by a direct coupling of Hb molecules and produces a very large polymer, which is easily purified to eliminate any of the smaller extravasation-prone polymers. Other useful attributes include a high oxygen affinity, which is believed to be more desirable, and a slightly negative charge, which reduces movement across the basement membrane. In animal models, zero-linked Hb lacks any vasoconstrictive effect [35].

Rather than creating large polymers, researchers at Wasada University have selected a large natural protein, albumin, and linked heme groups to it. Albumin does not extravasate and this new preparation does not scavenge NO [36,37].

SynZyme Technologies (Irvine, California) is developing a second-generation blood substitute called HemoZyme. It consists of an Hb carrier and a caged NO complex, which remains in blood vessels, delivers oxygen to tissues and catalytically removes reactive oxygen and reactive nitrogen species. Termed 'polymerized polynitroxyl hemoglobin' it contains caged NO, which is a stable, free radical referred to as nitroxide. In the bloodstream, free NO combines with reactive oxygen species to form peroxynitrate, a toxic radical. However, caged NO breaks down peroxynitrate into a nontoxic specie. Still in the early phase of development, SynZyme states that Hemo-Zyme can treat ischemia and postreperfusion phenomena, and has significant advantages over other HBOCs. These include dilation of blood vessels, anti-oxidant and anti-inflammatory properties.

Distinct from the physical and chemical properties of the HBOCs, it is important to recognize that a patient's underlying illness and clinical condition may also influence the physiologic responses to any of these agents.

HemoBioTech's product, HemoTech, was designed to diminish the toxic intrinsic effects of Hb and help eliminate the pathological reactions associated with hemorrhagic shock [38]. Beyond oxygen transport, HemoTech has additional pharmacological activities that eliminate blood vessel constriction, improve the release of oxygen and produce antioxidant and anti-inflammatory effects. HemoTech reacts pure bovine Hb with o-adenosine 5'-triphosphate (o-ATP), o-adenosine and reduced glutathione (GSH) to produce intra- and intermolecular linkage, resulting in a large molecule with high purity, favorable surface charge and antioxidant properties, which are bestowed by the presence of glutathione.

Since its initial development, HemoTech has been tested in different *in vitro* and *in vivo* models including preclinical studies conducted at the Research Toxicology Centre SpA (Rome, Italy) and a human clinical trial [39]. The results of these studies are favorable, indicating that this novel RBC substitute has vasodilation activity; reduces the vasoconstriction that follows hemorrhage; prolongs intravascular persistence; functions as a physiological oxygen carrier; and produces no adverse nephrotoxic, neurotoxic, oxidative or inflammatory reactions.

Oxygent – Alliance Pharmaceutical

Perfluorocarbons are lipophilic solutions that have a high solubility for all gases, including oxygen and carbon dioxide. In 1965 the world saw a dramatic demonstration of rats submerged in this liquid, yet still alive (Leland Clark). Equilibrated with 100% oxygen at the surface, the rats were able to breathe in this liquid and meet their metabolic requirements for oxygen and carbon dioxide transport. In 1968, a perfluorocarbons microemulsion was used to perform a complete exchange transfusion in a rat, which survived, breathing 100% oxygen, with a hematocrit (Hct) of zero. This experiment established the practical viability of pursuing the clinical application of these agents.

The first-generation perfluorocarbon (Fluosol) had poor oxygen-carrying characteristics and had to be stored frozen. Despite FDA approval for use with angioplasty in 1989, its production was terminated in 1994. A second-generation perfluorocarbon emulsion, perfluorooctylbromide, developed by Alliance Pharmaceuticals, San Diego, California, is called Oxygent and contains 45% perflubron (C8F17) by volume. This fluorocarbon is emulsified with lecithin, has a viscosity of 4.0 cP (about 30% thicker than blood) and is stable at room temperature for 6 years.

When the inspired atmosphere contains 90–100% oxygen, this solution releases about 10 ml of oxygen per 100 ml or about twice that of normal blood. No serious adverse events have been reported with the use of Oxygent. A 10–24% reduction in platelet account does occur on the second day after infusion, but no bleeding abnormalities have been noted. Oxygent elimination occurs first through the reticuloendothelial system and is followed by pulmonary excretion of the perfluorocarbon. The emulsion is typically cleared within 24 h.

An international, multicenter phase III transfusion avoidance study in noncardiac elective surgical patients was recently completed [40]. This study enrolled 492 patients with expected blood loss of 20–70 ml/kg. Control patients were transfused at an Hb of 8 g/dl, or at predefined physiologic triggers. Perfluorocarbon patients underwent hemodilution to an Hb of 8 g/dl, and then received perfluorocarbon and were given transfusions at an Hb of 5.5 g/dl, or at the same physiologic triggers as control patients. The perfluorocarbon patients required significantly less allogeneic blood. In the patient population specifically targeted by this study protocol (i.e. surgical procedures with an anticipated blood loss > 20 ml/kg), Oxygent treatment resulted in a highly significant ($p < 0.001$) reduction and avoidance of blood transfusion, which translated into an overall sparing of allogeneic units compared to the control group. Safety assessments, performed quarterly during the conduct of the study by an independent data safety monitoring board, indicated that Oxygent was well tolerated.

RSR13 – Allos Therapeutics

In the 1980s two antilipidemic drugs, clofibrate and benzofibrate, demonstrated an allosteric effect on the oxyhemoglobin dissociation curve by shifting it to the right [41,42]. Such a shift means there is a decreased affinity for oxygen resulting in a greater release or desaturation of oxygen in the tissue beds. This effect was an *in vitro* phenomenon and is extinguished by albumin when used *in vivo*. Nontheless the concept of creating an allosteric agent was born. Allos therapeutics has committed considerable efforts toward the development of a compound known as RSR13, which decreases the oxygen affinity of Hb [43]. This effect is dose-related, and current dosing regimens result in approximately a 10-mmHg shift in the P_{50}. Although the rightward shift of the oxyhemoglobin dissociation curve provides for an increased release of oxygen to the tissues, it also means that there is a corresponding decrease in the uptake of oxygen in the lungs. This can be compensated for by providing supplemental oxygen to ensure complete saturation of Hb. This agent is being evaluated as a radiation sensitizer for hypoxic tumors. Hypoxic tumors are notoriously radio-resistant. By providing a more complete release of oxygen within the tumor, the PO_2 is elevated, rendering the tumor more susceptible to radiation.

Using electron paramagnetic resonance to directly measure cortical PO_2, Miyake examined whether RSR13 would improve brain tissue PO_2 following hemorrhagic shock in rats. After a 30-min shock period, resuscitation was performed by infusion with Ringer lactate plus RSR13 or saline. Following hemorrhage, brain PO_2 decreased by 14 mmHg in both groups. Following crystalloid resuscitation, brain PO_2 remained depressed in the control group but returned to the prehemorrhage values in the RSR13 treated rats. RSR13 immediately increased and maintained the PO_2 while controls had a very gradual return to prehemorrhage values. There was no difference in the blood pressure or heart rate between groups. Whar *et al.* recently evaluated the safety and dosing schedules in surgical patients. A shift of 10 mmHg was achieved at 75 mg/kg. There were no adverse events and further studies are planned to more fully evaluate RSR13 for the management of acute blood loss anemia.

Myocardial and cerebral hypoxia in the setting of cardiopulmonary bypass (CPB) surgery is another potential application for allosteric modulation. RSR13 improves myocardial oxidative metabolism and contractile function in models of myocardial ischemia. In CPB patients, RSR13 improved PO_2 and reduced neuronal cell death following cerebral ischemia [44,45]. Allosteric modification of the oxyhemoglobin dissociation curve by RSR13 represents a unique therapeutic strategy.

Tables 12.1 and 12.2 summarize the characteristics and status of the major oxygen therapeutics.

Figure 12.1 illustrates the oxygen performance curves for various oxygen therapeutics. The typical oxygen requirements are 5 vol%. Assuming a tissue PO_2 of approximately 40 mmHg one can determine the arterial venous difference.

Table 12.1 Characteristics of major oxygen therapeutics.

Characteristic	Banked blood	HBOC*	Perfluoro-carbon	Allosterics	Hypberbaric oxygen
Shelf life	42 days	3 years	2 years	Years	Unlimited
Storage temperature	Refrigeration	Room temperature	Refrigeration	Room temperature	Room temperature
Size	7 μm	0.007 μm	0.2 μm	NA	NA
Crossmatching	Required	Not required	Not required	Not required	Not required
Risks	Disease transmission	NO scavenging	Mild decrease in platelet count	None apparent	Oxygen toxicity
	Immune depression				
	Transfusion reactions				
	RBC storage Defects				

Note: *HBOC, hemoglobin-based oxygen carrier.

Table 12.2 Status of major oxygen therapeutics.

Company	Product	Type	Status
Northfield	PolyHeme	Human	Phase III
			Elective surgery/trauma resuscitation
Biopure	Hemopure	Bovine	Phase III*
			Approved in South Africa/elective surgery
Hemosol	Hemolink	Human	Phase III
			Elective surgery
Alliance	Perflubron	Perfluorocarbon	Phase III
			Elective surgery
Allos	RSR13	Allosteric	Phase II
NA	Oxygen	Hyperbaric	Approved

Note: *FDA application filed October 2004. Approval for clinical use in South Africa granted in 2001.

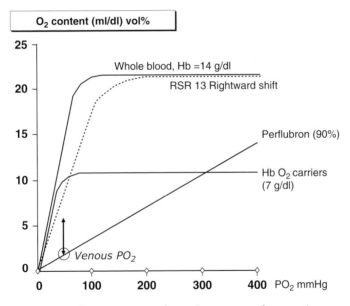

Figure 12.1 Oxygen performance curves for various oxygen therapeutics.

Hyperbaric oxygen

Hyperbaric oxygen (HBO) therapy is a 'physical' oxygen therapeutic. HBO therapy is the administration of pure oxygen to patients who are within pressurized vessels, referred to as hyperbaric chambers. Normally the amount of oxygen dissolved in plasma is quite small (0.003 ml/mmHg). However, at 3 atmospheres absolute (ATA), the arterial PO_2 is in excess of 2000 mmHg, which is more than 6 vol% of oxygen dissolved in the plasma. At this pressure the oxygen content of plasma will meet the body's resting requirement of 6 vol%. These mathematical considerations were put to a physiological test by Boerema using pigs. In a study entitled 'Life without Blood', he exchanged the pigs' whole blood with an acellular perfusate, lowering the pigs' Hb to 0.4 g/dl while they were inside a hyperbaric chamber [46]. Despite the near absence of blood, the pigs survived without complications. Based on Boerema's classic study, Ammonic was the first to demonstrate that HBO could also support human life at an extremely low Hct. Further use of HBO by Hart *et al.* extended the clinical experience greatly and established HBO's role in the management of acute blood loss anemia [47,48].

Experimental evidence

It is not surprising that HBO can be used to augment DO_2 in the setting of anemia. But can HBO still be effective when the patient is hypovolemic or has significant vasoconstriction? The answer appears to be 'yes'. Several shock models indicate that HBO provides significant protection against irreversible shock. In a hemorrhagic canine shock model employed by Doi *et al.*, the animals' blood pressure was lowered to 30 mmHg by removal of blood through the femoral artery into a reservoir bottle [49]. This pressure was maintained for 90 min. A control group breathed air during the 90 min while the experimental group received HBO at 2 ATA. At the end of the 90 min, their blood was reinfused. In the control group oxygen consumption (VO_2) was decreased to 2 ml/kg/min. An oxygen debt subsequently accrued during the hypotensive period. In the hyperbaric group, the decrease in VO_2 was negligible as was the change in lactate. In the control group, all animals with an oxygen debt in excess of 140 ml/kg died.

Similar findings were reported by Attar, utilizing a comparable hemorrhagic shock model. Animals were held at a mean arterial pressure (MAP) of 30 mmHg for $2\frac{1}{2}$ h. During that time the control group breathed air and the experimental group received HBO at 3 ATA. At the end of the $2\frac{1}{2}$-h period only 17% of the control animals were alive in contrast to 74% of the HBO group [50,51].

In a canine model of controlled hypotension of 40 mmHg for 2 h, Elliot investigated survival rates for animals on room air, 100% oxygen, 100% oxygen by ventilator and HBO at 3 ATA. Mortality rates were 90% in the control, 50% in those receiving normobaric oxygen with or without a ventilator, and 27% for those given HBO [52].

Our understanding of hemorrhagic shock as a cytokine trigger has grown considerably in recent years. Many shock-induced cytokines are responsible, in part, for the evolution of organ failure hours to days later. HBO has established benefit as an aid to recovery from reperfusion-mediated injury. Yamashita recently reported on the effect of HBO treatment on cytokine induction after hemorrhage in a rat model. The HBO treatment group had a significant reduction in TNF-α, IL-6 and mortality compared to the room air controls. It would appear that the benefits of HBO are far more substantial than the simple notion of oxygen as just a metabolite [53].

Clinical experience

Typically HBO is employed in those instances where the patient has religious convictions that proscribe the use of blood or blood products. In rare instances it may be required to temporarily support a patient when there are blood shortages, crossmatch problems or warm antibody hemolytic anemias. Hart summarized a series of 26 patients with severe anemia who were managed with HBO between 1970 and 1987. Clinical management consisted of replacing lost volume with dextran and later with hetastarch, giving generous doses of hematenics (vitamins B, C and iron) and intermittently wrapping of the lower extremities with ace bandages. The particular details of the patient treatment profiles were not published; however, the average survivor required HBO for 10 days. No instances of pulmonary or central nervous system oxygen toxicity occurred.

Concern is sometimes raised that HBO might blunt the erythropoietic response to anemia. This should not be a concern for two reasons. First, these patients should already be on high doses of erythropoietin (EPO), in which case endogenous production is not a factor. Second, Wright et al. demonstrated that HBO facilitates a more rapid recovery from hemorrhage, independent of any exogenous EPO. In their rabbit blood loss model involving 30% loss of Hb they found a faster recovery, with the HBO-treated group reaching the baseline level of Hb in 11 days as opposed to 14 days for the control group ($p < 0.001$) [54].

Historically HBO was administered according to Hart's criteria:
1 systolic blood pressure below 90 mmHg or patients requiring vasopressors;
2 disorientation or coma;
3 ischemic electrocardiogram (ECG) changes; and
4 ischemic gut.
Unfortunately these criteria have a number of limitations. Ischemic diarrhea is often a preterminal event where HBO may be 'too little, too late'. ECG changes in the form of flipped T waves can be caused by a variety of factors. Disorientation oftentimes cannot be assessed because paralysis, sedation and mechanical ventilation are continued postoperatively to reduce unnecessary VO_2, and finally, current concepts of shock no longer endorse a blood pressure–based definition.

Goal-directed oxymetric monitoring

On an individual basis, the tolerance for anemia is quite variable. For this reason the decision to transfuse should not be based solely on the Hb concentration. As already discussed, the current concept in transfusion medicine is to treat 'the physiology, not the lab' [55]. Where HBO is involved, a clear understanding of physiologic principles is required as a basis for determining the frequency and duration of therapy. Central to this understanding is an appreciation for the total amount of oxygen delivered and consumed.

In the past it was difficult to measure DO_2 and VO_2, but it was easy to measure blood pressure. This was unfortunate for the understanding of circulatory function. 'Blood pressure cuffs have had a fatal influence on clinical practice because blood pressure and blood flow are not equivalent. Organs respond to blood flow, and hence, DO_2, not blood pressure' [56]. In a large series of carefully monitored, critically ill, postoperative patients, over 50 000 values of the five most commonly measured variables were evaluated: MAP, heart rate, central venous pressure, pulmonary artery wedge pressure and cardiac output (CO). These values were restored to normal in 76% of nonsurvivors who, nevertheless, still died. Thus traditional indicators do not have a clear relationship with outcome. They are useful descriptors of end-stage circulatory failure, but are neither sensitive nor accurate as an *early warning* of circulatory impairment [57,58].

Shock is more appropriately characterized as a state in which DO_2 is inadequate. For this reason, responsible use of oxygen therapeutics requires an understanding of oxygen dynamics. Whether the etiology is anemia, hypovolemia, cardiogenic, respiratory, septic or toxic, the net effect is the same: tissue hypoxia, a cumulative oxygen debt and the cessation of oxidative metabolism. Failure to provide adequate amounts of oxygen will result in cellular injury owing to the loss of electrochemical gradients. When a critical mass of cells in an organ is injured, organ function is impaired, and an inflammatory process follows. Through the release of inflammatory mediators, cellular oxygen and substrate delivery suffer further, leading to the multiorgan failure syndrome. Early identification of failing physiology permits a more timely use of oxygen therapeutics.

A recent meta-analysis by Kern showed significant benefit when pulmonary artery catheter data are used as a guide to therapy during the intraoperative and immediate postoperative periods [59]. Goal-directed therapy is ineffective in the late stages of oxygen debt after the onset of organ failure. No amount of extra oxygen will restore irreversible oxygen debt, failed organs or dead cells. In the late stage of acute illness after organ failure has occurred, aggressive therapy directed to improve DO_2 is generally futile. *The goal of oxymetric monitoring is to detect significant changes earlier than by simple clinical observation* – early enough to permit timely interventions. The ability to monitor delivered and consumed oxygen permits a more timely intervention when these values are tending in the wrong direction. Early intervention prevents tissue ischemia and secondary organ dysfunction.

Tissue oxygen debt in the surgical setting

Postoperative multiorgan failure is a major problem associated with circulatory insufficiency. Because of the vital interdependence of organs, the failure of one organ almost invariably sets the stage for failure of other organs. When metabolic processes are limited by insufficient oxygen over prolonged periods, multiorgan failure ensues. First described by Baue, this condition has been regarded as a common intensive care unit (ICU) syndrome associated with postoperative death [60,61].

Shoemaker advanced the concept that a tissue oxygen debt is reflected by inadequate VO_2 in the intraoperative and immediate postoperative periods [62]. Oxygen debt is a common determinant of multisystem organ failure and death [62]. Earlier work by other investigators calculated the cumulative VO_2 deficit in dogs subjected to hemorrhagic shock [63]. When VO_2 was less than 100 ml/kg, there was no mortality; when it increased to 120 ml/kg, the mortality increased to 50%, and when it was greater than 140 ml/kg, mortality was greater than 95%. Shoemaker observed that the cumulative oxygen deficit averaged $33 L/m^2$ in patients who died, $27 L/m^2$ in survivors with one or more organ failures, and $8 L/m^2$ in survivors who had no shock-related complications. In addition, the temporal pattern of VO_2 was important. The duration of the oxygen deficit averaged 35 h for nonsurvivors, 24 h for survivors with organ failure and 8 h for survivors without any complications. All of these patients had normal preoperative hemodynamic values and did not have any existing handicaps such as trauma, sepsis, cirrhosis or major cardiovascular problems.

For the past 25 years intensivists have been studying the hemodynamic and oxygen transport responses to operative trauma [64]. Increased cardiac index (CI), DO_2 and VO_2 characterized the physiologic status of surviving high-risk patients. Relatively normal DO_2 and VO_2 values were associated with nonsurvivors who developed an early oxygen debt followed by progressive organ failure and death. The oxygen transport differences were sufficiently large and consistent to be used to predict outcome. An outcome predictor based on CI, DO_2, and VO_2 values was tested prospectively on a series of high-risk postoperative patients and found to be correct in 94% of the patients. It was most accurate in the first 24 h [65]. It was concluded that the 'supranormal' values of DO_2 and VO_2 were necessary compensatory responses for survival [66]. It seemed clear that the use of normal values as therapeutic goals in an abnormal situation (e.g. recovery from operative trauma) may not be appropriate. Compensatory increases in DO_2 and VO_2 are needed to quickly correct intraoperative oxygen debt, overcome impaired peripheral perfusion, and meet the increased metabolic demands or recovery from operative trauma.

Understanding DO_2/VO_2 relationships

To properly manage a patient with significant blood loss anemia physicians must understand the principle factors governing DO_2 and VO_2. The adequacy of tissue oxygenation depends upon the volume of oxygen delivered to the tissues and the volume consumed. This supply/demand balance is determined by five factors that are readily measured and a sixth that cannot be measured.

The five measured factors are (1) Hb concentration; (2) the affinity of Hb for oxygen (P_{50}); (3) the percentage of arterial Hb saturated with oxygen (SaO_2); (4) oxygen consumption (VO_2); and (5) cardiac output (CO). The sixth factor is the distribution of perfusion. If DO_2 is reduced by a partial loss in any of the five measurable factors, compensations will occur among the others.

Under normal conditions DO_2 or oxygen availability greatly exceeds VO_2. For this reason VO_2 is considered to be supply-independent. In other words, increasing the DO_2 does not cause an increase in VO_2. A change in DO_2 only results in a reciprocal change in oxygen extraction from blood. Increasing DO_2 results in less oxygen being extracted per unit volume. Conversely, decreasing DO_2 produces a higher oxygen extraction ratio. In a case where DO_2 is greatly reduced, there exists for tissue a critical DO_2 value after which the oxygen extraction ratio cannot increase enough to meet VO_2. At this point, VO_2 becomes 'supply-dependent'. When this occurs, VO_2 will vary directly with the DO_2. When VO_2 is supply-dependent, anaerobic metabolism begins, oxygen debt accrues and the patient is now in the first stage of shock [67,68].

The relationship between DO_2 and VO_2 has been the subject of numerous studies. As previously mentioned, under normal conditions there is an abundant oxygen supply, and VO_2 is a function of metabolic rate, not oxygen supply. As the supply of oxygen is reduced, there is a compensatory increase in the oxygen extraction ratio and VO_2 is unchanged. However, this extraction reserve can be exhausted when there are severe reductions in DO_2. At this point VO_2 becomes completely dependent on DO_2 and will directly fluctuate with the changes in DO_2. This state of affairs is pathologic and referred to as supply-dependent VO_2. The DO_2 value at which this occurs is termed the 'critical DO_2' (DO_2crit). Below the DO_2crit, the tissues begin to consume energy stores in the form of phosphocreatine, eventually turning to anaerobic glycolysis with lactate production. When perfusion is appropriately regulated and the oxygen requirements are met, VO_2 is maximal (VO_2 max). Basal VO_2 is approximately 2 ml/kg/min and is typically constant when the DO_2 is in the range of 7–9 ml/kg/min [69,70].

Understanding mixed venous blood gas analysis

Mixed venous blood gas analysis is the cornerstone for assessing the adequacy of global oxygen transport. So long as the patient maintains appropriate capillary regulation, venous oxygen saturation (SvO_2) will serve as a global index of oxygen supply/demand balance. Because a decrease in SvO_2 may indicate inadequate oxygen transport, continuous monitoring is desirable. It will not identify the precise cause but will bring to attention any change in supply and demand. The mixed venous saturation is a flow-weighted average of the oxygen extraction for all tissues. Some tissues such as skin, resting muscle or kidneys extract less oxygen than other tissues such as the heart. The magnitude of the effect of oxygen extraction by any organ on SvO_2 is proportional to the blood flow to that organ so that low-consumption, high-flow organs such as the kidneys have a greater effect on SvO_2 than do high-consumption organs like the heart.

Normally, SVO_2 is maintained within a narrow range. Decreases in SvO_2 occur frequently in patients with cardiopulmonary complications. The changes in SvO_2 often precede changes in blood pressure. The decrease may correlate with the magnitude of cardiopulmonary impairment, and decreases in SvO_2 that do not improve with therapy are associated with a poor prognosis. Severe venous hypoxemia has been associated with lactic acidosis and high mortality. In 20 patients with severe cardiac or pulmonary disease or both, mixed venous PO_2 (PvO_2) correlated better with both hyperlactemia and survival than did CO or arterial PO_2 (PaO_2). A PvO_2 below 28 mmHg was usually associated with death in this study [71].

Swan *et al.* measured PvO_2 during CPB and found a close correlation to increases in lactic acid [72]. They concluded that maintaining patient levels above 35 mmHg will ensure adequate tissue oxygenation and prevent lactic acidosis. Conversely, if the PvO_2 drifts below 30 mmHg, lactic acidemia will develop. In dogs, the lactate production threshold for PvO_2 was 27 mmHg whether caused by arterial hypoxemia, low CO or a combination of these variables. These observations suggest that when vasoregulation is intact, there is a threshold value, or critical PvO_2 of about 28 mmHg, below which anaerobic metabolism is usually manifest as an increase in blood lactate. Despite a general lack of knowledge regarding the precise relationships between PvO_2 levels and the adequacy of tissue oxygenation, there exists a strong interdependence.

These observations suggest that oxygen requirements are being met when PvO_2 is above 28 mmHg. However, metabolic compromise may occur at higher perfusion levels even when the PvO_2 is more than 28 mmHg. For example, lactate production by isolated tissues (muscle) might be compensated for with increased lactate consumption by heart, kidney and liver. The threshold value of 28 mmHg actually marks a metabolic level where lactate production is no longer compensated. In other words, tissue hypoxia may occur at higher levels; however, the lactate production is compensated for by increased liver consumption [73].

Extreme anemia may represent a unique state of affairs in the microcirculation [74,75]. Traditionally it was thought that mixed SVO_2 values would be similar during hypoxic hypoxia and anemic hypoxia. Using a pig model to duplicate conditions of hypoxic hypoxia and anemic hypoxia, van der Hoeven followed SvO_2, DO_2, oxygen extraction and determined critical values based on lactate and VO_2 [76]. In comparison with hypoxic hypoxia, critical values of SvO_2 are higher in anemic hypoxia (26% vs. 55%), indicating that oxygen unloading from blood to tissues is impaired in anemic hypoxia. Because the RBC velocity is increased and the RBC residence time is reduced during isovolemic hemodilution, a decrease in precapillary oxygen release and in diffusional oxygen transfer to other microvessels is thought to account for a higher critical SvO_2 value. These characteristics in oxygen transport and capillary hemodynamics should be taken into consideration when SvO_2 is used in clinical critical care.

Loss of vasoregulation

Early investigators evaluating DO_2, VO_2 or SVO_2 patterns in general ICU populations reported conflicting clinical outcomes. It was hoped that a relationship as fundamental as that of DO_2 and VO_2 would produce a set of universal parameters that would transcend any particular disease state. With the passage of time it became apparent that more meaningful relationships could be found when critically ill patients are divided into the following five categories: (1) posttraumatic and/or postoperative; (2) cardiogenic; (3) septic; (4) cirrhotic; and (5) adult respiratory distress syndrome (ARDS). This division reflects the observation that some diseases produce tissue hypoxia by limiting the ability to extract sufficient oxygen despite an adequate CO with normal arterial oxygen content. Specifically patients with sepsis, cirrhosis and ARDS have reduced extraction capacity, which reflects disordered regulation of capillary beds [77,78].

Although SvO_2 is an indicator of the supply/demand balance for perfused tissues, its value as a threshold marker for anaerobic metabolism depends on appropriate vasoregulation. When vasoregulation is impaired due to multiorgan failure, sepsis, etc., the utility of using SVO_2 to guide therapy is greatly diminished. On the other hand, oxygen extraction relationships appear to remain intact for the critically ill posthemorrhagic or postoperative patients. The oxygen requirements of these patients are of particular interest because 90% of exceptional blood loss cases will either be going into surgery or coming out of surgery.

Beyond data from a pulmonary artery catheter, physical examination findings and urine output, several other gauges of shock and perfusion have been promoted. Of these, serum lactate levels have emerged as the simplest and possibly the most useful, and should be considered part of the decision process for frequency and duration of HBO therapy. In patients with poor tissue oxygenation, cells increase anaerobic metabolism and lactate levels rise. The clinician may, therefore, monitor serial lactate levels in patients with normal hepatic function as measures of global perfusion. Waxman *et al.* followed sequential perioperative lactate levels in 12 high-risk surgical patients [79]. There was a marked increase in lactate values intraoperatively. This increase did not correspond to decreases in either MAP or CO, but did correlate with VO_2. Postoperatively, lactate levels remained elevated, and this elevation correlated with the intraoperative oxygen deficit. Rashkin *et al.* had similar findings in 44 critically ill patients with and without ARDS [80]. Blood lactate was used as an indicator of tissue hypoxia independent of CO. Survival was good (55%) and blood lactate was near normal for those with DO_2 greater than 8 ml/kg/min. Below this level, survival was poor (14%) and blood lactate markedly increased [81].

In summary, the physiologic concepts relevant to postoperative circulatory failure can be summarized as follows:

1 among the metabolic substances transported by the circulatory system, oxygen has the highest extraction ratio and is the most flow-dependent;
2 the general adequacy of the circulation system can be evaluated by the mass movement of oxygen in terms of the DO_2;
3 the VO_2 reflects the sum of all oxidative metabolism; thus DO_2 and VO_2 provide the best measure of the functional adequacy of both circulation and metabolism;
4 the pattern of oxygen transport (DO_2 and VO_2) correlates with survival or death.

The hyperbaric implications of the foregoing should be clear – if the postoperative survival goals for DO_2/VO_2 cannot be reached using conventional therapies, HBO should be added to the regimen. Other factors to weigh into the decision process would include ischemic ECG changes as an indicator of isolated cardiac failure and lactate levels. These general considerations of oxygen dynamics may also serve as a guide to the use of other oxygen therapeutics.

Potential applications

The short half-life, side-effects and expense of oxygen therapeutics preclude the indiscriminate use of these agents based simply on an Hb level. In recent years it has become clear that the singular use of an Hb level is overly simplistic and does not accurately predict whether the patient is compensating for the anemic state.

FDA licensure of an oxygen therapeutic requires a demonstration of safety and efficacy. Safety and the concept of adverse events is easily defined. However, the definition of efficacy is quite nebulous given the lack of consensus on a transfusion trigger, especially when comorbid problems exist. The efficacy end points may include transfusion avoidance, mortality and organ perfusion. Because the FDA has focused more on transfusion avoidance, manufacturers have designed trails with that index as a primary outcome variable. Although the oxygen therapeutics will make their greatest contribution in the management of trauma patients, the majority of the clinical studies have been performed in the more controlled setting of elective surgery.

Accordingly, the first area of licensure will probably be for transfusion avoidance during elective orthopedic or cardiovascular surgery. However, once a product is clinically available it will most likely be used in a variety of off-label scenarios. Several different applications could be considered.

Trauma
The popularization of the 'golden hour' of trauma management underscores the importance of rapidly restoring oxygen transport. The ability to provide these agents at the scene would be invaluable. In addition, there could be a

substantial saving of banked blood when these agents are given during the initial resuscitation [82]. It is far more desirable to have a patient 'bleeding' oxygen therapeutics as opposed to RBCs. This would conserve the use of banked blood for transfusion after bleeding has been controlled. As noted earlier, other potential benefits for the use of oxygen therapeutics in trauma include possible reduction in multiorgan failure syndrome and the elimination of RBC storage defects, thereby, insuring an immediate improvement in DO_2 [83,84].

Remote settings

The long shelf life of these agents would be of immediate value in first aid stations, which provide care in locations that are in remote settings. A second 'delayed care' scenario would be disaster relief where neither bank blood nor definitive care are readily available. The elimination of crossmatching further contributes to the practical aspects of having these agents readily available to buy time for patient transport.

Elective surgery

To completely avoid allogeneic blood use in this setting will require several different strategies. The first would be to conserve the patient's red cell mass by using an enhanced form of acute normovolemic hemodilution (ANH) (see Chapter 5) [85]. At present, ANH is limited by the amount of blood that can be safely withdrawn into a holding reservoir [86]. If large amounts are withdrawn, the patient is at risk for accruing a significant intraoperative oxygen debt, myocardial infarction or stroke [87]. However, if the hemodilutional agent is an oxygen therapeutic, substantially more blood can be withdrawn without the risk of hypoxia-related events [88]. In essence these agents will afford the patient an 'oxygen bridge' to carry him or her through the operative bleeding, after which the RBCs can be safely returned [89–91]. Because oxygen therapeutics have a short half-life ($< 24\,h$), multiple administrations will be required for 5–7 days if ANH is not performed or is inadequate. During this time the use of recombinant EPO will accelerate the endogenous replacement of RBCs. Ideally, 'EPO therapy' would be initiated prior to surgery to compensate for the reticulocytosis production time (see Chapter 3).

Acute vascular occlusions

The small particle size and reduced viscosity of these agents offer therapeutic promise to enhance both direct and collateral DO_2 following acute obstructions such as myocardial infarctions, strokes and failing flaps [92–94]. Several favorable reports have been published that substantiate this area to be worthy of further investigation.

Sickle cell anemia

Sickle cell anemia is well known for the sickling phenomenon that may occur whenever the tissue PO_2 drops. As the cells sickle, they cause obstruction, which could be compensated for by oxygen carriers smaller than RBCs. A number of reports have detailed the use of Hb-based substitutes in the management of painful crisis, aplastic crisis and acute chest syndrome [95]. All of the investigators believed there was a beneficial effect. Clearly, further work needs to be done in this area.

Radiation sensitizer

The relationship of radiation and oxygen is an important determinant of successful tumor kill [96]. It is well recognized that hypoxic tumors are notoriously resistant to radiation. Some of the earliest applications of hyperbaric therapy were directed toward tumor oxygenation. Although there was limited success, there has been a resurgence of interest in recent years for HBO and brain tumors. Oxygen therapeutics is technically easier to administer and has also shown promise as a radiation sensitizer.

Septic shock

Although the mechanisms of septic shock are complex, recent work has focused on the unregulated production of NO by an endotoxin-inducible form of NO synthase. This observation has led investigators to speculate on the utility of using NO-scavenging attributes of HBOCs in a therapeutic capacity. Unlike synthetic NO synthase inhibitors, HBOCs are capable of downregulating NO concentrations while maintaining physiological levels of this important messenger. Curacyte (Durham, North Carolina) has employed this strategy using its pyridoxalated hemoglobin polyoxyethylene (PHP) product. PHP is a natural human Hb, which is chemically modified in order to preserve its physiological functions and to deliver them to locations affected by inflammation. Curacyte has just completed a phase IIc study in patients suffering from distributive shock. Although promising, the application of HBOC in septic shock is still largely theoretical.

Summary

The development of oxygen therapeutics parallels man's quest for flight. It took less than 100 years since the achievement of the first flight to lunar landing. In a similar fashion it was only 100 years since Karl Landsteiner's description of blood types, which made transfusion possible, to the commercial release of the first 'blood substitute', Hemopure, in South Africa. Because the four classes of oxygen therapeutics have different delivery mechanisms and side-effect profiles, each can be expected to have its own unique clinical applications as the characteristics of the individually designed products are better understood. Increasing volunteer–blood donor shortages, coupled with increasing blood transfusion needs, as well as an expanding list of pathogens and adverse effects continue to fuel the demand for further development of these products.

References

1 Moore FA, Moore EE. Evolving concepts in the pathogenesis of postinjury multiple organ failure. *Surg Clin North Am* 1995; **75**: 257–77.

2 Zallen G, Moore EE, Ciesla DJ. Stored red blood cells selectively activate human neutrophils to release IL-8 and secretory PLA2. *Shock* 2000; **13**: 29–33.

3 Ghio M, Contini P, Mazzei C *et al.* In vitro immunosuppressive activity of soluble HLA class I and Fas ligand molecules: do they play a role in autologous blood transfusion? *Transfusion* 2001; **41**: 988–96.

4 Gould SA, Moore EE, Moore FA *et al.* Clinical utility of human polymerized hemoglobin as a blood substitute after acute trauma and urgent surgery. *J Trauma* 1997; **43**: 325–32.

5 Phillips WT, Lemen L, Goins B *et al.* Use of oxygen-15 to measure oxygen-carrying capacity of blood substitutes in vivo. *Am J Physiol* 1997; **272**: H2492–H2499.

6 Gulati A, Sharma AC, Singh G. Role of endothelin in the cardiovascular effects of diaspirin-crosslinked and stroma-reduced hemoglobin. *Crit Care Med* 1996; **24**: 137–47.

7 Hindman BJ, Dexter F, Cutkomp J *et al.* Diaspirin-crosslinked hemoglobin does not increase brain oxygen consumption during hypothermic cardiopulmonary bypass in rabbits. *Anesthesiology* 1995; **83**: 1302–11.

8 Jia L, Bonaventura J, Stamler JS *et al.* S-nitrosohemoglobin: a dynamic activity of blood involved in vascular control. *Nature* 1996; **380**: 221–6.

9 Gould SA, Moss GS. Clinical development of human polymerized hemoglobin as a blood substitute. *World J Surg* 1996; **20**: 1200–7.

10 Matheson B, Razynaka A, Kwansa H, Bucci E. Vascular response to infusions of a nonextravasating hemoglobin polymer. *J Appl Physiol* 2002; **93**: 1479–86.

11 Winslow RM. Alternative oxygen therapeutics: products, status of clinical trials, and future prospects. *Curr Hematol Rep* 2003; **2**: 503–10.

12 Intaglietta M, Johnson P, Winslow R. Microvascular and tissue oxygen distribution. *Cardiovasc Res* 1996; **32**: 632–43.

13 Homer L, Weathersby P, Kiesow L. Oxygen gradients between red blood cells in the microcirculation. *Microvascular Res* 1981; **22**: 308–23.

14 Biro G, Anderson P, Curtis S, Cain S. Stroma-free hemoglobin: its presence in plasma does not improve oxygen supply to the resting hindlimb vascular bed of hemodiluted dogs. *Can J Physiol Pharmacol* 1991; **69**: 1656.

15 Scholander P. Oxygen transport through hemoglobin solutions. *Science* 1960; **131**: 585–90.

16 Vlahakes GJ, Lee R, Jacobs EE Jr *et al.* Hemodynamic effects and oxygen transport properties of a new blood substitute in a model of massive blood replacement. *J Thorac Cardiovasc Surg* 1990; **100**: 379–88.

17 Looker D, Abbott-Brown D, Cozart P, Durfee S, Hoffman S, Mathews AJ, Miller-Roehrich J, Shoemaker S, Trimble S, Fermi G, Komiyama NH, Nagai K, Stetler GL. A human recombinant haemoglobin designed for use as a blood substitute. *Nature* 1992; **356**: 258–60.

18 Resta TC, Walker BR, Eichinger MR, Doyle MP. Rate of NO scavenging alters effects of recombinant hemoglobin solutions on pulmonary vasoreactivity. *J Appl Physiol* 2002; **93**: 1327–36.

19 Sakai H, Tsai A, Rohlfs R *et al.* Microvascular responses to hemodilution with Hb vesicles as red blood cell substitutes: influence of O2 affinity. *Am J Physiol* 1999; **276**: H553–H562.

20 Sakai H, Horinouchi H, Tomiyama K, Ikeda E, Takeoka S, Kobayashi K, Tsuchida E. Hemoglobin-vesicles as oxygen carriers: influence on phagocytic activity and histopathological changes in reticuloendothelial system. *Am J Pathol* 2001; **159**: 1079–88.

21 Hoag H. Blood substitute from worms shows promise: haemoglobin from sea creature could replace red cells. *Nature* 2003; 4 June.

22 Zal F, Lallier F, Toulmond A. Utilisation comme substitut sanguin d'une hémoglobine extracellulaire de poids moléculaire élevé. French Patent No. 00 07031, granted 2 August 2002.

23 Amberson WR, Mulder AG, Steggerda FR *et al.* Mammalian life without red blood corpuscles. *Science* 1933; **78**: 106–7.

24 Amberson WR, Jennings JJ, Rhode CM. Clinical experience with hemoglobin-saline solutions. *J Appl Physiol* 1949; **1**: 469–89.

25 Gould SA, Moore EE, Hoyt DB *et al.* The first randomized trial of human polymerized hemoglobin as a blood substitute in acute trauma and emergent surgery. *J Am Coll Surg* 1998; **187**: 113–20.

26 Gould SA, Moore EE, Hoyt DB *et al.* The life-sustaining capacity of human polymerized hemoglobin when red cells might be unavailable. *J Am Coll Surg* 2002; **195**: 445–52.

27 Sprung J, Kindscher JD, Wahr JA *et al.* The use of bovine hemoglobin glutamer-250 (Hemopure) in surgical patients: results of a multicenter, randomized, single-blinded trial. *Anesth Analg* 2002; **94**: 799–808.

28 Mullon J, Giacoppe G, Clagett C *et al.* Brief report: transfusions of polymerized bovine hemoglobin in a patient with severe autoimmune hemolytic anemia. *N Engl J Med* 2000; **342**: 1638–43.

29 Chang TMS. Future generations of red blood cell substitutes. *J Intern Med* 2003; **253**: 527–35.

30 Powanda DD, Chang TM. Cross-linked polyhemoglobin-superoxide dismutase-catalase supplies oxygen without causing blood-brain barrier disruption or brain edema in a rat model of transient global brain ischemia-reperfusion. *Artif Cells Blood Substit Immobil Biotechnol* 2002; **30**: 23–37.

31 Chang TM. Modified hemoglobin-based blood substitutes: cross-linked, recombinant and encapsulated hemoglobin. *Vox Sang* 1998; **74**: 233–41.

32 Winslow RM. Alternative oxygen therapeutics: products, status of clinical trials, and future prospects. *Curr Hematol Rep* 2003; **6**: 503–10.

33 Tsai AG, Vandegriff KD, Intaglietta M *et al.* Targeted O_2 delivery by low-P_{50} hemoglobin: a new basis for O_2 therapeutics. *Am J Physiol Heart Circ Physiol* 2003; **285**: H1411–H1419.

34 Wettstein R, Tsai A, Erni D *et al.* Resuscitation with polyethylene glycol-modified human hemoglobin improves microcirculatory blood flow and tissue oxygenation after hemorrhagic shock in awake hamsters. *Crit Care Med* 2003; **31**: 1824–30.

35 Matheson B, Razynaka A, Kwansa H, Bucci E. Vascular response to infusions of a nonextravasating hemoglobin polymer. *J Appl Physiol* 2002; **93**: 1479–86.

36 Huang Y, Komatsu T, Nakagawa A, Tsuchida E, Kobayashi S. Compatibility in vitro of albumin-heme (O_2 carrier) with blood cell components. *J Biomed Mater Res* 2003; **66A**: 292–7.

37 Zunszain PA, Ghuman J, Komatsu T, Tsuchida E, Curry S. Crystal structural analysis of human serum albumin complexed with hemin and fatty acid. *BMC Struct Biol* 2003; **3**: 6 (Epub. 7 July 2003).

38 Simoni J, Simoni G, Wesson DE, Griswold JA, Feola M. A novel hemoglobin-adenosine-glutathione based blood substitute: evaluation of its effects on human blood ex vivo. *ASAIO J* 2000; **46**: 679–92.

39 Feola M, Simoni J, Angelillo R *et al*. Clinical trial of a hemoglobin-based blood substitute in patients with sickle cell anemia. *Surg Gynecol Obstet* 1992; **174**: 379–86.

40 Spahn DR, Waschke KF, Standl T *et al*. Use of perflubron emulsion to decrease allogeneic blood transfusion in high-blood-loss non-cardiac surgery: results of a European phase 3 study. *Anesthesiology* 2002; **97**: 1338–49.

41 Perutz MF, Poyart C. Bezafibrate lowers oxygen affinity of haemoglobin. *Lancet* 1983; **2**: 881–2.

42 Poyart C, Marden MC, Kister J. Bezafibrate derivatives as potent effectors of hemoglobin. *Methods Enzymol* 1994; **232**: 496–513.

43 Wahr JA, Gerber M, Venitz J *et al*. Allosteric modification of oxygen delivery by hemoglobin. *Anesth Analg* 2001; **92**: 615–20.

44 Miyake M, Grinberg OY, Hou H, Steffen RP, Elkadi H, Swartz HM. The effect of RSR13, a synthetic allosteric modifier of hemoglobin, on brain tissue PO_2 (measured by EPR oximetry) following severe hemorrhagic shock in rats. *Adv Exp Med Biol* 2003; **530**: 319–29.

45 Grinberg OY, Miyake M, Hou H, Steffen RP, Swartz HM. The dose-dependent effect of RSR13, a synthetic allosteric modifier of hemoglobin, on physiological parameters and brain tissue oxygenation in rats. *Adv Exp Med Biol* 2003; **530**: 287–96.

46 Boerema I, Meijne NG, Brummelkamp WH *et al*. Life without blood. *J Cardiovasc Surg* 1960; **182**: 133–46.

47 Hart G. Exceptional blood loss anemia: treatment with hyperbaric oxygen therapy. *JAMA* 1974; **228**: 1028–9.

48 Hart GB. Hyperbaric oxygen in exceptional acute blood-loss anemia. *J Hyperbaric Med* 1987; **2**: 205–10.

49 Doi Y, Onji Y: Oxygen deficit in haemorrhagic shock under hyperbaric oxygen. Proceedings of the 4th International Congress on Hyperbaric Medicine. Japan, September 1969; 181.

50 Attar S, Esmond WG, Cowley RA. Hyperbaric oxygenation in vascular collapse. *J Thor and Cardio Surg* 1962; **44**: 759.

51 Attar S, Esmond WG, Blair E *et al*. Experimental aspects of the use of hyperbaric oxygen in hemorrhagic shock. *Am Surg* 1964; **30**: 243–6.

52 Elliott DP, Paton BC. Effect of 100% oxygen at one and three atmospheres on dogs subjected to hemorrhagic hypotension. *Surgery* 1965; **57**: 401–8.

53 Yamashita M. Hyperbaric oxygen treatment attenuates cytokine induction after massive hemorrhage. *Am J Physiol* 2000; **278**: 811–16.

54 Wright JK, Ehler W, McGlasson DL, Thomson W. Facilitation of recovery from acute blood loss with hyperbaric oxygen. *Arch Surg* 2002; **137**: 850–3.

55 Spahn DR. Perioperative transfusion triggers for red blood cells. *Vox Sang* 2000; **78**(Suppl): 163–6.

56 Shoemaker WC, Kram HB. Effects of crystalloids and colloids on hemodynamics, oxygen transport, and outcome in high-risk surgical patients. In: Simmons RL, Udekwu AO, eds. *Debates in General Surgery*. Chicago: Year Book Medical Publishers, 1990: 263–302.

57 Schwartz S, Frantz A, Shoemaker WC. Sequential hemodynamic and oxygen transport responses in hypovolemia, anemia, and hypoxia. *Am J Physiol* 1981; **241**: 864–71.

58 Cone JB. Monitoring of tissue oxygenation. In: Snyder JV, Pinsky JR, eds. *Oxygen Transport in the Critically Ill*. ISBN 0-8151-7903-0. Chicago: Year Book Medical Publishers, 1987: 164–76.

59 Kern JW, Shoemaker WC. Meta-analysis of hemodynamic optimization in high-risk patients. *Crit Care Med* 2002; **30**: 1686–92.

60 Baue AE. Multiple, progressive or sequential system fauilure: a syndrome of the 1970s. *Arch Surg* 1975; **110**: 779.

61 Baue AE, Chaudry IH. Prevention of multiple systems failure. *Surg Clin North Am* 1980; **60**: 1167–78.

62 Shoemaker WC, Appel PL, Kram HB. Tissue oxygen debt as a determinant of lethal and nonlethal postoperative organ failure. *Crit Care Med* 1988; **16**: 1117–20.

63 Crowell JW, Smithe EE. Oxygen deficit and irreversible hemorrhagic shock. *Am J Physiol* 1964; **106**: 313.

64 Shoemaker WC, Czer L, Chang P *et al*. Cardiorespiratory monitoring in postoperative patients – I: prediction of outcome and severity of illness. *Crit Care Med* 1979; **7**: 237.

65 Shoemaker WC, Appel PL, Kram HB. Measurement of tissue perfusion by oxygen transport patterns in experimental shock and high-risk surgical patients. *Intens Care Med* 1990; **16**: S135.

66 Shoemaker WC, Appel PL, Kram HB *et al*. Oxygen transport measurements to evaluate tissue perfusion and titrate therapy: dobutamine and dopamine effects. *Crit Care Med* 1991; **19**: 672–88.

67 Schumacker PT, Cain SM. The concept of a critical oxygen delivery. *Intens Care Med* 1987; **13**: 223–9.

68 Reinhart K, Hannemann L, Kuss B. Optimal oxygen delivery in critically ill patients. *Intens Care Med* 1990; **16**(Suppl.): S149–S155.

69 Shibutani K, Komatsu T, Kubal K, Sanchala V, Kumar V, Bizzarri DV. Critical level of oxygen delivery in anesthetized man. *Crit Care Med* 1983; **11**: 640–3.

70 Buran MJ. Oxygen consumption. In: Snyder JV, Pinsky JR, eds. *Oxygen Transport in the Critically Ill*. ISBN 0-8151-7903-0. Chicago: Year Book Medical Publishers, 1987: 16–23.

71 Kasnitz P, Druger GL, Yorra F *et al*. Mixed venous oxygen tension and hyperlactatemia. *JAMA* 1976; **236**: 570.

72 Swan H, Sanchez M, Tyndall M, Koch C. Quality control of perfusion: monitoring venous blood oxygen tension to prevent hypoxic acidosis. *J Thorac Cardiovasc Surg* 1990; **99**: 868–72.

73 Cain SM. Assessment of tissue oxygenation. *Crit Care Med* 1986; **2**: 537.

74 Trouwborst A, Tenbrinck R, van Woerkens ECSM. Blood gas analysis of mixed venous blood during normoxic acute isovolemic hemodilution in pigs. *Anesth Analg* 1990; **70**: 523–9.

75 Kuo L, Pittman RN. Effect of hemodilution on oxygen transport in arteriolar networks of hamster striated muscle. *Am J Physiol* 1988; **254**: H331–H339.

76 Van der Hoeven MAHBM, Maertzdorf WJ, Blanco CE. Relationship between mixed venous oxygen saturation and markers of tissue oxygenation in progressive hypoxic hypoxia and in isovolemic anemic hypoxia in 8- to 12-day-old piglets. *Crit Care Med* 1999; **27**: 1885–92.

77 Weg JG. Oxygen transport in adult respiratory distress syndrome and other acute circulatory problems: relationship of oxygen delivery and oxygen consumption. *Crit Care Med* 1991; **19**: 650–7.

78 Dantzker DR, Foresman B, Gutierrez G. Oxygen supply and utilization relationships. *Am Rev Respir Dis* 1991; **143**: 675.

79 Waxman K, Nolan LS, Shoemaker WC. Sequential perioperative lactate determination: physiological and clinical implications. *Crit Care Med* 1982; **10**: 96.

80 Rashkin MC, Bosken C, Baughman RP. Oxygen delivery in critically ill patients: relationship of blood lactate and survival. *Chest* 1985; **87**: 580–3.

81 Komatsu T, Shibutani K, Okamoto K *et al*. Critical level of oxygen delivery after cardiopulmonary bypass. *Crit Care Med* 1987; **15**: 194.

82 Knudson MM, Lee S, Erickson V, Morabito D *et al*. Tissue oxygen monitoring during hemorrhagic shock and resuscitation: a comparison of lactated Ringer's solution, hypertonic saline dextran, and HBOC-201. *J Trauma* 2003; **54**: 242–52.

83 Moore EE. Blood substitutes: the future is now. *J Am Coll Surg* 2003; **196**: 1–17.

84 Standl T, Freitag M, Burmeister MA *et al*. Hemoglobin-based oxygen carrier HBOC-201 provides higher and faster increase in oxygen tension in skeletal muscle of anemic dogs than do stored red blood cells. *J Vasc Surg* 2003; **37**: 859–65.

85 Spahn DR, van Brempt R, Theilmeier G, Reibold JP *et al*. Perflubron emulsion delays blood transfusions in orthopedic surgery. European Perflubron Emulsion Study Group. *Anesthesiology* 1999; **91**: 1195–208.

86 Levy JH, Goodnough LT, Greilich P *et al*. Polymerized bovine hemoglobin solution as a replacement for allogeneic red blood cell transfusion after cardiac surgery: results of a randomized, double-blind trial. *J Thorac Cardiovasc Surg* 2002; **124**: 35–42.

87 Hill SE, Gottschalk LI, Grichnik K. Safety and preliminary efficacy of hemoglobin raffimer for patients undergoing coronary artery bypass surgery. *J Cardiothorac Vasc Anesth* 2002; **16**: 695–702.

88 Hill SE, Leone BJ, Faithfull NS *et al*. Perflubron emulsion (AF0144) augments harvesting of autologous blood: a phase II study in cardiac surgery. *J Cardiothorac Vasc Anesth* 2002; **16**: 555–60.

89 Krieter H, Hagen G, Waschke KF *et al*. Isovolemic hemodilution with a bovine hemoglobin-based oxygen carrier: effects on hemodynamics and oxygen transport in comparison with a nonoxygen-carrying volume substitute. *J Cardiothorac Vasc Anesth* 1997; **11**: 3–9.

90 Schubert A, Przybelski RJ, Eidt JF *et al*. Diaspirin-crosslinked hemoglobin reduces blood transfusion in noncardiac surgery: a multicenter, randomized, controlled, double-blinded trial. *Anesth Analg* 2003; **97**: 323–32.

91 Levy JH. The use of haemoglobin glutamer-250 (HBOC-201) as an oxygen bridge in patients with acute anaemia associated with surgical blood loss. *Exp Opin Biol Ther* 2003; **3**: 509–17.

92 Niquille M, Touzet M, Leblanc I, Baron JF. Reversal of intraoperative myocardial ischemia with a hemoglobin-based oxygen carrier. *Anesthesiology* 2000; **92**: 882–5.

93 Saxena R, Wijnhoud AD, Carton H *et al*. Controlled safety study of a hemoglobin-based oxygen carrier, DCLHb, in acute ischemic stroke. *Stroke* 1999; **30**: 993–6.

94 Claudio C, Schramm S, Wettstein R *et al*. Improved oxygenation in ischemic hamster flap tissue is correlated with increasing hemodilution with Hb vesicles and their O_2 affinity. *Am J Physiol Heart Circ Physiol* 2003; **285**: H1140–H1147.

95 Lanzkron S, Moliterno AR, Norris EJ. Polymerized human Hb use in acute chest syndrome: a case report. *Transfusion* 2002; **42**: 1422–7.

96 Teicher BA, Schwartz GN, Alvarez Sotomayor E *et al*. Oxygenation of tumors by a hemoglobin solution. *J Cancer Res Clin Oncol* 1993; **120**: 85–90.

CHAPTER 13

Basic Principles of Bloodless Medicine and Surgery

Nicolas Jabbour

Questionnaire

Choose the correct statement(s) for each question (one or more are possible).

1 Blood utilization in the USA:
   (a) Over 12 million units of blood are used annually
   (b) Over 40% of blood used is prescribed by surgeons
   (c) Over 50% of blood is used in patients over 60 years of age
   (d) Blood utilization is expected to increase in the future

2 Blood donors:
   (a) In the USA, blood donors can be paid in order to increase the donor pool
   (b) The donor pool is increasing on a consistent basis due to the awareness of blood shortages
   (c) Donors may be excluded if they spend significant time in certain countries
   (d) The safest blood donation is from a directed-donor, i.e. family members or friends

3 Cost of blood products:
   (a) Currently the average cost of packed red blood cells (PRBCs) is approximately $200–250
   (b) This cost does not include costs related to type and crossmatching, blood administration and banking
   (c) Indirect costs of blood products should include the costs of its complications, i.e. fever or viral transmission

4 Potential risks of blood transfusion:
   (a) The risk of hepatitis C transmission is less than 1 per 100 000 units
   (b) Some clinical studies have shown that blood transfusion may increase the risk of tumor recurrence

   (c) Blood transfusion may increase the risk of postoperative infection
   (d) As many as 1% of patients may experience fever as a result of blood transfusion

5 Preoperative autologous donation (PAD):
   (a) May decrease the need for homologous blood transfusion
   (b) Requires one or more preoperative visits to the blood bank
   (c) Does not decrease the risk of clerical error associated with blood transfusions
   (d) Significant amount of blood collected is not used perioperatively

6 Acute normovolemic hemodilution (ANH):
   (a) Does not eliminate the risk of clerical error when the blood is given to the patient
   (b) Can be used even in severely anemic patients
   (c) Unlike banked blood, the blood collected during ANH contains normal platelets and clotting factors
   (d) ANH has no effect on blood conservation

7 Intraoperative cell salvage (cell saver):
   (a) Cell saver is contraindicated in patients with gross contamination in the surgical field
   (b) Can be used in trauma with major bleeding such as hemothorax or major vascular injury
   (c) Blood saved is depleted from platelets and coagulation factors
   (d) May cause severe coagulopathy in patients with large amounts of blood loss
   (e) Can be performed without heparinization
   (f) May cause disseminated intravascular coagulation (DIC) or air embolism if not set up appropriately

8 Erythropoietin (Procrit, Epogen):
   (a) Erythropoietin is a recombinant factor available as an intravenous (IV) or subcutaneous (SC) injection
   (b) It stimulates the bone marrow to produce more RBCs
   (c) Requires the use of therapeutic doses of iron to be more effective
   (d) May yield up to 3 units of blood within 3 weeks of administration
   (e) Although it was originally used in patients with chronic renal failure (CRF), erythropoietin is currently approved in selective patients preoperatively

9 Legal aspects of blood transfusion in Jehovah's Witness (JW) patients:
   (a) In the USA, adult JW patients have the right to refuse blood transfusion at the risk of their life

    (b) If the patient is unknown to be a JW and is seen in a trauma or emergency situation, physicians must administer blood, if necessary, without consent

    (c) Pediatric patients of JW families should be transfused, if medically necessary, with or without court order depending on the urgency of the situation

    (d) In adult patients, if appropriate consent is signed prior to surgery, transfusions cannot be administered even if the patient became incapacitated postoperatively

    (e) If standard of care is applied appropriately when treating adult JW patients, the physician and the institution are not liable in case of patient demise from severe anemia

10 The following are some of the contraindications to ANH:

    (a) Hemodynamic instability

    (b) Low hematocrit

    (c) Underlying severe cardiovascular disease

    (d) Older than 75 years of age

11 Activated factor VII (NovoSeven):

    (a) Is a recombinant protein produced from hamster renal cells

    (b) Enhances coagulation cascade at the site of vascular injury

    (c) Its only FDA approved indication is for the treatment of hemophilia with inhibitors

    (d) Has proven beneficial in conditions such as severe trauma, liver disease and transplantation in off-label use

12 Bleeding disorders in surgical patients:

    (a) History of prior bleeding during minor surgery or minor trauma is one of the most important details regarding underlying bleeding disorders

    (b) Normal platelet count, prothrombin time (PT) and activated partial thromboplastin time (APTT) do not eliminate the potential risks for medical bleeding

    (c) Platelets may need to be transfused even with normal platelet counts in patients treated with nonsteroidal anti-inflammatory drugs (NSAIDs) who have medical bleeding

    (d) Thromboelastogram offers information regarding the quality of the clotting system

13 The following products may have some value in limiting surgical bleeding:

    (a) Aprotinin in cardiac surgery, orthopedic surgery and liver transplantation

    (b) Epsilon-aminocaproic acid (Amicar) in the face of fibrinolysis

  (c) Desmopressin (DDAVP), especially in patients with chronic kidney disease
  (d) NovoSeven (factor VIIa) in patients with severe coagulopathy from massive blood transfusion

14 These anesthetic techniques may decrease surgical blood loss:
  (a) Controlled hypotension in surgeries such as liver resection
  (b) The use of thromboelastogram to evaluate the coagulation system, especially in liver transplantation
  (c) The use of ANH
  (d) The use of cell saver

15 Blood transfusion in the intensive care unit (ICU):
  (a) A significant percentage of blood transfusions given in the ICU is due to excessive blood testing
  (b) Randomized clinical trials have shown that a higher hematocrit enhances patient survival
  (c) Erythropoietin is very effective in ICU patients even in the presence of underlying sepsis
  (d) Maintaining a high level of hematocrit is more important than maintaining normal intravascular volume status

16 Pathophysiology of acute anemia:
  (a) Decreasing the hematocrit to a level of 20% is well tolerated in healthy patients
  (b) Perioperative mortality is significantly increased in severely anemic patients with underlying vascular disease
  (c) Oxygen delivery is maintained in moderate anemia as long as the patient has normal intravascular volume
  (d) The physiologic response to acute anemia consists of decreased peripheral vascular resistance, increased heart rate and increased oxygen extraction

17 Tissue oxygen consumption/need:
  (a) Increases significantly with fever
  (b) Decreases in patients on artificial ventilation and paralyzed
  (c) Increases with shivering
  (d) May be decreased in hypothermic patients

18 Oxygen delivery:
  (a) Is directly proportional to hemoglobin concentration
  (b) Is directly proportional to cardiac output and heart rate
  (c) Can be maintained in anemic patients by increased cardiac output
  (d) Mechanical ventilation and increased inhaled oxygen concentration may increase oxygen delivery

19 Severely anemic patients may benefit from the following:
   (a) Increased oxygen delivery by increasing inhaled oxygen delivery and/or mechanical ventilation
   (b) Decreased oxygen consumption by artificial ventilation
   (c) Decreased oxygen consumption by the use of paralytics to avoid shivering in patients on the ventilator
   (d) Maintaining euvolemia
   (e) Potential benefits with hypothermia

20 Artificial blood products:
   (a) They are derived from hemoglobin, old blood or perfluorocarbon molecules
   (b) They have a long shelf life
   (c) They do not require refrigeration for banking
   (d) They have small-sized particles that can potentially deliver oxygen beyond critical obstruction such as in cardiac or cerebrovascular disease

21 The pitfalls of artificial blood product usage:
   (a) Has a high affinity for oxygen
   (b) Requires high FiO_2 to deliver significant oxygen to the tissues
   (c) Has shorter half-life in comparison to autologous blood once transfused
   (d) Requires the infusion of large volume to adequately increase oxygen delivery

22 The potential benefits of artificial blood products:
   (a) Can be used on site in trauma and in the military
   (b) Its use in the operating room increases the safety of ANH by maintaining close-to-normal oxygen delivery in the presence of severe anemia
   (c) May be used in JW patients with severe anemia while the RBCs are being synthesized by the bone marrow

23 Transfusion-free surgery in pediatric patients:
   (a) Techniques used in adult patients cannot be applied to pediatric patients
   (b) Transfusion in children should be avoided since the transmission of some diseases manifests itself many years following blood product transfusion
   (c) Erythropoietin has been used successfully in pediatric patients

24 Major surgery in JW patients:
   (a) Major surgery can be done safely in JW patients without blood product transfusion

Chapter 13

  (b) Liver transplantation in JW patients has been done successfully in specialized centers such as University of Southern California/USC University Hospital
  (c) Large studies have shown that severe anemia (hemoglobin < 6 g/dl) significantly affects postoperative mortality in patients with underlying cardiovascular disease
  (d) Techniques used in treating JW patients can be applied to non-JW patients to decrease overall blood utilization

25 Refractory conditions to erythropoietin therapy:
  (a) Patients with underlying inflammatory disease from cancer
  (b) Patients with severe sepsis
  (c) The presence of iron deficiency
  (d) Bone marrow disease

26 Reasons for surgeons to initiate transfusion-free program:
  (a) More than half of blood transfusions are prescribed by surgeons
  (b) Elective surgery cannot proceed without available blood products
  (c) Blood savings decrease the overall costs of surgical care
  (d) Blood loss is a reflection of the quality of surgeons

27 These pathogens can be transmitted via blood transfusions:
  (a) Human immunodeficiency virus (HIV)
  (b) Mad cow disease
  (c) West Nile virus (WNV)
  (d) Hepatitis B and C virus (HBV and HCV)

28 Despite donor testing, disease transmission via blood transfusion is still possible due to the following reasons:
  (a) Most testing detects antibodies rather than antigens
  (b) There are still potentially unknown pathogens that escape testing and can be transmitted through blood
  (c) There is always a small window between infection and disease detection in potential donors

29 The benefits of blood product transfusion:
  (a) Increases oxygen delivery to the tissues
  (b) Enhances coagulation by transfusion of fresh frozen plasma and platelets
  (c) Serves as intravascular volume expander similar to colloids or crystalloids

30 These products can only be derived from human blood:
  (a) Factor VIII concentrate
  (b) Factor IX concentrate

(c) Fresh frozen plasma

(d) Cryoprecipitate

(e) Factor VIIa

31 Drugs that may affect platelet function:

(a) Aspirin

(b) Dextran

(c) Steroids

(d) Cox II inhibitors

32 The basics for successful transfusion-free surgery:

(a) Starting the surgery at a higher hematocrit level by preoperative bone marrow stimulation

(b) Careful surgical technique

(c) Selective hypotensive anesthesia

(d) The use of cell saver and ANH during surgery

33 Iron use along with erythropoietin:

(a) Can enhance bone marrow production of RBCs

(b) Very well tolerated orally and almost completely absorbed

(c) Can be safely used intravenously in gluconate form

(d) If not used with erythropoietin, may decrease the bone marrow response or lead to the production of hypochromic RBCs

34 Current shelf life of blood products:

(a) Packed red cells = 42 days at 0–6°C

(b) Platelets = 5 days at room temperature

(c) Fresh frozen plasma = 1 year at −18°C

(d) Cryoprecipitate = 1 year at −18°C

(e) Frozen red cells = over 1 year

35 Potential perioperative complications that may lead to post-operative bleeding disorders:

(a) Thrombotic thrombocytopenic purpura (TTP) induced by surgery

(b) Thrombocytopenia from use of heparin, even as a flush solution

(c) Sepsis

(d) The presence of large intra-abdominal clot with local fibrinolysis that promotes localized bleeding

36 These interventions may decrease the side-effects of blood transfusion:

(a) Pretreatment with benadryl and oral Acetaminophene

(b) The use of white cell filters that may eliminate or decrease the risk of febrile reaction to blood transfusion

(c) Careful verification by two persons of the crossmatch between the blood being transfused and the patient receiving the transfusion

37 Signs and symptoms of potential transfusion reactions:
  (a) Hematuria
  (b) Severe back pain
  (c) Chills and fever
  (d) Hypotension

38 The optimal threshold for red cell transfusion:
  (a) Hematocrit level of 30% (hemoglobin of 10 g/dl) is the optimal accepted threshold
  (b) A precise threshold cannot be used universally in any patient and in any situation
  (c) Threshold is lower in younger, healthy patients
  (d) The threshold of 30% or higher is appropriate in patients with underlying cardiovascular disease

39 Absolute contraindications to cell saver:
  (a) Presence of amniotic fluid at the surgical site
  (b) Presence of gastrointestinal (GI) fluid at the surgical site
  (c) Cutting through tumor during the surgery
  (d) The use of certain local hemostatic products that may lead to intra-vascular coagulopathy

40 The following are local hemostatic agents used in surgery to decrease blood loss:
  (a) Fibrin glue (Tisseel, Floseal, etc.)
  (b) Surgicel
  (c) NovoSeven (factor VIIa)
  (d) Avitene
  (e) Amicar

41 Indirect costs of blood transfusion include:
  (a) Type and screen testing
  (b) Type and crossmatching
  (c) Blood dispensing and administration
  (d) Work-up for transfusion reaction

42 The calculation of the increase in oxygen delivery as a result of blood transfusion should take into consideration the following:
  (a) Old RBCs may lose some elasticity with negative effect on tissue perfusion
  (b) RBC affinity for oxygen increases with aging
  (c) The rbc half-life is lower in banked blood than in native RBCs
  (d) 1 unit of blood transfusion administered to an adult is expected to yield a 3% increase in the hematocrit level

43 Contraindications to the use of erythropoietin:
   (a) Known sensitivity to antibiotics
   (b) Recent coronary surgery
   (c) Uncontrolled hypertension
   (d) Anemia

Index

Page numbers in *italic* refer to figures; those in **bold** refer to tables.

abciximab 118
ABO incompatibility **49**
acetylsalicylic acid 77
activated clotting time 128
activated partial thromboplastin
    time 99, 128
acute hemolytic reaction **49**
acute lung disease, transfusion-
    associated 44
acute normovolemic hemodilution *62*,
    198–9, *198*
  neonatal and pediatric surgery
    221–2
acute renal failure 171
agents transmitted by blood
    transfusion **48**, **239**
albumin 78
alloimmunization **49**
allosteric modifiers 259
aminocaproic acid *see* epsilon-
    aminocaproic acid
anaphylaxis **49**
anemia 144–57
  causes and compensatory
    mechanisms 144–7
  ICU-acquired 158–60, *160*,
    170–2
    prevention of 177–80
  in neonates **219**
  of oncologic disease 229–30
  physiologic response to 147–51
  of prematurity 228–9, **229**
  refractory to erythropoietin
    therapy 188–90, *190*
  risk benefit of blood
    transfusion 151–4
  sickle cell 147, 276–7
  tolerance of 179–80, 203
anesthesia management 199–200
antifibrinolytics 136–7
antithrombin 33
APACHE II score 172, 173, 175
aprotinin *62*, 96–9, 136–7, 200, 222

cost **250**
arenicola hemoglobin 259
artificial blood *see* oxygenation
    therapy
autologous transfusion 2–4, 60, *62*,
    87–90, **88**
  contraindications **88**
  cost **250**
  neonatal and pediatric surgery
    221–2
Avitene **197**

Babesia microti **48**
bacterial contamination **61**
bleeding time 127
blood conservation 94–101
  aprotinin 96–9
  DDAVP 94–5
  epsilon-aminocaproic acid 95–6
  erythropoietin 100–1
  recombinant factor VIIa 99–100
  tranexamic acid 95–6
  see also autologous transfusion
blood gas measurement 153, 272–4
blood lactate 165
bloodless programs 15–17
  early pioneers 16
  evolution of 16–17
  future extension of 21–2
  legal structure 17–22
    confirmation of patient's decision
      to refuse blood 17–20, *18–19*
    consent, liability of physician and
      hospital 17–18
    policies and procedures 20
  see also restrictive transfusion
    practice
blood products, cost-effectiveness
    of 185–7
  see also individual products
blood salvage *see* cell salvage
blood shield laws 243
blood viscosity 149
Borrelia burgdorferi **48**
bovine hemoglobin 258
burn surgery 227–8

cardiac output 162–3
  increasing 166
cardiac surgery 225–6
  cost **248**
cardiopulmonary bypass 126
cell salvage *62*, 90–3, **91**, **92**, 194–8,
    193, *195*, **197**
  complications **92**
  contraindications **91**
  hemostatic agents **197**
  neonatal and pediatric surgery 223
central nervous system, effects of
    erythropoietin 69–70
Chagas' disease 186
circulating anticoagulants 126
circulatory overload **50**
coagulation factors 118–20
coagulation management 133–6,
    200–2, *201*
coagulation system *see* hemostasis
coagulation tests 126–8
  activated clotting time 128
  activated partial thromboplastin
      time 127
  bleeding time and platelet count
      127
  platelet function analyzer 128
  platelet function tests 128
  prothrombin time 126–7
  thrombin time and reptilase
      time 127
coagulopathy 93
cold-induced thrombopathy **50**
colloids 78, 80
Collostat **197**
competent adults 6
consent
  hospital's liability 17–18
  informed 5–6
  physician's responsibility 17–18
controlled hypotension 101–5
convection 147
Cooley, Denton 16
cost-effectiveness of blood
    products 185–7
cost of transfusion therapy 237–53
  blood transfusion as service 243–4
  case studies 248–9, **249**
  difficulties in estimation 240–2
  hospital costs 245–6, **245**
  leukoreduction 246–8, **247**, **248**
  oxygenation therapy and
      pharmacologic agents 249, **250**

reasons for 242–3, **243**
  regulatory environment 244–5
  supply of donated blood 237–40
craniosynostosis surgery 226–7
Creuztfeldt–Jakob disease 47, 186
critical hemoglobin value 147–51
critically ill patients 170–84
  clinical relevance of blood
      transfusions 173
  experience with Jehovah's Witness
      patients 180–1
  ICU-acquired anemia 170–2
    prevention of 177–80
  ICU transfusion practice 172–3
  restrictive transfusion practice
    efficacy of 173–6
    safety of 176–7
cryoprecipitate 24, 33–4, 75, 200
  clinically appropriate situations 36
  cost **243**, **245**
  under-dosing 39–40
cryoprecipitate-reduced fresh frozen
    plasma 247
crystalloids 80
cyclic AMP 118
cytomegalovirus **48**
cytomegalovirus-negative
    components 247

darbopoietin 70
  cost **255**
DDAVP 94–5
deamino-8-D-arginine vasopressin *see*
    DDAVP
delayed hemolytic reaction 45–6, **49**
desmopressin *62*, 137, 222
  cost **250**
diffusion 147–8
disagreeing family members 13–14
disseminated intravascular
    coagulation 75, 152
donor room 237–8, *238*
Drew, Charles 24
drug-induced coagulation
    disorders 125

elective surgery 276
electrolyte imbalances **50**
emergency situations 7–14
  known Jehovah's Witnesses 7–11
  no information available 11–13
encapsulated hemoglobin 258–9
epoietin alfa *see* erythropoietin

epsilon-aminocaproic acid *62*, 95–6, 136, 222
   cost **250**
Epstein–Barr virus **48**
eptifibatide 118
erythropoiesis 144
   optimization of 179
erythropoietin *2*, 60, *62*, 144, 188
   central nervous system effects 69–70
   cost **250**
   low circulating concentrations 171
   neonatal and pediatric surgery 219–21, **219**, **220**
   postoperative 166, 203–5, *204*
   preoperative 62–5, *63*, *64*
   safety issues 67–9, **68**

febrile nonhemolytic transfusion reaction **49**, 152
fibrin 120–1
free radicals 257
fresh frozen plasma 24, 32–3, 75, 200
   cost 243, 245
   cryoprecipitate-reduced 247

gastrointestinal bleeding 145
gelatin 78
Gelfoam **197**
goal-directed oxymetric monitoring 269–70
graft versus host disease, transfusion-associated 45, **49**, 75

Harvey, William 24
Helistat **197**
hematocrit 144, 171
hemochromatosis 65
hemoglobin 144–5, 257–8
   arenicola 259
   bovine 258
   encapsulated 258–9
   in ICU patients 160
   recombinant 258
   zero-linked 263
hemoglobin-based oxygen carriers 255–67
   free radicals 257
   half-life 256
   hypertension and smooth muscle effects 256–7
   next generation 262–7
      Oxygent 264–5

RSR13 265–7, **266**, **267**
   oncotic properties 255–6
   oxygen affinity 255
   physiological challenges 255
   products under clinical investigation 260–2
      Hemopure 262
      Hemosol 261–2
      PolyHeme 261
   types of 257–60
      allosteric modifiers 259
      arenicola hemoglobin 259
      bovine hemoglobin 258
      encapsulated hemoglobin 258–9
      human hemoglobin 257–8
      perfluorocarbons 259–60
      recombinant hemoglobin 258
hemoglobinopathies 148
hemoglobinuria 146
Hemolink **267**
hemolytic transfusion reaction syndrome 46, 152
Hemopad **197**
hemophilia 33, 123
Hemopure 262, **267**
Hemosol 261–2
hemostasis 114–43
   abnormal 122–6
      acquired disorders 124–6
      congenital disorders 123
   coagulation phase 118–20
   evaluation of 126–31
      coagulation tests 126–8
      history and physical examination 126
      preoperative screening tests 128
      thromboelastography 129–31
   fibrin formation 120–1
   fibrinolysis 121
   platelet phase 115–8
   regulation of 121–2
   vascular phase 115
hemostatic agents 136–7
   antifibrinolytics 136–7
   cell salvage **197**
   desmopressin *62*, 137, 222, **250**
   neonatal and pediatric surgery 222–3
   recombinant factor VIIa 99–100, 137, 200–2, **250**, 272
   see also individual agents
HemoTech 264
HemoZyme 263

heparin-induced
thrombocytopenia 30, 125
hepatic surgery 227
hepatitis **48**, 186
hetastarch 81
hospital
charges 245–6, **245**, **247**
liability of 17–19
human immunodeficiency virus **48**,
186
human T-lymphotrophic viruses
48
hydroxyethyl starches 78
hyperbaric oxygen 267–9
clinical experience 269
experimental evidence 268–9
hyperbilirubinemia 146
hypothermia
and increased blood loss 77
transfusion-associated 153

iatrogenic blood loss, minimization
of 178
ICU-acquired anemia 158–60, *160*,
170–2
prevention of 177–80
minimization of iatrogenic blood
loss 178
minimization of oxygen
consumption 179
optimization of erythropoiesis 179
optimization of oxygen
delivery 178
prevention and arrest of
bleeding 177–8
tolerance of anemia 179–80
idiopathic thrombocytopenia
purpura 30
immune-mediated adverse effects
49
imported blood 239
incompetent adults 7–13
known Jehovah's Witnesses
7–11
no information available 11–13
infectious disease testing **239**
informed consent 5–6
Instat **197**
intensive care unit *see* critically ill
patients; postoperative
management
International Normalized Ratio 33

intraoperative cell salvage *see* cell
salvage
intraoperative strategies 75–113,
191–202
acute normovolemic
hemodilution 198–9, *198*
anesthetic management 199–200
blood conservation 94–101
aprotinin 96–9
DDAVP 94–5
epsilon-aminocaproic acid 95–6
erythropoietin 100–1
recombinant factor VIIa 99–100
tranexamic acid 95–6
clinical coagulation 131–3
coagulation management 133–6,
200–2, *201*
controlled hypotension 101–5
general considerations 76–8
hemostatic drug therapy 136–7
antifibrinolytics 136–7
desmopressin 137
recombinant factor VIIa 137
intraoperative cell salvage 90–3, **91**,
92, 194–8, *193*, *195*, **197**
isovolemic hemodilution 78–87
clinical applications 86–7
physiologic consequences 81–6
technique 79–81, **79**
preoperative autologous
donation 60, *62*, 87–90, **88**
surgical judgement 191–2
surgical technique 193–4
iron deficiency anemia 147
iron therapy, preoperative 65–6
irradiation of blood products 153–4
isovolemic hemodilution 78–87
clinical applications 86–7
contraindications **79**
physiologic consequences 81–6
technique 79–81, **79**

Jehovah's Witnesses 1–4
acceptable products, treatments
and procedures 2–4, *3*
autologous procedures and
equipment 2–4
critically ill paients 180–1
legal principles 6–15
competent adults 6
disagreeing family
members 13–14

emergency/incompetent adults
7–13
mature and emancipated
minors 15
minors 14–15
organ transplantation 4
Refusal To Permit Blood
Transfusion *12*

kallikrein-inhibiting units 97, 200
legal principles 4–15
Jehovah's Witnesses 6–15
competent adults 6
disagreeing family
members 13–14
emergency/incompetent
adults 7–13
mature and emancipated
minors 15
minors 14–15
refusal of blood as life-saving
treatment 4–6

Leishmania spp. **48**
leishmaniasis 186
leukoreduction 246–8, **247**, **248**
freezing and deglycerolizing 246
irradiation 246
washing 246
liver disease 124
liver transplantation 200–2, 206–11,
207, *208*, **209**, **210**
cost **249**
lysine analogs
epsilon-aminocaproic acid *62*,
95–6, 136, 222, **250**
tranexamic acid *62*, 95–6, 136, 222,
250

Malnutrition Inflammation Score 189
manufacturing center 239
massive transfusion 124–5
mature minors 15
mechanical hemolyzation **50**
minors 14–15
mature and emancipated 15
mixed venous blood gas analysis
272–4

necrotizing enterocolitis 224
neonatal and pediatric surgery 218–36
anemia of oncologic disease 229–30
anemia of prematurity 228–9, **229**

burn surgery 227–8
cardiac surgery 225–6
craniosynostosis surgery 226–7
hepatic surgery 227
limitation of transfusion 219–24
autotransfusion 221–2
erythropoietin 219–21, **219**, **220**
hemostatic agents 222–3
perioperative approaches 223
physician awareness 223–4
neonatal surgery 224–5
orthopedic surgery 226
trauma surgery 228
nicardipine 104–5
nonimmune-mediated adverse
effects **61**
nonsteroidal anti-inflammatory
drugs 77
normothermia 77–8
nucleic acid testing 237

O_2ER 163–4, *164*
organ transplantation 4
orthopedic surgery 226
osmotic hemolysis **50**
oxygenation, monitoring of 162–5
blood lactate 165
cardiac output 162–3
O_2ER 163–4, *164*
regional markers of tissue
oxygenation 165
SvO_2 163
oxygenation therapy 249–50, **250**,
254–82
DO_2/VO_2 relationships 271–2
goal-directed oxymetric
monitoring 269–70
hemoglobin-based oxygen
carriers 255–67
free radicals 257
half-life 256
hypertension and smooth muscle
effects 256–7
next generation 262–7
oncotic properties 255–6
oxygen affinity 255
physiological challenges 255
products under clinical
investigation 260–2
types of 257–60
hyperbaric oxygen 267–9
clinical experience 269
experimental evidence 268–9

oxygenation therapy (*cont'd*)
  loss of vasoregulation 274–5
  mixed venous blood gas
      analysis 272–4
  need for 254–5
  potential applications 275–7
    acute vascular occlusion 276
    elective surgery 276
    radiation sensitizer 277
    remote settings 276
    septic shock 277
    sickle cell anemia 276–7
    trauma 275–6
  tissue oxygen debt 270–1
oxygen consumption, minimization
      of 165–6, 179
oxygen delivery, optimization of 178
Oxygent 264–5
oxyhemoglobin dissociation curve 148

partial prothrombin time 200
patient
  confirmation of decision to refuse
      blood 18–9, 19–20
  informed consent 5–6
  refusal of blood as life-saving
      treatment 4–6
Paul Gann Blood Safety Act, Health
      & Safety Code 17, 18–19
pediatric surgery *see* neonatal and
      pediatric surgery
Perflubron **267**
perfluorocarbons 212, 259–60, **266**
phlebotomy, and blood loss 159
physician, liability of 17
plasma, clinically appropriate
      situations 36–7
plasmapheresis, volume overload 42–3
plasminogen 33
Plasmodium spp. **48**
platelet count 127, 200
platelet function analyzer 128
platelet function tests 128
platelets 24, 30–2
  bacterial contamination 44
  clinically appropriate situations 35
  cost **243**, **245**
  overdosing 40
  role in coagulation 115–8
  transfusion without clinical need 41
  volume overload 43
Polk, Hiram C 16
PolyHeme 261, **267**

postoperative management 158–69,
      202–6, *204*
  adequacy of oxygenation
      162–5
    blood lactate 165
    cardiac output 162–3
    O_2ER 163–4, *164*
    regional markers of tissue
        oxygenation 165
    SvO_2 163
  anemia 158–60, *160*
  restrictive transfusion practice
      165–6
    erythropoietin 166
    increased cardiac output 166
    minimization of oxygen
        requirement 165–6
  role of transfusion in
      resuscitation 160–2
posttransfusion purpura 30, **49**
preoperative autologous donation 60,
      62, 87–90, **88**
  contraindications **88**
preoperative management 60–74
  assessment 60–1, **61**
  optimization of red cell mass 61–70,
      62, 187–91, *188*, *190*
    central nervous system effects
        69–70
    darbopoietin alfa 70
    erythropoietin therapy 62–5, **63**,
        64
    iron therapy 65–6
    safety issues 67–9, **68**
preoperative screening tests 128
process risks 48–51, **49**, **50**, *51*
product/component risks 47–8, **48**
protein C 33
protein S 33
prothrombin time 126–7, 200
pure red cell aplasia 69
pyruvate kinase deficiency 147

radiation sensitizers 277
recombinant factor IX **250**
recombinant factor VIIa 99–100, 137,
      200–2, 272
  cost **250**
recombinant factor VIII **250**
recombinant hemoglobin 258
recombinant human erythropoietin
      see erythropoietin
red blood cells 24, 26–30, *27*, **29**

clinically appropriate situations
        34–5
    cost **243**, **245**
    regulation of 144
    transfusion without clinical need 40
red cell mass, optimization 61–70, *62*
    central nervous system
        effects 69–70
    darbopoietin alfa 70
    erythropoietin therapy 62–5, **63**, *64*
    iron therapy 65–6
    safety issues 67–9, **68**
refusal of blood as life-saving
        treatment 4–6
Refusal To Permit Blood
        Transfusion *12*
regional markers of tissue
        oxygenation 165
regulation of blood transfusion 244–5
relative iron deficiency 65
reptilase time 127
restrictive transfusion practice
    critically ill patients 172–3
    efficacy of 173–6
    neonatal and pediatric
        surgery 219–24
        autotransfusion 221–2
        erythropoietin 219–21, **219**, **220**
        hemostatic agents 222–3
        perioperative approaches 223
        physician awareness 223–4
    postoperative management 165–6
        erythropoietin 166
        increased cardiac output 166
        minimization of oxygen
            requirement 165–6
    safety of 176–7
    see also blood conservation
retinopathy of prematurity 219
risks of transfusion therapy 25–6, *26*,
        46–51
    process risks 48–51, **49**, **50**, *51*
    product/component risks 47–8, **48**
RSR13 265–7, **266**, **267**

SARS 47
septic shock 277
Sequential Organ Failure Assessment
        (SOFA) score 175
sickle cell anemia 147, 276–7
Surgicel **197**
SvO$_2$ 163

thalassemia 147
thermal hemolyzation **50**
thrombin time 127
thrombocytopenia, heparin-
        induced 30, 125
thromboelastography 129–31, 201
Thrombogen **197**
thrombomodulin 115
Thrombostat **197**
thrombotic thrombocytopenia
        purpura 30
tissue oxygen debt 270–1
tissue plasminogen activator 33
tranexamic acid *62*, 95–6, 136, 222
    cost **250**
transfusional hemosiderosis **50**
transfusion-associated graft versus host
        disease 45, **49**, 75
transfusion-associated sepsis **50**
transfusion-free surgery
    intraoperative management *see*
        intraoperative strategies
    postoperative management *see*
        postoperative management
    preoperative management *see*
        preoperative management
    results 206–11, **207**, *208*,
        209, **210**
    trends in 211–2
    see also restrictive transfusion
        practice
transfusion-related acute lung
        injury 44, **49**, 75
Transfusion Requirements in Critical
        Care study 174–6
transfusion service 240
transfusion therapy
    in anemia 151–4
    benefits of 25–6, *26*, 151–4
    clerical errors 41–2
    clinically appropriate 34–7
    clinical utility 26–34
        cryoprecipitate 33–4
        fresh frozen plasma 32–3
        platelets 30–2
        red blood cells 26–30, *27*, **29**
    cost of 237–53
        blood transfusion as service 243–4
        case studies 248–9, **249**
        difficulties in estimation 240–2
        hospital costs 245–6, **245**
        leukoreduction 246–8, **247**, **248**

transfusion therapy (*cont'd*)
    oxygenation therapy and
      pharmacologic agents 249, **250**
    reasons for 242–3, **243**
    regulatory environment 244–5
    supply of donated blood 237–40
  critically ill patients 173
  errors of commission 40–1
  errors of omission 37–40
  inadvertent adverse clinical
    outcomes 42–6
  neonates 228
  possible harm **29**
  reactions to 46
    febrile nonhemolytic transfusion
      reaction **49**, 152
    hemolytic transfusion reaction
      syndrome 46, 152
    hypothermia 153
  reduced requirement for 165–6
    erythropoietin 166
    increased cardiac output 166
    minimization of oxygen
      requirement 165–6
  in resuscitation 160–2
  risks of transfusion therapy 25–6,
    26, 46–51, 151–4

    process risks 48–51, **49**, **50**, *51*
    product/component risks 47–8,
      48
transfusion triggers 145
trauma surgery 228, 275–6
Treponema pallidum **48**
Trypanosoma cruzi **48**

USC University Hospital Program
  17
  highlights of 20–1, *21*
utility of transfusion practice
  25–6, *26*

viral transmission **48**
vitamin K deficiency 124
volume overload
  plasmapheresis 42–3
  platelets 43
von Willebrand disease 123
von Willebrand factor 33, 78
  cost **250**
  deficiency 202

West Nile virus 47

zero-linked hemoglobin 263